Health under Fire

Health under Fire

MEDICAL CARE DURING AMERICA'S WARS

James R. Arnold, Editor

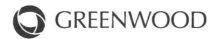
GREENWOOD

AN IMPRINT OF ABC-CLIO, LLC
Santa Barbara, California • Denver, Colorado • Oxford, England

616.98023
Mea .

Copyright © 2015 by ABC-CLIO, LLC

Publ.
11/24/14

Library of Congress Cataloging-in-Publication Data

Health under fire : medical care during America's wars / James R. Arnold, editor.
    pages cm
Includes bibliographical references and index.
    ISBN 978–1–61069–747–7 (hard copy : alk. paper) — ISBN 978–1–61069–748–4 (ebook)
1. Medicine, Military—History. 2. Medicine, Military—Moral and ethical aspects. I. Arnold,
James R., 1952–
RC971.H39   2015
616.9'8023—dc23   2014024409

ISBN: 978–1–61069–747–7
EISBN: 978–1–61069–748–4

19 18 17 16 15   1 2 3 4 5

This book is also available on the World Wide Web as an eBook.
Visit www.abc-clio.com for details.

Greenwood
An Imprint of ABC-CLIO, LLC

ABC-CLIO, LLC
130 Cremona Drive, P.O. Box 1911
Santa Barbara, California 93116-1911

This book is printed on acid-free paper ∞

Manufactured in the United States of America

Contents

Introduction

When medical care providers accompanied European colonists to North America, they brought with them detailed knowledge of human anatomy and physiology. However, because of deep holes in their knowledge, they were unable to translate this information into clinically useful techniques. Military forces of the 18th century relied upon physicians and surgeons to provide medical care. No one knew what caused contagious diseases or how infections developed. Physicians administered a variety of drugs ranging from useful, including opiates and quinine, to harmful, such as strychnine and arsenic. They relied upon centuries of handed-down information as well as personal observation. But, since they were ignorant of the underlying chemical and medical processes, their ability to provide effective care was exceedingly limited. Surgeons, in turn, treated wounds by probing with unsterile fingers and performed amputations with unsterile knives and saws. In combat conditions, as soon as they completed one operation they began another. Washing surgical instruments between operations, at best, meant a quick plunge into a bucket of water. Because of these practices, military medical care had a well-deserved notorious reputation among soldiers and sailors.

Slowly, the knowledge base expanded and medical care advanced. For example, in 1775, the year of revolution in the 13 colonies, France established its first military medical school. However, from the beginning of the revolutionary war in 1775 until the end of active military operations in 1781, American armies struggled to assemble and maintain men and material sufficient to contest Great Britain's vastly superior resources. The difficulties establishing an effective medical military service mirrored the tremendous problems associated with building from scratch a military force. One of the few bright spots came when George Washington mandated smallpox inoculation with live virus for his army. Controversial at the time, this approach evolved until smallpox, which had always been a dreaded and recurring plague, was virtually eliminated.

Other diseases, notably typhus and dysentery, continued to afflict thousands of soldiers. Mortality statistics showed that far more men died of disease than from combat in all of America's wars until.... When American soldiers landed on the

Mexican Coast in 1847, they entered a region prone to yellow fever, which joined the ranks of deadly, soldier-killing diseases. The American Civil War witnessed some advances, particularly with the expanded use of anesthesia and, among Federal armies, the use of a well-organized casualty clearing system. But there was still no control of operative infection, so surgical results remained dismal. Unless wounds could be managed by simple dressing, splinting, or amputation, patients were generally beyond help. Continued ignorance of the cause of disease, the lack of basic sanitation, and poor nutrition caused thousands to die from dysentery, typhus, typhoid, and malaria.

Finally, in the 1860s came scientific breakthroughs that discovered the role of microorganisms in disease. Nonetheless, when American forces mobilized for the Spanish-American War in 1898, an extraordinary number of men died of typhoid while at the training camps. Meanwhile, yellow fever and malaria afflicted soldiers campaigning in Cuba and Puerto Rico. Military surgeons tackled these problems, with Walter Reed and his famous Yellow Fever Commission proving that this dreaded disease was mosquito borne. This was the first scientific documentation of the viral causation of a human disease and its transmission by mosquitoes. In addition, the postwar Dodge Commission investigated the sicknesses and deaths that had occurred in the training camps. The result was a complete overhaul of the U.S. Army Medical Department. The Spanish-American War represented a turning point in medical care and knowledge. Advances included the limited use of X-ray and the general adoption of surgical asepsis.

Medical care in World War I built on these advances. During the war, monitored, safe anesthesia and aseptic surgery lead to the successful treatment of wounds that had previously been untreatable. A new vaccine almost eliminated tetanus. The role of sanitation was better understood. Yet, even as these beneficial trends occurred, military technology advanced, with the widespread use of more lethal artillery, machine guns, chemical agents, and the like.

With the introduction of antibiotics, military medicine beginning in World War II started to approach modern standards. Because infection could be controlled, surgeons could operate successfully on parts of the body that previously they could enter only at great peril, such as the chest, head, and abdomen. Disease became a minor contributor to military morbidity and mortality. Simultaneously, however, aerial bombardment produced civilian casualties on an unprecedented scale culminating with the use of atomic weapons in 1945. Thereafter, nations have refrained from using nuclear weapons and, with some notable exceptions, not employed biological or chemical weapons.

In the Korean and Vietnam wars, battlefield casualty evacuation accelerated with the employment of helicopters. Wounded soldiers were removed from inhospitable terrain and taken to first-class surgical hospitals with astonishing alacrity. Survival rates soared accordingly. Whereas in World War II the percentage of deaths from wounds among Army soldiers admitted to a medical facility was 4.5 percent, in Korea it declined to 2.5 percent. By the time of the Gulf wars, the full range of surgical equipment and technique proved able to save the lives of countless combatants who previously would have died. The flip side of this medical success is, and probably will continue to be, an increasing number of survivors with extensive and often incapacitating injuries. Perhaps the next great medical breakthroughs will come in the fields of rehabilitation and regeneration.

■ CHAPTER 1
Colonial Conflicts and the American Revolutionary War

INTRODUCTION

The First Continental Congress convened in Philadelphia on September 5, 1774. It petitioned King George III and Parliament to resolve peacefully differences between the 13 colonies and the British government. Simultaneously, the Congress adopted trading restrictions designed to coerce the British government into repealing various acts of Parliament that regulated commerce in the colonies. To enforce these restrictions, the Congress formed committees throughout the colonies that effectively superseded the constituted authorities. These de facto governments took over control of the militia.

Massachusetts was the focal point of the growing crisis. In anticipation of armed conflict, the Massachusetts Provincial Congress established a military depot at Concord, some 20 miles outside of Boston. In turn, the British commander in Boston dispatched an expedition to destroy the depot. On April 19, 1775 while en route to Concord, British soldiers and American militia clashed at Lexington. The British proceeded to Concord where they encountered increasing numbers of militia. During the return march to Boston, the militia harassed the British, inflicting some 273 casualties. Although Massachusetts had established the first general military hospital of the war at Cambridge, Massachusetts, it lacked adequate medicine, supplies, and leadership. Consequently, although the British had an established medical service, the 90 wounded rebels had to rely upon relatives, friends, or upon the kindness of strangers for care.

News of the outbreak of fighting spread rapidly throughout the colonies. Thousands of New England militia formed a ring around Boston whereas others secured British forts at Ticonderoga and Crown Point located on the route between New York and Canada. The Second Continental Congress assembled in Philadelphia on May 10, 1775. Its members addressed the problems of organizing, controlling, and supplying a military effort. Before it could exercise control over the New England militia, the June 17, 1775 Battle of Bunker Hill, the bloodiest single engagement of the entire Revolution, took place. Here, on the Charleston peninsula overlooking Boston harbor, American militia stoutly resisted two British attacks before yielding the high ground. They inflicted a staggering 1,054 casualties while suffering about 440 killed and wounded. King George III and his ministers responded to the Battle of Bunker Hill with a determined effort to put down the American rebellion by force.

The ensuing Revolutionary War was fought over the next eight years. Fighting took place in all 13 colonies, extended west to the Mississippi River to embroil numerous Indian tribes, and north into Canada. After France entered the war on the American side in 1778, the conflict became a world war. From the beginning to end, American rebels struggled to assemble and maintain men and material sufficient to contest Great Britain's vastly superior resources. The difficulties establishing an effective medical military service mirrored the tremendous problems associated with building a military force from scratch.

When the Revolutionary War began, there were only two hospitals in all the colonies and only about 200 physicians who practiced in the colonies had a medical degree. The vast majority of the 3,500 physicians were mere apprentices, often with no more than one year of formal study as an apothecary. Yet, these poorly prepared men had to provide medical care to the sick and wounded soldiers while also serving the civilian population. At first there were no formal provisions regulating military medical care. During the 1775–1776 Siege of Boston, pneumonia, dysentery, smallpox, malnutrition, and frostbite afflicted General George Washington's army. The medical corps, which the Continental Congress had established on July 27, 1775, proved woefully inadequate to address these afflictions. Trouble began at the top. Benjamin Church, the army's first medical director general, lasted only three months before being charged with treason and cashiered. Thus began a history of the Medical Department that featured medical quarrels, charges of incompetency, and bureaucratic conflict. Church's replacement, John Morgan, inherited a sick, scattered army so lacking in medical supplies that Morgan had to appeal to the public for basic necessities such as blankets and bandages. Although Morgan was able to institute useful reforms, he engaged in a political battle that cost him his post in January 1777. Under William Shippen, Jr., Morgan's successor, the medical service was reorganized on April 7, 1777. Henceforth, each of four military districts had its own director general who was responsible for hospitals, medical supplies, and the care of his district's sick and wounded. Like Morgan, Shippen fell to political bickering and retired in 1780. His replacement, John Cochran, served until the war ended in 1783.

Bureaucratic feuding and lack of resources seriously impaired American medical care during the war. However, ignorance played a much larger role. No one yet understood how disease and infection spread. The importance of basic hygiene was unrealized. Wounded soldiers were most commonly transported in open carts where they were exposed to the weather. They entered field stations or hospitals that were, by modern standards, filthy. Care providers could deal with fractures and cuts by time-honored splinting and bandaging techniques. They had few options for more complex wounds, with amputation being the surgical approach of choice. However, surgeons routinely operated with the same instruments on patient after patient without washing either their tools or their hands. Half of men subjected to mid-thigh amputations died. Overall, about one-quarter of the wounded who reached a hospital subsequently died, usually because of an infection. A total of about 25,000 American soldiers died during the war, out of approximately 250,000 who served. Only 6,500 were battle deaths. The rest died from various diseases. Care for disabled veterans was uneven. The concepts of reconstruction, reconditioning, and rehabilitation did not emerge until nearly 50 years had passed.

The war's most notable success in dealing with disease involved the practice of *variolation*; it meant intentionally exposing uninfected people to infectious material taken from people afflicted with mild cases of smallpox. Variolation was controversial since about 10 percent of the people so treated died. Regardless, Washington ordered both soldiers and nearby citizens to be inoculated. Washington's order to immunize all new recruits marks the first American use of institutional preventive medicine.

In contrast to the practice of variolation were punitive attempts to control venereal diseases, another widespread disease afflicting the American army. Officers and men hospitalized with venereal diseases had their pay docked, which, whereas it discouraged some, did nothing to treat the underlying disease. Indeed, most of this era's medical treatment of diseases was either ineffective or harmful. The practice of bleeding a patient, deliberately draining significant quantities of blood, was widespread. A typical physician's medical chest contained mostly herbal remedies, with an emphasis of purgatives like ipecac and toxic compounds such as mercurials. The sporadic use of opium to treat pain and quinine to treat fever were two of the few treatment approaches that satisfy modern standards.

The high death and complication rates experienced by American soldiers during the Revolutionary War led to widespread post-war demands for better medical training. This encouraged the formation of a number of new American medical schools that provided improved medical education in the years ahead.

James R. Arnold

ENTRIES

Cochran, John (1730–1807)

A doctor in the Continental Army and a close associate of Dr. William Shippen, John Cochran joined Shippen in proposing a reform of the army medical services

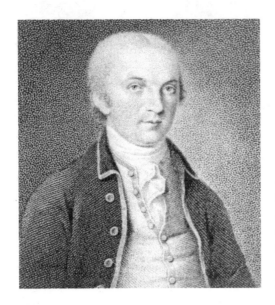

After examining the deficiencies in medical care in the Continental Army, John Cochran reorganized the medical department in 1777 and was appointed Chief Physician and Surgeon of the Army in October 1780. (National Library of Medicine)

and became chief of the army's medical services toward the end of the American Revolutionary War.

Cochran was born to Irish parents in Sadsbury, Pennsylvania, in 1730. He began his education with Dr. Francis Allison; studied medicine with doctors in Lancaster, Pennsylvania; and increased his medical expertise by serving with the British Army as a surgeon's mate during the Seven Years' War. Cochran married in 1760 and moved to New Brunswick, New Jersey, in 1763, where he helped found the New Jersey Medical Society in 1766.

At the beginning of the Revolutionary War, Cochran joined the Continental Army as a doctor. The army's medical services at the beginning of the war were a mess. The situation was not helped by the fact that the first head of the medical services, Dr. Benjamin Church, was of dubious loyalty to the rebel cause. His replacement, Dr. John Morgan, became involved in fights between individual regimental surgeons and supervisory personnel, such as himself, over who should control the medical services. Morgan was replaced by Dr. William Shippen, who also spent a lot of time and energy fighting both the regimental doctors and Dr. Benjamin Rush, his rival for the position.

On February 14, 1777, Cochran and Shippen submitted a plan that they had developed for reorganizing the Continental Army's medical department. Congress approved the plan on April 7, 1777 and appointed Cochran physician and surgeon general in the Middle Department. There Cochran focused on his duties as a medical director and not on political maneuvering like some of the other physicians. For the remainder of the war he labored to improve the operations of military hospitals and the conditions of the sick and wounded.

On January 17, 1781, Congress promoted him to the top position in the medical services of the Continental Army. On April 11, 1783, Cochran resigned his post and left the army.

After the war Cochran moved to New York City, and in 1790 President George Washington appointed him to the position of commissioner of loans. Cochran later suffered a stroke and retired to Palatine, New York, where he died in 1807.

Dallace W. Unger Jr.

Further Reading

Blanco, Richard L., ed. *The American Revolution, 1775–1783: An Encyclopedia.* New York: Garland, 1993.

Boatner, Mark. *Encyclopedia of the American Revolution.* Mechanicsburg, PA: Stackpole, 1994.

Purcell, L. Edward. *Who Was Who in the American Revolution.* New York: Facts On File, 1993.

Columbian Exchange

Initiated by Christopher Columbus's voyage to the New World in 1492, the Columbian Exchange involved the exchange of people, flora, fauna, diseases, and ideas between the Eastern and Western Hemispheres. This changed the New World's ecosystems and gave Europeans distinct advantages over Native Americans, ultimately helping European peoples to conquer and subdue the New World. Native American plants such as maize (corn), squash, beans, potatoes, and tomatoes were introduced to Europeans. In return, Europeans and Africans introduced wheat, rice, bananas, sugar, and wine grapes to the Americas.

Many European colonists used these Old World crops along with the New World cultivation of tobacco as cash crops to create viable economies that sustained their colonies. Europeans also introduced domesticated animals such as cattle, fowl, horses, hogs, and sheep to the New World. Unfortunately, disease proved to be perhaps the most significant element introduced to the New World, and it was also the single most destructive aspect of the Columbian Exchange for Native Americans. Europeans unintentionally brought with them influenza, malaria, measles, plague, and smallpox. Because Native Americans had no previous exposure to these diseases and had not acquired immunities to them, they suffered very high mortality rates once infected. Often, aspects of colonialism such as warfare and the Native American slave trade helped spread diseases and contributed to the devastating impact they had on native societies.

Dixie Ray Haggard

Further Reading

Alchon, Suzanne Austin. *A Pest in the Land: New World Epidemics in Global Perspective.* Albuquerque: University of New Mexico Press, 2003.

Crosby, Alfred W. *The Columbian Exchange: Biological and Cultural Consequences of 1492.* Westport, CT: Greenwood Press, 1972.

"Virgin Soil Epidemics as a Factor in the Aboriginal Depopulation in America." *William and Mary Quarterly*, 3rd ser., 3 (1976): 289–299.

Viola, Herman J., and Carolyn Margolis. *Seeds of Change: A Quincentennial Commemoration.* Washington, DC: Smithsonian Institution Press, 1991.

Disease and Mortality in Colonial America

As North America's original European settlers arrived over long distances in small, underprovisioned vessels, disease was the primary cause of mortality.

Under the best of circumstances, the voyage from England in the early 1600s took more than six weeks; rations consisted mostly of meat, bread, and dried legumes, and passengers were crowded into small, poorly ventilated spaces. Seasickness, scurvy, smallpox, dysentery, and various febrile diseases were common. Of John Blackwell's 150 Puritans who sailed in 1618, 130 died in transit. Of 100 Pilgrims who landed at Plymouth in 1620, only 50 were still alive three months later, most having died of scurvy or infections acquired onboard the ship. Of the initial 4,170 settlers who came to Jamestown in 1621, more than 2,000 succumbed to disease, and survivors complained that moaning from the sick and dying made it impossible to sleep at night.

Ironically, disease itself was not altogether detrimental to the colonists. It is likely that the Pilgrims were saved from annihilation by local Indian tribes because the native population had been cut by 90 percent in the previous four years by epidemic disease.

Scurvy had been the primary killer of sailors and nautical passengers since improvements in navigation made long voyages possible. The disease results from lack of vitamin C (ascorbic acid), which is normally acquired from citrus fruits and to a lesser extent from leafy vegetables such as cabbage or from onions and potatoes. In the absence of an ongoing supply of dietary vitamin C, symptoms of scurvy appear within two weeks and include weakness, swelling of the legs, softening of the gums culminating in loss of teeth, bleeding from mucous membranes, and, ultimately, death from heart failure. British naval surgeon James Lind had proved that the disease could be prevented by prophylactic ingestion of lemon juice in 1747, but the practice did not become routine in the Royal Navy until 179. Scurvy was a plague to both military and civilian sailors through the 18th century. In British ships posted to the West Indies during that time, about one man in seven died of scurvy while on post.

Close quarters aboard ship made transmission of infections likely. Typhus, which was transmitted by omnipresent lice, was pervasive and infected nearly every prisoner held by the British in hulks anchored in New York Harbor during the American Revolution. Epidemics of measles, scarlet fever, influenza, and diphtheria also recurred regularly. Seasickness was significant both because of the direct misery it caused and because it weakened passengers and left them susceptible to more lethal diseases.

Smallpox was a particular problem, with cyclical epidemics beginning in 1663 in New Netherlands and recurring every few years thereafter. William Penn's ship alone lost 30 settlers to the disease in 1682. Soldiers often carried the disease, and Pennsylvania suffered a disastrous outbreak when British troops brought it to Philadelphia in 1756. A smallpox epidemic in Boston after the British Army retreated from the city in 1776 affected local citizens far more than the revolution.

In 1721, Lady Mary Wortley Montague brought the Turkish practice of inoculating people who had not had smallpox with matter acquired from the sores of people with relatively mild cases. Inoculation (also known as variolation) caused real cases of the disease but carried a much lower mortality than naturally acquired smallpox. After smallpox forced troops under General Benedict Arnold to withdraw from their Canadian invasion, General George Washington mandated that all Continental Army soldiers be inoculated. Smallpox remained a significant problem until 1798, when Edward Jenner demonstrated that inoculation with the almost entirely safe cowpox virus conveyed lasting immunity against the disease.

Dysentery was a problem both on shipboard and on land. A British official complained in 1607 that the Jamestown settlement was being destroyed by "swellings, fluxes, and burning fevers" as much as by wars with the Indians. Ships might bring contaminated water aboard and repeatedly distribute it through a voyage. Settlements were often built with little concern for drainage and with latrines close to water used for washing and drinking. The more concentrated the population became; the higher was the likelihood of water supplies becoming contaminated. Wherever a military expedition went, dysentery followed the troops. A 1709 British expedition against French Canada had to be abandoned when dysentery broke out near Wood Creek, New York. The disease was widespread in the earliest Continental Army encampments in 1775 and 1776.

Yellow fever, although less common than other febrile diseases, was uniquely terrifying because it carried a mortality rate approaching 30 percent. The disease came from West Africa with the slave trade and was especially well adapted to transmission over the sea-lanes. The disease is carried by the *Aedes aegyptii* mosquito that reproduces only in standing fresh water such as that found in ships' water barrels. It first appeared in Barbados in 1647 and, beginning with 1699 epidemics in Philadelphia and Charleston, repeatedly struck port cities from Boston to New Orleans throughout the colonial period. A single episode in New York in 1702 cost the city 10 percent of its population.

Jack McCallum

Further Reading

Garrison, Fielding. *Notes on the History of Military Medicine*. Washington, D.C.: Association of Military Surgeons, 1922.

Packard, Francis. *History of Medicine in the United States*. New York: Paul B. Hoeber, Inc., 1931.

Reiss, Oscar. *Medicine and the American Revolution: How Diseases and Their Treatment Affected the Colonial Army*. Jefferson, NC: McFarland & Co., Inc., 1998.

Roddis, Louis. *A Short History of Nautical Medicine*. New York: Paul B. Hoeber, Inc., 1941.

Jones, John (1729–1791)

The author of *Plain, Concise, Practical Remarks on the Treatment of Wounds and Fractures*, the only American medical text prior to the start of the Revolutionary War, John Jones, was born in Jamaica, Long Island. He was the grandson of Welsh physician Edward Jones, who came to Pennsylvania with William Penn, and the son of physician Evan Jones, who brought the family to New York. John Jones began his studies under Thomas Cadwalader in Philadelphia before traveling to Europe, where he studied under William Hunter and Percival Pott in London, Jean-Louis Petit and Henri-François LeDran in Paris, and the elder Alexander Monro in Edinburgh before taking his degree at the University of Rheims in 1751.

He returned to the United States to practice in New York and served as military surgeon to the British troops in the 1755 war against France. After the war, he served as professor of surgery at the Medical School of New York before moving to Philadelphia and the Pennsylvania Hospital in 1780, where he was one of the founders of Philadelphia's College of Physicians. Jones was a severe chronic asthmatic and, although he helped organize the American medical corps in the Revolutionary War, he was unable to serve himself. After the revolution, he remained a respected physician and attended both George Washington and Benjamin Franklin in their final illnesses. He was particularly close to the latter and was remembered in his will. Jones died in his sleep in Philadelphia at the age of 62.

Jack McCallum

Further Reading

Kelly, Howard, and Walter Burrage. *Dictionary of American Medical Biography*. Boston: Milford House, 1971.

Packard, Francis. *History of Medicine in the United States*. New York: Paul B. Hoeber, Inc., 1931.

Military and Naval Medicine

As virtually all naval and military forces operating in colonial North America were of western European origin, their medical care closely mirrored the practices in their home countries. The 18th century was the first time that military medicine became a governmental responsibility, a change that can be traced to England in 1660, when King Charles II created a professional corps of military surgeons. As with their counterparts in the regimental officer corps, military surgeons purchased their commissions. Many functioned both as doctors and as warriors, holding rank in both capacities and collecting salaries in each. A standing army also necessitated screening recruits and housing, feeding, and dressing them in a manner that would promote their health, and all of those responsibilities fell to a lesser or greater extent on the military surgeons.

Professional training in an era when surgeons were separate from and inferior to physicians was a recurring problem. In the first half of the 18th century, the only place in Europe where surgery was being formally taught was Paris, and the Prussian king approached French military surgeon Louis Petit in 1744 asking for trained surgeons to help educate his military medical corps. His new Prussian physicians established field dressing stations near the front, as well as intermediate level field hospitals and rear area facilities for those with the most severe wounds. They also generally improved transport and care of those wounded in the battle.

The Prussians and Austrians eventually established their own schools of military medicine and even published periodicals devoted to military medicine. They promulgated printed regulations for camp sanitation and administration of military hospitals. France had already done much the same under King Louis XIV

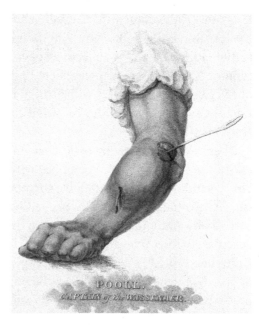

Introduction of a long probe in the forearm to counteract formation of an abscess due to gunshot wound. In the absence of knowledge about infection, such early nineteenth century procedures often proved lethal. (Wellcome Images, London)

(1643–1715), who ordered that his army have a regular medical staff chosen by examination and who built military hospitals in 51 French cities where the surgeons were annually required to take and pass courses in anatomy.

The British were slower to change, although by the War of the Spanish Succession (1701–1714) the Duke of Marlborough had issued regulations dealing with health and sanitation for his armies and by the Battle of Blenheim (1704) he had placed collecting stations for the wounded just out of musket range of the front lines. British articles of war mandated that one day's pay a year be withheld from a soldier's wages to pay for military hospitals and that any spoils taken after a battle be set aside for maintenance of the sick and wounded.

In 1752, Sir John Pringle published his *Observations on Diseases of the Army*, which contained rules for sanitation and ventilation of military hospitals and took the radical point of view that cleanliness decreased the rate of hospital-acquired infections. Prior to Pringle's reforms, military hospitals were crowded, poorly ventilated, and filthy. They were major sources of infection and death. Typhus, or "jail fever," was recognized as identical to the "hospital fever" that plagued military facilities.

Shortly after the publication of Pringle's book, James Lind's A treatise of the scurvy (1753), Baron von Swieten's *Camp Diseases* (1758), and Richard Brocklesby's *Observations on Military Hospitals* (1764) offered major improvements in military medical care at a time when soldiers and sailors were fed diets almost entirely lacking fruits and vegetables, when water was often drawn from contaminated streams next to open latrines, and when woolen uniforms sold to the troops by their officers sometimes led to death from heat stroke during summer marches.

By the 18th century, the musket had become the primary weapon of set-piece battles. Since the bulk of training in military surgery was still obtained on the battlefield, treatment of gunshot wounds assumed primary importance during that century. John Hunter, the preeminent English surgeon of the 1700s, obtained much of his experience serving with British forces in the Belle Isle invasion and the Portuguese campaign and returned to write his landmark *Observations on Gunshot Wounds* (1794).

There was still a general belief that gunpowder was, of itself, poisonous and that musket wounds should be cauterized with hot oil and dressed with a variety of salves. The ointments were often the surgeon's closely guarded secret and were never sterile. Wounds were usually probed with unsterile instruments in an effort to extract any foreign material and were then washed with antiseptics such as mercury based corrosive sublimate, chalk, camphor, myrrh, or hot turpentine. They were then typically packed with charpie (unraveled linen cloth) soaked in wine or brandy. Infection was the rule rather than the exception and was so common that production of "laudable pus" was viewed as an essential phase of healing.

The most common operation performed by military surgeons in the 18th century was amputation. It was a routine remedy for not only gangrene but also serious trauma that defied easy repair, injuries to major vessels, and open fractures or penetration of a joint.

Naval medicine was, like its land-based counterpart, a combination of health maintenance composed mostly of sanitary and dietary considerations and wound surgery. Although James Lind had demonstrated in 1747 that scurvy could be prevented by regular intake of citrus juice, the disease remained the plague of sailing ships because the Royal Navy did not mandate citrus supplements until 1793. Diseases such as typhus, smallpox, yellow fever, and dysentery were fostered by close quarters, poor hygiene, unsanitary food and water, and visits to areas where infectious agents were endemic. Ships were notoriously dangerous places in which to work, with injuries quite common as a result of falls from rigging and blows from heavy tackle.

The sick and wounded were typically housed in the forward area of the ships' gun decks. The decks were divided by the vessel's ribs into bays. Those bays in the main part of the ship contained guns, whereas those in the bow, where hammocks were hung for the patients, came to be known as "sick bays." During battle, the ship's surgeon set up shop below the water line, where he and his patients were less likely to be struck by cannon balls. Surgery was performed on chests laid side by side beside barrels for wash water and for collecting amputated body parts. Ships' boys were responsible for feeding and washing the sick and injured and for mopping the blood that accumulated around surgeries.

Physicians and surgeons were among the first colonists in both Massachusetts and Virginia. John Winthrop brought a barber surgeon to the Massachusetts Bay Colony in 1645, but the man left after three years, complaining he was unable to make a living. Jamestown had a surgeon general (Thomas Wooten) in 1607, and two doctors, Walter Russell and Anthony Bagnall, served with John Smith in 1608. Wooten treated Smith for an injury and a local Indian for a gunshot wound that year, but both returned to England in 1609 so that when Smith was injured by exploding gunpowder, he had to return to London for treatment.

Samuel Fuller came to Plymouth on the *Mayflower* as surgeon to the colony, although he probably lacked a medical degree. In one of the few instances when Plymouth and the Massachusetts Bay Colony cooperated, Fuller helped treat an outbreak of scurvy in Charles Town (present-day Charleston, South Carolina). Fuller died of fever in 1633. In 1636, Plymouth Colony did pass a law requiring that veterans injured in Indian wars be supported for life. Virginia and Rhode Island followed with provisions for lifetime half pay for disabled soldiers.

Still, for much of the 17th century, American colonists were forced to rely on their own resources, on ministers doubling as medical practitioners, or on doctors from passing ships for the majority of their care. As late as 1775 and the coming of the American Revolutionary War, there was still a dearth of trained physicians and surgeons in the colonies. On May 8 of that year, the Provincial Congress of the Massachusetts Bay Colony authorized a committee of physicians to examine the qualifications of potential military surgeons. What they found was primarily a collection of men trained by apprenticeship with little more than knowledge gained by practice. Although the Continental Army medical corps was formalized after the Battle of Bunker Hill in 1775, medical care in the colonies remained well below European military medical standards throughout the war.

Jack McCallum

Further Reading

Garrison, Fielding. *Notes on the History of Military Medicine*. Washington, DC: Association of Military Surgeons, 1922.

Packard, Francis. *History of Medicine in the United States*. New York: Paul B. Hoeber, 1931.

Reiss, Oscar. *Medicine and the American Revolution: How Diseases and Their Treatment Affected the Colonial Army*. Jefferson, NC: McFarland & Co., Inc., 1998.

Roddis, Louis. *A Short History of Nautical Medicine*. New York: Paul B. Hoeber, 1941.

Rush, Benjamin (1745–1813)

Benjamin Rush, a signer of the Declaration of Independence, was known variously as "the American Sydenham" and "the American Hippocrates." Rush was born in Byberry Township near Philadelphia on December 24, 1745. He was educated at Nottingham Academy. He entered New Jersey College at Princeton at the age of 15 and graduated the following year. Rush then spent five years apprenticed to Dr. John Redmond, during which time he translated the *Aphorisms* of Hippocrates into English and wrote a classic account of the 1762 Philadelphia's yellow fever epidemic.

After finishing his apprenticeship, Rush went to England, where he studied in London and received his medical degree from the University of Edinburgh in 1768. He returned to Philadelphia the following year to become professor of chemistry at John Morgan's new College of Philadelphia medical school where he, along with Morgan, William Shippen, Jr., and Adam Kuhn comprised the faculty. Rush was active in Philadelphia society and politics; was a member of the Continental Congress, and signed the Declaration of Independence. He chaired the Congress's medical committee and served as physician and surgeon general of the middle department of the Continental Army from April 1777.

Rush became involved in General Thomas Conway's attempt to have George Washington relieved of his command and Morgan's failed attempt to discredit Shippen. He resigned under pressure in 1778, but not before publishing the *Directions for Preserving the Health of Soldiers*, a useful compendium of recommendations on military hygiene and camp sanitation.

Rush returned to a prosperous, genteel life of teaching and practice. He fathered 13 children and is said to have educated 2,872 physicians in his career. However, he promoted the notion that vigorous purging with calomel and bleeding was beneficial and is accused of having cost the lives of tens of thousands through a combination of personal influence and misguided ideas. During his life, though, his reputation remained unchallenged and he died in April 1813, the subject of general adoration and respect.

Jack McCallum

Further Reading

Gillet, Mary. *The Army Medical Department, 1775–1818.* Washington, D.C.: Center of Military History, 1981.

Packard, Francis. "[Benjamin Rush]." In Howard Kelly and Walter Burrage, *Dictionary of American Medical Biography: Lives of Eminent Physicians of the United States and Canada, from the Earliest Times.* Boston: Milford House, 1928.

Packard, Francis. *History of Medicine in the United States.* New York: Paul B. Hoeber, Inc., 1931.

Reiss, Oscar. *Medicine and the American Revolution.* Jefferson, NC: McFarland & Co., Inc., 1998.

Scurvy

Scurvy is both the greatest scourge and the greatest triumph of naval medicine. Although the disease is best known for causing soft, bleeding gums and loss of teeth, its effects are protean and, if untreated, fatal. Scurvy causes ulceration and bleeding from mucous membranes such as the gums and an associated foul breath. It also leads to bleeding elsewhere, including under the skin (bruises); in joints and muscles; and from the bladder, bowels, and lungs. Bleeding between the bones and surrounding periosteum causes knots and swelling in the arms and legs. Blood loss can be enough to result in anemia and lethargy. Headache, delirium, and coma characterize scurvy's final stages.

Scurvy is caused by lack of dietary vitamin C, an essential nutrient that humans are incapable of manufacturing and that, consequently, must come from food. An appropriate supply of vitamin C will completely prevent the disease, and supplying the vitamin to a patient with scurvy will reverse its effects.

Scurvy became a maritime concern when sailing ships and navigation techniques allowed protracted voyages away from land. Meats and carbohydrates were less perishable than fruits and vegetables and comprised almost the entire seagoing diet in the first three centuries of transoceanic voyages. During Sir Francis Drake's circumnavigation in 1585, 300 of his original 2,300-man crew died of scurvy within three months of leaving England. Commodore George Anson, who sailed around the world from 1740 to 1744, lost 1,050 of his 1,955 men to scurvy.

A

TREATISE

OF THE

SCURVY.

IN THREE PARTS.

CONTAINING

An inquiry into the Nature, Caufes,
and Cure, of that Difeafe.

Together with

A Critical and Chronological View of what
has been publifhed on the fubject.

By JAMES LIND, M. D.

Fellow of the Royal College of Phyficians in *Edinburgh*.

EDINBURGH:

Printed by SANDS, MURRAY, and COCHRAN.
For A. KINCAID & A. DONALDSON.
MDCCLIII.

In 1847, British naval surgeon James Lind scientifically showed that citrus juice cured scurvy. In spite of his "Treatise of the Scurvy", naval authorities were slow to reform naval diet. (Wellcome Images, London)

Ironically, Anson's logs noted that the men improved after eating Tahitian oranges, but the observation was ignored. That was not the only time the observation was made and ignored. East India Company physicians, at the time of the Company's 1600 expedition to India, suspected that citrus fruits might prevent scurvy. One of their four ships was supplied with lemons and oranges, and, although only the crew given the fruit remained free of scurvy, the practice still did not become general for nearly 200 years.

In May 1747, British naval surgeon James Lind designed what may have been scientific medicine's first controlled experiments: He divided 12 sailors with scurvy into six groups; each assigned one of the commonly accepted treatments for the disease. Only the group given lemons and oranges benefited and they were cured. In spite of the strength of Lind's experiment, general acceptance of citrus juice to prevent and treat scurvy was slow. Even Lind continued to believe that "good air" was at least as important as lemons in treating the disease. The Royal Navy finally introduced lemon juice as a treatment for scurvy in the early 1790s. First Lord of the Admiralty Earl Spencer ordered that it be a mandatory part of the British sailor's diet in 1795. Lemons and oranges were replaced by cheaper—but less effective—West Indian limes shortly thereafter, leading to the sobriquet "limey."

As late as 1900, Sir William Osler still believed overcrowding, damp quarters, prolonged fatigue, and depression contributed to scurvy, especially in a military setting. It was not until well into the 20th century that the exact nature of the vitamin deficiency leading to scurvy was delineated, by which time Lind's empirical treatment had long since eliminated the disease as a factor in naval medicine.

Jack McCallum

Further Reading

Gordon, Maurice Bell. *Naval and Maritime Medicine during the American Revolution.* Ventnor, NJ: Ventnor Publishing, 1978.

Hudson, Robert P. *Disease and Its Control: The Shaping of Modern Thought.* Westport, CT: Greenwood Press, 1983.

Osler, William. *Practice of Medicine.* New York: D. Appleton & Co., 1899.

Shippen, William (1712–1808)

Dr. William Shippen of Philadelphia, sometimes called "the father of American anatomy and midwifery," had a brilliant but tumultuous career as a military surgeon and administrator during the American Revolutionary War. Unlike most colonial physicians, Shippen had earned a medical degree from the University of Edinburgh, one of the most prestigious centers for medical education in Great Britain. This training gave him the organizational skills he used to overhaul America's military hospitals when he became director general of the army's Hospital Department in 1777. The nation's military hospitals were plagued with overcrowded conditions, inadequate ventilation, and meager sanitation, which contributed heavily to the high mortality rates during the war.

In April 1775, Massachusetts established the first general military hospital of the war at Cambridge, Massachusetts. From its inception, however, it lacked adequate medicine, supplies, and leadership. The Continental Congress, which quickly recognized the disarray in available military medical care, established an Army Medical Department in May 1775, with Massachusetts's Dr. Benjamin Church as director general and chief physician, and created a Hospital Department in July. But although Congress created departments and administrative positions, it failed to enact operational guidelines for such vital matters as the provision of medical supplies. Church's tenure as the first director general lasted only a few months; in the fall he was court-martialed for corresponding with the enemy.

In October 1775, Dr. John Morgan of Philadelphia succeeded to the position of director general. Morgan initiated clear procedural rules that included sending wounded militiamen to the Continental Army General Hospital along with injured Continental soldiers. He also attempted to gain control over the regimental surgeons, who were known to request more rum and wine than other staples and supplies. But Morgan soon acquired enemies in the heavily politicized Hospital Department, including Shippen, and his tenure as director general was brief.

Shippen began his military service in June 1776, when he was appointed medical director of the flying camp based in Trenton, New Jersey. Despite the establishment of the Hospital Department, the Continental Congress was still receiving reports of the sick being neglected, and the delegates were appalled at the high mortality rate during the disastrous New York Campaign. A congressional resolution in November 1776 gave Shippen the supervision of all military hospitals west of the Hudson River, whereas Director General Morgan supervised hospitals east of the Hudson, a region that the retreating Continental Army had largely abandoned by that date. This geographical division gave Shippen the greater share of the hospital stores and medicines along with half the department's surgeons. Consequently, Morgan was left with few resources to tend the sick and wounded left to his care. Coupled with this division of authority, Shippen's criticism of Morgan soured their once friendly relationship. In January 1777 Congress, responding to persistent criticisms of the director general, dismissed Morgan, but he was later exonerated from all charges of misconduct.

At this juncture Shippen joined Dr. John Cochran, another military surgeon, to devise a complex reorganization plan modeled on the British Army's medical service. After George Washington reviewed the plan, which contained a pay increase for regimental surgeons, he forwarded it to Congress. After some prodding, Congress finally enacted the new plan and elected Shippen as director general in April 1777, with Cochran serving as physician and surgeon of the army. The reorganization established four military districts—middle, eastern, northern, and southern—each with a physician general and a surgeon general who reported to the director general. As head of the entire department and commander of its middle district, the director general set up hospitals and supervised the procurement of all hospital stores and medical supplies, and the payment of the salaries of all departmental personnel.

When Shippen began his tenure, money and medical supplies were scarce. Overcrowded conditions in the General Hospital rapidly spread communicable diseases such as typhus, influenza, impetigo, and smallpox. Smallpox had decimated American troops during their invasion of Canada in 1776 and was a major factor in the collapse of that campaign. Inoculation for smallpox was available but still encountered considerable suspicion and resistance. At first Shippen, with the full support of Washington, was to inoculate all Continental troops, but he later amended the program to include only those recruits who had never had smallpox. For other diseases and injuries, few drugs were available to treat the sick and wounded. A medical equipment assessment in New York that included the regimental surgeons' personal medical equipment revealed the lack of surgical instruments and bandages.

Less than a year after Shippen's appointment, Dr. Benjamin Rush, an army surgeon, began to criticize the Hospital Department. Rush believed that an inspector general and chief physician should only visit the hospitals in each district, examine the medical stores and instruments, and report on the sick and wounded. And he insisted that an appointed purveyor, rather than the director general, should supply the hospitals with all necessities. Initially, these criticisms were directed against the hospital system as a whole, but Rush later attacked Shippen directly. At the time of these complaints, Washington and his troops were suffering through the harsh winter of 1777–1778 at Valley Forge. After Congress directed Rush's suggestions for changes to a committee, the committee recommended that Director General Shippen be relieved of his purchasing duties, and Congress agreed.

The bitterness between Rush and Shippen escalated to the point where Rush accused Shippen of malpractice and neglect. Rush charged that there was overcrowding and a high rate of infection at the Princeton Hospital, which Shippen denied. Washington presented the charges to Congress, but Congress took no action. In June 1779, Morgan, the previous director general, joined with Rush to press the issue and seek the court-martial of Shippen. Congress believed that Shippen had not committed any wrongdoing, but in May 1780, after much delay, Shippen was subjected to a formal court-martial trial. Although many persons strongly believed the charges against him, Shippen was acquitted in July of speculation and the illegal sale of hospital stores because of a lack of evidence.

The Hospital Department that Congress's medical committee had been overseeing following Shippen's arrest, however, needed complete reform. Congress soon overhauled the department by eliminating its geographical districts and reducing the number of officers. At the same time, it retained Shippen as director general, but in January 1781, feeling that his reputation had been heavily damaged by the inconclusive court-martial, Shippen resigned his office to resume his private medical practice and his teaching in Philadelphia. Cochran succeeded him as director general and completed the reorganization of the Hospital Department. In his later years, Shippen helped found the College of Physicians of Philadelphia and served as its president until his death in 1808.

Suzanne M. Carter

Further Reading

Bell, Whitfield. *John Morgan, Continental Doctor.* Philadelphia: University of Pennsylvania Press, 1965.

McDonald, Walter J. "Physician Revolutionaries of 1776—Patriots, Opportunists, or Both?" *Transactions of the American Clinical and Climatological Association* 108 (1996): 286–297.

Risch, Erna. "The Hospital Department." In *Supplying Washington's Army.* Washington, DC: Center of Military History, United States Army, 1981. http://www.army.mil/cmh-pg/books/RevWar/risch/chpt-13.htm.

Toledo-Pereyra, Luis H. "William Shippen, Jr.: Pioneer Revolutionary War Surgeon and Father of American Anatomy and Midwifery."*Journal of Investigative Surgery* 15 (July–August 2002): 183–184.

Wilbur, C. Keith. *Revolutionary Medicine: 1700–1800.* Old Saybrook, CT: Globe Pequot, 1980.

Smallpox

A systemic viral disease that occurs in two forms: variola major, which carries 25 percent mortality, and variola minor, with a 1 percent mortality. The disease is caused by an orthopoxvirus. This deoxyribonucleic acid (DNA) based organism is the largest virus that infects animals. The virus initially multiplies in the bloodstream before infecting internal organs, especially the lungs, liver, and spleen. About 12 days after exposure there is a secondary viremia at which time the organism infects the skin causing a rash that develops into vesicles after two to three days. Fluid from either infected lungs or from weeping vesicles carries viral particles and can spread the infection, although human-to-human transmission is usually by inhalation of infected airborne fluids. The disease is relatively contagious, with one drop of pulmonary secretion typically carrying 1,000 or more viral particles than are needed to cause an infection, although a carrier is typically infectious for only three to four days.

There is no treatment for an established infection, however smallpox was the first disease successfully prevented by creating immunity in potential hosts. For centuries the Chinese and later the Turks intentionally exposed susceptible people to infectious material from patients suffering from mild forms of smallpox. This "variolation" or "buying the pox" carried a mortality of some 1–10 percent but conferred permanent immunity. In 1796, English physician Edward Jenner proved that exposure to cowpox (vaccinia) was almost universally safe and, in 99 percent of cases, conferred lasting immunity to the genetically related smallpox virus.

Smallpox has played an intentional and an unintentional military role over the centuries. Native Americans had no previous exposure to this disease, Europeans unintentionally brought with them influenza, malaria, measles, plague, and smallpox. Because the Native Americans had no previous exposure to this disease and had not acquired any immunity, they suffered very high mortality rates once infected. In 1763, the British commander-in-chief, Major General Jeffery Amherst, attempted to use smallpox as a weapon by ordering that infected blankets be distributed to Native Americans during Pontiac's Rebellion.

Jack McCallum

Further Reading

Levine, Arnold, *Viruses*. New York: Scientific American Library, 1992.

McNeill, William. *Plagues and Peoples*. New York: Doubleday, 1977.

Syphilis

Syphilis is a venereal disease caused by *Treponema pallidum* and has accompanied armies at least since the 15th century. Syphilis is transmitted by human sexual contact and begins as a painless genital ulcer that typically arises within a few weeks of exposure and resolves spontaneously. If untreated, syphilis can progress to a secondary stage characterized by skin rash and fever. The organism can again become dormant to reemerge years later in its tertiary form with infection of the meninges, brain, spinal cord, and nerves; with masses in various organs known as gummas; and with damage to the heart and blood vessels—all potentially lethal complications. Syphilis is sensitive to penicillin, which remains the primary means of treatment.

The exact history of syphilis is clouded by its confusion with leprosy and scabies, although, of the three, only syphilis is sensitive to mercurials. For unexplained reasons, the clinical nature of syphilis underwent a fundamental change in the late 15th century. In 1495, physicians described what they thought was a new disease characterized by pain so severe that patients drowned themselves

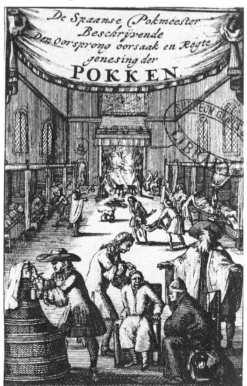

Syphilis has afflicted military personnel since at least the 15th century. This image shows treatment for syphilis in a seventeenth century hospital. (National Library of Medicine)

attempting to decrease the burning in their limbs accompanied by a red rash that progressed to foul-smelling, black pustules. The first epidemic of the "new" disease came during the Italian Wars (1494–1559) and spread across Northern Europe as either the *Mal Francese* or the Great Pox. The French understandably attributed the disease either to the Italians or the Spanish. By 1505, the pox had accompanied the Portuguese to India, China, and Japan. The virulence and easy transmissibility suggest that the disease, if not altogether new, was at least a significant bacterial mutation.

As it coincided temporally with Christopher Columbus's return from the New World, medical authorities after 1539 credited his sailors with having imported the illness. Regardless of where the disease originated, syphilis remained a major European problem for the next two centuries, especially in areas frequented by migrating armies. It affected all levels of society. With general acceptance of the bacterial nature of infectious disease in the second half of the 19th century, control of venereal disease among soldiers became largely a matter of policing and controlling prostitutes. The British Contagious Diseases Act of 1866 required that all prostitutes around naval or military stations be periodically examined in a government dispensary and be hospitalized for treatment if found to be infected. This law was singularly effective although it was repealed in 1883 in favor of the self-control advocated by Victorian morality.

Although prophylactics were issued to soldiers during World War I, American officials, like their English predecessors, preferred to emphasize "education" and self-restraint. Syphilis was the seventh most common disease in the American Expeditionary Force, and, between April 1917 and December 1919, the incidence of venereal disease in the U.S. Army was 87 per 1,000 with a total of 259,621 cases treated or hospitalized. Many of these cases were, however, present at the time of enlistment, since 5 percent of all draftees were found to have a venereal disease.

During World War II, the incidence of syphilis among American troops was 16 per 1,000, and venereal disease overall accounted for 1,250,846 admissions during the conflict.

Jack McCallum

Further Reading

Arrizabalaga, Jon, John Henderson, and Roger French. *The Great Pox: The French Disease in Renaissance Europe*. New Haven, CT: Yale University Press, 1997.

Lada, John, ed. *Medical Statistics in World War II*. Washington, D.C.: Office of the Surgeon General, 1975.

McNeill, William H. *Plagues and Peoples*. Garden City, NY: Anchor Press, 1976.

Sun, Sue. 2004. "Where the Girls Are: The Management of Venereal Disease by United States Military Forces in Vietnam." *Literature and Medicine* 23 (1): 66–87.

Warren, John (1753–1815)

John Warren, a physician and brother to the martyred General Joseph Warren, spent the Revolutionary War serving as a surgeon to the Continental Army and operating the army hospital at Boston.

The youngest of four sons of a Roxbury, Massachusetts, farmer and physician, Warren graduated from Harvard College in 1771. Upon leaving school, he spent two years studying medicine with his brother Joseph, one of the leading physicians in Boston. A two-year internship was the only requirement at the time to qualify a student for the practice of medicine.

Warren then settled in Salem, Massachusetts, and began his medical practice there. He aided the Revolutionary cause with his tongue and his pen, but not with his purse. Perhaps scarred by the early death of his father, Warren gained a reputation for carefully watching his coins and refused financial assistance to Joseph when the latter's medical practice suffered because of his Revolutionary activities.

Warren's medical skill and political leanings, however, did make him one of the first medical men to aid the Revolutionary cause. At the time of the battles at Lexington and Concord, he served as surgeon to Colonel Timothy Pickering's Salem regiment. After Joseph's death at Bunker Hill, Warren accepted the post of a hospital surgeon at the Continental Army General Hospital in Cambridge. Eager to avenge his brother's death, he was persuaded in part to take this job by his mother's distress at the thought of losing another son in battle. General hospitals received the sick of the garrison, the corps of invalids, the regiment of the train, the vagrant troops, new recruits, and all Continental prisoners. Warren remained in Cambridge from July 1775 to April 1776.

During the New York–New Jersey Campaign of 1776 to 1777, Warren served as senior surgeon in several Continental Army general hospitals, including those at Long Island, Trenton, and Hackensack. By April 1777, he had left the army and returned to Boston. In July 1777, however, he was chosen to head the army hospital being set up in Boston. He remained in this post until the end of the Revolution.

In 1780, Warren became a medical pioneer by teaching the first anatomical classes in Boston that used actual specimens of the human body. In this era, considerable opposition existed toward dissection, but Warren took advantage of his position within the hospital to obtain bodies. Appointed the first professor of anatomy and surgery at Harvard Medical School in 1782, he would be the first surgeon to amputate at the shoulder joint, perform an abdominal resection, and remove the parotid gland. In 1781, he helped found the Massachusetts Medical Society. Warren died of heart failure on April 4, 1815.

Caryn E. Neumann

Further Reading

Truax, Rhoda. *The Doctors Warren of Boston: First Family of Surgery.* Boston: Houghton Mifflin, 1968.

Warren, Edward. *The Life of John Warren, M.D.* Boston: Noyes, Holmes, 1874.

DOCUMENTS

William Trent was the son of a prominent merchant involved with the founding of the colony of Pennsylvania. Trent resided on the frontier where he worked as a trader, Indian agent, and land speculator. During Pontiac's Rebellion, Trent served in the colonial military. The following excerpt from Trent's journal, written in 1763 during the Siege of Fort Pitt, relates his plan to infect hostile Indians with smallpox. As Trent explained to his superior, "Could it not be contrived to send the Small Pox among those disaffected tribes of Indians? We must on this occasion use every stratagem in our power to reduce them." In this early attempt to use biological warfare, Trent had chosen a particularly deadly virus. Smallpox passed directly from human to human, and there was no treatment for infected victims. Smallpox occurs in two forms. About one-quarter of those infected with variola major died.

22th Between 9 and 10 o'clock in the morning a smoke was seen rising on the back of Grants Hill where the Indians had made a fire and about 2 o'clock several of them appeared in the Spelts field moving of the horses and cattle. About 5 o'clock one James Thompson who it was supposed was gone after a horse was killed and scalped in sight of the fort on this a great number of Ind[ian]s appeared on each river and on Grants Hill shooting down the cattle and horses.

23th about 12 o'clock at night two Delawares called for Mr McKee and told him they wanted to speak to him in the morning.

24th The Turtles Heart a principal warrior of the Delawares and Mamaltee a chief came within a small distance of the Fort. Mr McKee went out to them and they made a speech letting us know that all our [ ] as Ligonier was destroyed, that great numbers of Indians [were coming and] that out of regard to us, they had prevailed on 6 Nations [not to] attack us but give us time to go down the country and they desired we would set of immediately. The Commanding Officer thanked them, let them know that we had everything we wanted, that we could defend it against all the Indians in the Woods, that we had three large Armies marching to chastise those Indians that had struck us, told them to take care of their women and children, but not to tell any other natives, they said they would go and speak to their chiefs and come and tell us what they said, they returned and said they would hold fast of the chain of friendship. Out of our regard to them we gave them two blankets and an handkerchief out of the smallpox hospital. I hope it will have the desired effect.

Source: William Trent's Journal at Fort Pitt, 1763. Edited by A.T. Volwiler. Mississippi Valley Historical Review, Vol XI, No. 3, 390–413, December 1924.

When the American Revolution began, the difficulties establishing an effective medical military service mirrored the tremendous problems associated with building a military force from scratch. There were only two hospitals in all the colonies and only about 200 practicing physicians had a medical degree. The vast majority of the 3,500 physicians were mere apprentices, often with no more than one year of formal study as an apothecary. Yet, these poorly prepared men had to provide medical care to the sick and wounded soldiers while also serving the civilian population. The Continental Congress established a Medical Corps on July 27, 1775. It proved inadequate to address wartime needs. Five years later, Congress passed a revised law that was much more comprehensive. The progression of requirements from 1775 to 1780 demonstrate the young nation's increasing understanding of the complexities associated with creating and administering an effective military medical service.

Law of 27 July 1775

The Congress took into consideration the report of the committee on establishing an hospital, and the same being debated, was agreed to as follows:

That for the establishment of a hospital for an army consisting of 20,000 men the following officers and other attendants be appointed, with the following allowance or pay, viz.

1 Director general and chief physician, his pay per day	4 dollars
4 Surgeons, per diem, each	1 1/3 do.
1 Apothecary	1 1/3 do.
20 Mates, each	2/3 do.
1 Clerk	2/3 do.
2 Storekeepers, each	4 dollars per month
1 Nurse to every 10 sick labourers occasionally	1/15 of a dollar per day, or 2 dollars per month

The duty of the above officers: viz.

Director to furnish medicines, bedding and all other necessaries, to pay for the same, superintend the whole, and make his report to, and receive orders from, the commander-in-chief.

Surgeons, apothecary and mates: To visit and attend the sick and the mates to obey the orders of the physicians, surgeons and apothecary.

Matron: To superintend the nurses, bedding, etc.

Nurses: To attend the sick, and obey the matron's orders.

Clerk: To keep accounts for the director and storekeepers.

Storekeeper: To receive and deliver the bedding and other necessaries by order of the director.

The Congress then proceeded to the choice of officers for the hospital, when Benjamin Church was unanimously elected as director of, and chief physician in, the hospital.

Resolved, That the appointment of the four surgeons and the apothecary be left to Dr Benjamin Church.

That the mates be appointed by the surgeons; that the number do not exceed twenty; that the number be not kept in constant pay, unless the sick and wounded should be so numerous as to require the attendance of twenty, and to be diminished as circumstances will admit; for which purpose, the pay is fixed by the day that they may only receive pay for actual service.

That one clerk and two storekeepers and one nurse to every ten sick be appointed by the director.

Source: Worthington Chauncey Ford; Gaillard Hunt; and others, eds. *Journals of the Continental Congress.* 2: 209–10, 211. Washington: Government Printing Office, 1904–37.

Law of 30 September 1780

Whereas, the late regulations for conducting the affairs of the general hospital are in many respects defective; and it is necessary that the same be revised and amended, in order that the sick and wounded may be properly provided for and attended, and the business of the hospitals conducted with regularity and economy; therefore,

Resolved, That there be one director of the military hospitals, who shall have the general direction and superintendance of all the hospitals to the northward of North Carolina; that, within the aforesaid limits, there be three chief hospital physicians, who shall also be surgeons; one chief physician, who shall also be a surgeon, to each separate army; fifteen hospital physicians, who shall also be surgeons; twenty surgeons mates for the hospitals; one purveyor, with one assistant; one apothecary; one assistant apothecary; and to each hospital a steward, matron, orderly men and nurses, as heretofore:

That the director, or, in his absence, one of the chief hospital physicians, be empowered and required, with the advice and consent of the commander-in-chief, or commander of a separate army, to establish and regulate such a number of hospitals, at proper places, for the reception of the sick and wounded of the army, as may be found necessary:

That the director be authorized and instructed to enjoin the several chief hospital physicians, and other officers of the hospitals under his superintendence, to attend at such posts or stations as he may judge proper, and also to attend and perform such duties, at any post or place, as a change of the position of the army, or other circumstances, may from time to time make necessary, and shall be required by the commander-in-chief; and that, in case of any dispute concerning their seniority or precedence, the director shall determine the same in the first instance, the party supposing himself aggrieved being at liberty to appeal for redress to the Medical Committee.

That in time of action, and on any other emergency, when the regimental surgeons are not sufficient in number to attend properly to the sick and wounded that cannot be removed to the hospitals, the director, or, in his absence, the nearest chief hospital physician, be empowered and required, upon request of the chief physician and surgeon of the army, to send from the hospitals under his care, to the assistance of such sick and wounded, as many surgeons as can possibly be spared from the necessary business of the hospitals:

That the director, or, in his absence, two of the chief hospital physicians, shall make out and deliver, from time to time, to the purveyor, proper estimates of hospital stores, medicines, instruments, dressings, and such other articles as may be judged necessary for the use of the hospitals; also direct the apothecary or his assistant, to prepare and deliver medicines, instruments, dressings, and other articles in his possession to the hospitals and surgeons of the army and navy, as he or they may judge necessary:

That the director authorize and instruct the purveyor and apothecary to supply, for the use of the regimental surgeons, such medicines and refreshments as may be proper for the relief of the sick and wounded, before their removal to a general hospital, and to be dispensed under the care, and at the direction of the chief physician of the army:

That the director, or, in his absence, the chief hospital physicians, respectively, be empowered occasionally to employ second mates, when the number of the sick shall increase so as to make it necessary, and to discharge them as soon as the circumstances of the sick will admit:

That the director, or, in his absence, the chief hospital physicians, respectively, shall appoint a ward master for each hospital, to receive the spare regimental clothing, arms, and accoutrements of each soldier admitted therein, keeping entries of and giving receipts for every article received, which, when the soldier shall be discharged, shall be accounted for by the said ward master with the commanding officer of the regiment to which such soldier belonged, or the officer directed to take charge of the convalescents from the said hospital; or, in case of the death of the soldier, shall be accounted for with, and delivered to the quartermaster of the regiment to which the said soldier belonged; and the ward master shall receive and be accountable for the hospital clothing, and perform such other services as the chief hospital physician shall direct.

That the director shall make returns of all the sick and wounded in the hospitals, once every month, to the medical committee, together with the names and ranks of all the officers and others employed in the several hospitals:

That the director be required to employ such part of his time as may be spared from the duties before pointed out to him, in visiting and prescribing for the sick and wounded of the hospitals; and that he pay particular attention to the conduct of the several officers in the hospital department, and arrest, suspend and bring to trial, all delinquents within the same:

That the duty of the chief hospital physicians shall be, to do and perform all the duties herein before enjoined them to do in the absence of the director; to receive and obey the orders of the director, made and delivered to them in writing, to superintend the practice of the sick and surgery in the hospitals put under their particular care by the director, or which, by the order of the commander-in-chief or the commander of a separate army, may be by them established; to see that the hospital physicians and other officers attending the same, do their duty; and make monthly returns to the director, of the state and number of the sick and wounded in the hospitals under their care; and also make returns to the director, and to the medical committee, of all delinquent officers, in order that they may be speedily removed or punished; and to take measures that all such sick and wounded as are recovered and fit for duty be delivered weekly to the officer of the guard, to be conducted to the army: when present at any hospital, to issue orders to the proper officers for supplying them with necessaries; and generally, in the absence of the director, to superintend and control the business of such hospitals, suspend delinquent and remove unnecessary non-commissioned officers, making report to the director; and, when in their power, to attend and perform or direct all capital operations:

That the hospital physicians shall take charge of such particular hospitals as may be assigned them by the director: They shall obey the orders of the director, or in his absence, of the chief hospital physician: They shall have power to suspend officers under them, and to confine other persons serving in the hospitals under their charge, for negligence or ill-behavior, until the matter be regularly inquired into: They shall diligently attend to the cases of the sick and wounded of the hospitals under their care, administering at all times proper relief, as far as may be in their power: They shall respectively give orders, under their hands, to the assistant purveyor or steward at the hospital, for the issuing provisions and stores, as well as for the procuring any other small articles that the exigencies of the hospital may require, and which the store is not provided with, having always a strict regard to economy, as well as the welfare of the sick then to be provided for: They shall make weekly returns to the nearest chief hospital physician, of the state of the hospitals under their respective care.

The mates shall each take charge of and attend the patients assigned them and perform such other duties as shall be directed by the director, chief or other physicians and surgeons.

The chief physician and surgeon of the army shall be subject to the orders and control of the director: His duty shall be to superintend the regimental surgeons and their mates, and to see that they do their duty: To hear all complaints against the said regimental surgeons and mates, and make report of them to the director, or, in his absence, to the commander-in-chief or commanding officer of a separate army, that they may be brought to trial by court-martial for misbehavior: To draw for and receive from the purveyor a suitable number of large strong tents, beds, bedding and hospital stores, and from the apothecary, or his assistant, proper medicines, for such sick and wounded persons as cannot be removed to the general hospital with safety, or may be rendered fit for duty in a short time. He shall also see that the sick and wounded, while under his care, are properly attended and provided for, and conveyed, when fit to be removed, to the general hospital; for which last purpose, he shall be supplied by the quartermaster general, with a proper number of convenient wagons and drivers; he shall have a steward, which he is to appoint, to receive and properly dispense such articles of diet and refreshment as shall be procured for the sick; and also shall appoint such a. number of nurses and orderly men as may be necessary for the attendance of the sick and wounded under his care. He shall cause daily returns to be made to him of all the sick and wounded which have been removed to the hospitals, all that remain in the hospital tents, all that are become fit for duty, all that are convalescent, and all who may have died, specifying the particular maladies under which the sick and wounded labor, and shall make a monthly return thereof to the director, who shall add it to his general hospital returns, to be transmitted monthly to the Medical Committee.

That whenever any regimental surgeon or mate shall be absent from his regiment, without leave from the chief physician and surgeon or commander of the army where his duty lies, the said chief physician and surgeon shall have power to remove such surgeon or mate and forthwith appoint another in his stead.

That the purveyor provide, or cause to be provided, all hospital stores, medicines, instruments, dressings, utensils, and such other articles as shall be prescribed by the written order of the director, or two of the chief hospital physicians, and deliver, or cause the same to be delivered, upon written orders, under the hands of the director, or chief hospital physician, or one of the hospital physicians, having the charge of a particular hospital, or of a chief physician and surgeon of the army, which, with receipts thereon for delivery of the same, shall be his sufficient vouchers. He shall be allowed a clerk, and as many store keepers as occasion may require, and the director shall approve of. He shall also pay the salaries of the officers, and all other expenses of the hospitals. He shall render his accounts every three months to the Board of Treasury for settlement, and make application for money to the Medical Committee, before whom he shall lay estimates of articles necessary, which shall previously have been approved and signed by the director or two of the chief hospital physicians; at the same time he shall render to them an account of the expenditure of the last sum of money advanced to him; and the said Medical Committee shall lay such estimates before Congress, with their opinion thereon:

That the assistant purveyor shall procure such supplies, and do and perform such parts of the purveyor's duty, as by him shall be particularly assigned to him.

That the apothecary and his assistant receive, prepare and deliver medicines, instruments and dressings, and such other articles of his department, to the hospitals and army, on orders in writing from the director or either of the chief hospital physicians, or chief physician and surgeon of the army; and that he be allowed as many mates as occasion may require, and the director shall approve of:

That the director, or in his absence, the chief hospital physician, shall appoint a steward for each hospital, whose duty it shall be to purchase vegetables and other small articles, under the direction of the purveyor, and to receive hospital stores from the purveyor, and provisions from the commissary general, and issue the same for the use of the sick and wounded, agreeably to the order of the physician and surgeon attending such hospital; the steward to account with the purveyor for all such issues:

That the director, or, in his absence, the chief hospital physician, appoint a proper number of matrons, nurses, and others, necessary for the regular management of the hospitals, and fix and ascertain their pay, not exceeding the sums heretofore allowed; and point out and prescribe their particular duties and employments, in writing, which they are enjoined to observe and obey:

That the director, with two chief hospital physicians, be empowered to fix the pay of second mates, and of such clerks, store keepers, and other persons, as may occasionally be employed; and also make such regulations, and point out and enjoin, in writing, such further particular duties for the several officers in the hospital department, as they may judge necessary for the regular management of the same; which duties shall always be consistent with, and in no wise contradictory to any of the duties herein before particularly enumerated, and which being reported to, and approved of by the Medical Committee, shall thereupon become obligatory to all those concerned:

That the quartermaster general furnish the hospital department, from time to time, as occasion may require, with such a number of horses and wagons as may be necessary for removing the sick and wounded, and for transporting the hospital stores; but that no other horses than those belonging to the officers of the department, for which forage may be herein allowed, be kept separately and at the expense of the department.

That no person concerned in trade, on his own account, shall be suffered to act as an officer in the hospital or medical department of the army:

That no officer or other person in the hospital department, except the sick and wounded, be permitted to use any of the stores provided for the sick:

That the director, chief hospital physicians, and the chief physicians and surgeons of the army, physicians and surgeons, purveyor, apothecary, assistant purveyor, and assistant apothecary, be appointed and commissioned by Congress; the regimental surgeons and mates to be appointed as heretofore:

That the director, with the advice and concurrence of two of the chief hospital physicians, appoint all hospital mates, which appointments shall be certified by warrants under the hand of the director; in which appointments no person shall be admitted under the age of twenty-one years:

That all the officers in the hospital or medical departments, shall be subjected to trial by courts-martial for all offences, in the same manner as officers of the line of the army.

Resolved, That the pay and establishment of the officers of the hospital department, and medical staff, be as follows:

Director, one hundred and fifty dollars per month, two rations for himself, and one for his servant, per day, and forage for two horses:

Chief physicians and surgeons of the army and hospitals, each, one hundred and forty dollars per month, two rations per day, and forage for two horses:

Purveyor and apothecary, each, one hundred and thirty dollars per month:

Physicians and surgeons of the hospitals, each, one hundred and twenty dollars per month, one ration per day, and forage for one horse:

Assistant purveyors and apothecaries, each, seventy-five dollars per month:

Regimental surgeons, each, sixty-five dollars per month, one ration per day, and forage for one horse:

Surgeons' mates in the hospitals, fifty dollars per month, one ration per day:

Surgeons' mates in the army, forty-five dollars per month, one ration per day:

Steward for each hospital, thirty-five dollars per month, one ration per day:

Ward master for each hospital, twenty-five dollars per month, one ration per day:

Resolved, That none of the aforesaid officers, or other persons employed in any of the hospitals, be entitled to rations of provisions or forage when on furlough.

Resolved, That the chief physician of the army be allowed a two horse covered wagon for transporting his baggage:

That the several officers abovementioned shall receive their pay in the new currency, emitted pursuant to a resolution of Congress of the 18th day of March last; and that they be allowed and paid at the rate of five dollars of said currency per month for every retained ration; and shall each be entitled annually to draw clothing from the stores of the clothier general, in the same manner and under the same regulations as are established for officers of the line, by a resolution of Congress of the 25th November, 1779:

That the returns for clothing for officers in the medical staff (regimental surgeons and their mates, who are to draw with the regimental staff, excepted) be signed by the directors, or one of the chief hospital physicians; and such clothing shall be delivered either by the clothier general or any sub-clothier in the state in which the officer to receive clothing shall reside, in the same manner as is provided in the cases of other staff officers not taken from the line:

That the several officers whose pay is established as above (except the stewards and ward masters) shall at the end of the war be entitled to a certain provision of land, in the proportion following, viz.

The director to have the same quantity as a brigadier-general;

Chief physicians and purveyor, the same as a colonel;

Physicians and surgeons and apothecary, the same as a lieutenant colonel;

Regimental surgeons and assistants to the purveyor and apothecary, the same as a major;

Hospital and regimental surgeons' mates, the same as a captain;

That the former arrangements of the hospital department, and all resolutions heretofore passed touching the same, so far as they are inconsistent with the foregoing, be repealed, excepting that the hospitals in the southern department, from North Carolina to Georgia, inclusive, be continued under the same regulations as heretofore, until the further order of Congress.

Source: Worthington Chauncey Ford; Gaillard Hunt; and others, eds. *Journals of the Continental Congress.* 18: 878–88. Washington: Government Printing Office, 1904–37.

◼ CHAPTER 2
War of 1812

INTRODUCTION

Following the Revolutionary War, Congress retained only a very small military force. Most of that force provided garrisons for forts located on the western frontier. In 1798, war with France appeared imminent. Congress expanded the army and authorized a medical corps lcd by a physician general. The threat of war soon receded, so Congress discharged all but a skeleton force with a medical corps composed of only six surgeons and twelve surgeon's mates. Another reduction occurred in 1802, leaving the medical corps with only two surgeons and twenty-five surgeon's mates.

Growing tensions with Great Britain in 1808 led to a slight increase in authorized medical personnel. More importantly, for the first time since the Revolutionary War, the position of chief surgeon for the whole army was created. Congress declared war on Great Britain on June 18, 1812. Both the army and navy experienced a tremendous expansion. The medical corps witnessed a parallel expansion. However, there was neither a centralized medical command nor standard procedures for administration and treatment. Medical care depended upon the abilities of regimental surgeons. The militia provided their own surgeons while the Regular Army was responsible for medical supplies. This proved a formula for bureaucratic inefficiency.

Finally, in the summer of 1813 came the appointments of a physician general, surgeon general, and apothecary general.

James Tilton, a Revolutionary War veteran, assumed the combined position of physician and surgeon general of the army. Frances LeBaron became apothecary general. Tilton's poor health contributed to his poor performance. He contemplated reforms but failed to implement them. He was particularly poor at administration. Consequently, medical care in the American army was little better than it had been at the end of the American Revolution. After Tilton's retirement in 1815, Congress abolished the separate offices of physician general and surgeon general, replacing them with a single surgeon general of the army. LeBaron confronted different problems. The commissary general had the mission of purchasing supplies and then turning them over to LeBaron for distribution. National distrust of paper money made the supplies difficult and expensive to purchase. A disorganized bureaucracy, poor roads, and long distances impaired delivery of the purchases. Consequently, LeBaron's apothecaries stocked limited amounts of poor supplies. The resultant quality of the medicines on hand was inconsistent.

As a group, the doctors who relied upon the federal apothecaries were worse than the supplies themselves. At the beginning of the war there were three classes of medical officers. Hospital surgeons and their mates stood at the top. Regulations stated that all hospital surgeons were either medical school graduates or capable of passing an examination by an army board. Garrison surgeons and their mates were a step below the hospital surgeons. At the bottom stood regimental surgeons and their mates. Given that the lower two classes were distinctions with little actual difference, in 1814 these two classes were combined into one. But, such bureaucratic shuffling did little to improve performance.

Medical knowledge had barely progressed since the Revolution. Ignorance of the role of sanitation and the methods of disease transmission allowed fevers, gastrointestinal diseases, and pulmonary diseases to kill far more men than died in battle. Typhus and malaria were the most common fevers. Bacterial infections caused by contaminated food and water afflicted soldiers' gastrointestinal tracts. Pulmonary infections included everything from common upper respiratory infections to much more lethal pneumonia and tuberculosis. Medical personnel had no effective medicines to administer for these ailments. Consequently, sickness was so widespread that by August 1813, more than one-third of serving soldiers were on sick report. Although contemporary European armies, particular Napoleon's French army, had begun employing more modern casualty clearing techniques, American attempts to imitate them failed. Poor roads and long distances conspired to prevent the widespread use of wheeled ambulances.

Once a wounded man arrived at a field hospital, he faced the same lethal conditions experienced by Revolutionary War soldiers. Confined to filthy, damp, poorly ventilated huts, the wounded had to be strong and lucky to survive. The mistaken notion that smoke limited the risk of infection contributed to the misery of the wounded. Reforms at the end of 1814 sought to ensure that bed clothes be aired daily and bed straw changed once a month. In the all too common event that a patient died, the bed straw was supposed to be burned immediately. The reforms required privies to be cleaned twice daily. Each outhouse was to contain water or charcoal to limit odor. In the inchoate recognition that cleanliness mattered, each hospital ward had a cleaning woman assigned.

The 800-bed hospital at Burlington, Vermont stood out for its attention to cleanliness. Workers regularly scrubbed the whitewashed walls with soap and water.

White sand covered the floors with workers changing the sand when it became soiled. The wounded and sick received a bath upon admission and thereafter had to wash their faces and hands daily. A shave every other day and twice weekly distribution of clean shirts further encouraged hospital sanitation.

However, surgical practice still put contaminated dressings on contaminated wounds. Unsterile amputation remained the most common surgical intervention. Surgeons dealt with head traumas by drilling into the skull to relieve pressure.

The treatment of disease relied upon medicines ranging from ineffective to positively harmful. Most American physicians were adherents of Revolutionary-era Benjamin Rush. Rush recommended purgatives such as calomel and tartar emetic and copious bloodletting for anyone not already in shock. These treatments badly weakened already stressed patients. Cauterization and swabbing a wound with alcohol somewhat limited infection. Practitioners had no idea why these practices were beneficial. Physicians used digitalis to stimulate the heart, which was effective although often used inappropriately, and administered opium for pain.

In sum, during the War of 1812 soldiers recognized that falling into the hands of the medical corps was a high-stake roll of the dice with lethal outcomes all too likely. But there was progress as slowly hospitals became cleaner and the medical corps became more efficient. The medical corps' trials and tribulations during the War of 1812 led to the establishment of a permanent peacetime Army Medical Department in 1818, three years after the war ended.

James R. Arnold

ENTRIES

Abdominal Injuries in War

Because of the risk of damage to multiple organs, penetrating injuries of the abdomen have been a major cause of battlefield death. Prior to the 16th century, most such injuries were caused by bladed weapons that could perforate the digestive tract; major blood vessels; or solid viscera such as the kidney, liver, or spleen. The advent of gunpowder weapons made penetrating abdominal injuries more common and more lethal.

Prior to the 18th century, patients with penetrating abdominal injuries were essentially untreatable, and most died from their injuries. A common course involved penetration of the intestine, and spillage of feces into the peritoneal cavity followed—often after days of excruciating pain—by sepsis and death. In the late 1700s, scattered reports of exploration and repair of punctured viscera, especially the stomach, appeared. A historic case involved American army surgeon William Beaumont. After serving in the War of 1812, Beaumont published a landmark study of gastric physiology based on observations of a gastric fistula that resulted from a shotgun blast to the abdomen.

The advent of anesthesia and antiseptic technique made surgical exploration and repair of damaged organs practical and gave surgery for intra-abdominal trauma a reasonable chance of success. In 1881, American gynecologist James Marion Sims, a medical volunteer in the Franco-Prussian War, recommended early operation for all abdominal penetrations. In the absence of antibiotics, however, the death rate from secondary infection caused by fecal spillage from the perforated bowel remained high. In a monograph describing his experience with abdominal wounds in the Boer War, George Makins persisted in recommending nonoperative management, although 33 percent of the patients who survived long enough to come under his care still died. Nicholas Senn had a similar experience with American soldiers at Santiago during the Spanish-American War in 1898.

At the onset of World War I, there was still a debate as to whether patients with abdominal wounds were more likely to survive with or without exploratory surgery. Mortality from abdominal wounds in that war was an estimated 53 percent. In World War II, even with the advent of antibiotics, mortality ranged from 18 to 36 percent. In a series of soldiers wounded in Vietnam, mortality was said to have been 10 percent, but if one includes all patients who did not live to come to the hospital, the estimate ranges as high as 42 percent. Of those who died, 60 percent succumbed to hemorrhage; 25 percent died from sepsis; and 15 percent died in pulmonary failure (presumably related to shock).

In recent conflicts in southeastern Europe and in the Middle East, an estimated 20 percent of battle casualties had an abdominal wound, and approximately half of those died. Because infection is most often averted with early surgery or controlled with broad-spectrum antibiotics, sepsis has become a relatively rare cause of death after abdominal wounds. Most deaths are now because of blood loss and its complications.

Jack McCallum

Further Reading

Coupland, R. 1996. "Abdominal Wounds in War." *British Journal of Surgery* 83: 1505–1511.

Makins, George. *Surgical Experiences in South Africa, 1899–1900*. Philadelphia: Blakiston, 1900.

Rignault, Daniel. 1992. "Abdominal Trauma in War." *World Journal of Surgery* 16 (September): 940–946.

Senn, Nicholas. *Medico-surgical Aspects of the Spanish American War*. Chicago: AMA Press, 1900.

Wangensteen, Owen, and Sarah Wangensteen. *The Rise of Surgery from Empiric Craft to Scientific Discipline*. Minneapolis: University of Minnesota Press, 1978.

Amputation

The term "amputation" generally refers to the removal of all or part of an extremity which has been deemed impossible to save either because of the extent of injury or the risk of spreading disease such as infection or tumor from the injured limb to the rest of the body.

After dressing of wounds and removal of foreign bodies, amputation was the military surgeon's most important operation from ancient times until well into the 19th century. In the days before transfusion, anesthesia, and antisepsis, the surgeon's speed was the primary determinant of a patient's survival, and operating time of three to four minutes for amputation through the thigh were typical. Early amputations were performed with a single sweeping, circular cut through the skin, muscle, tendons, nerves, and vessels, followed by a quick transection of the bone with a specially designed saw. The inevitable hemorrhage was then controlled by applying hot pitch or oil and a pressure dressing.

The earliest surviving detailed description of amputation dates to the 1st century A.D. and was used to stop the spread of infection from gangrene. Early Roman practice stressed the importance of avoiding undue blood loss, of making the incision well within the margin of healthy tissue and never through a joint, and of leaving enough skin to cover the end of the remaining extremity to allow the fitting of effective prostheses. Although some authorities described ligating vessels, finding and tying a bleeding artery took time. Since speed was essential in operations

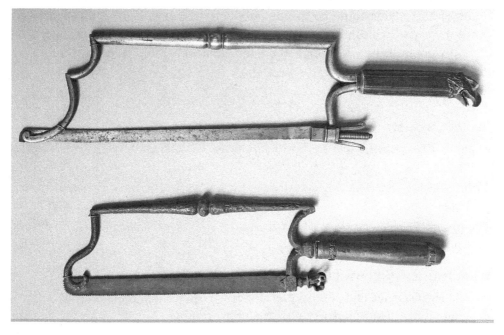

Amputation, using bone saws, was the military surgeon's most important operation until well into the 19th century. (Wellcome Images, London)

being done without anesthesia, hot oil long remained the preferred method of hemostasis.

The technique of amputation changed little through the mid-19th century. Most military physicians considered it an operation best done with only three instruments: a scalpel to cut the skin; a long, double-edged amputation knife to cut the muscle, tendons, vessels, and nerves; and a sharp saw to cut the bone. The sole exception to this approach was Ambroise Paré's reintroduction of the ligature for hemostasis in the late 16th century. Napoleon's surgeon, Baron Dominique-Jean Larrey, brought amputation directly to the battlefield, arguing that shock from the initial injury lessened the pain of surgery and that patients had better chance of recovery if they were not allowed to lose large amount of blood during transport to a hospital for surgery.

Speed remained the cardinal consideration well into the 1800s, and English surgeon Robert Liston became world famous for his ability to amputate a limb in an astoundingly short time. Liston was also the first to use anesthesia for amputation. He referred to the technique as a "Yankee dodge" but was ultimately forced to admit it was an irreplaceable advance. Anesthesia may have removed the suffering from the operation, but the death rate from postoperative infection following amputation still approached 60 percent, and it would not be until Joseph Lister's introduction of antisepsis late in the 19th century that amputation would finally become both tolerable and safe.

With the advent of anesthesia and antisepsis, most limbs that had previously required amputation could be saved, and the importance of the operation faded. Since the early 20th century, even limbs beyond salvage usually heal better after carefully controlled amputation and are more amenable to prosthesis. Death from the procedure is now rare.

Jack McCallum

Further Reading

Bennion, Elisabeth. *Antique Medical Instruments*. Berkeley: University of California Press, 1979.

Sachs, Michael, Jorg Bojunga, and Albrecht Encke. 1999. "Historical Evolution of limb Amputation." *World Journal of Surgery* 23: 1088–1093.

Thompson, C. J. S. *The History and Evolution of Surgical Instruments*. New York: Schuman's, 1942.

Beaumont, William (1785–1853)

A military physician and clinical physiologist, William Beaumont was born into a farming family in Lebanon, Connecticut, on November 21, 1785. As a young man, he refused his father's offer of an adjoining farm and moved to upstate New York, where he worked briefly as a teacher before entering an apprenticeship with a physician in St. Albans, Vermont.

When the War of 1812 began, Beaumont, then 27 years of age, enlisted as a surgeon's mate, an assistant position below the rank of surgeon. He participated in both the Battle of Niagara and the siege of Plattsburgh, where he took a particular interest in the pleurisy and other pulmonary infections that plagued the American force.

After the war, Beaumont entered private practice in Plattsburgh, but he found the practice of civilian medicine boring. In 1820, he convinced his friend Army Surgeon General Joseph Lovell to appoint him physician to the military base on Mackinac Island in the territory that later became Michigan.

In 1822 he was called on to treat 19-year-old French trapper Alexis St. Martin, who had suffered an accidentally self-inflicted shotgun wound to the stomach. Beaumont dressed the wound and waited for the trapper to die, but, over several months, the young man surprisingly recovered, although with a fistula that left his stomach lining visible through the skin of his upper abdomen. Beaumont took St. Martin into his home and began a series of experiments in which he introduced various substances directly into the trapper's stomach and documented the resulting gastric movements and secretions. He was able to show for the first time that gastric secretions only occurred after the stomach was presented with food and that hydrochloric acid and an unknown additional substance (later shown to be the enzyme pepsin) were responsible for breaking down of food. When Beaumont was transferred to Fort Niagara in 1825, he took St. Martin with him, employed him as an orderly and personal servant, and continued his experiments. The relationship between the two men was less than cordial, and St. Martin repeatedly ran away to Canada, particularly when Beaumont insisted on displaying him during public lectures. Beaumont retrieved St. Martin several times, but the Frenchman disappeared for good shortly after Beaumont published his epochal *Experiments and Observations on the Gastric Juice and the Physiology of Digestion* in 1825.

Beaumont left the army soon after his book was published and practiced medicine in St. Louis until his death in 1853. St. Martin lived with his fistula to age 83 and died in 1881.

Jack McCallum

Further Reading

Edelson, Edward. *Healers in Uniform.* Garden City, NY: Doubleday & Company, Inc., 1971.

Epstein, Sam. *Dr. Beaumont and the Man with the Hole in His Stomach.* New York: Coward, McCann & Geoghegan, Inc., 1978.

Gillet, Mary. *The Army Medical Department, 1775–1818*. Washington, D.C.: Center of Military History, 1981.

Myer, Jesse. *Life and Letters of Dr. William Beaumont, including Hitherto Unpublished Data Concerning the Case of Alexis St. Martin*. St. Louis: C. V. Mosby Company, 1912.

Cutbush, Edward (1772–1843)

Edward Cutbush was a surgeon who has been called the father of American naval medicine. Cutbush was born in Philadelphia, the son of a British immigrant. He entered Philadelphia College at the age of 12 and went on to study medicine at the Pennsylvania Hospital, where he worked under William Shippen. While still a student, he was honored by the city of Philadelphia for his services during the 1793 yellow fever epidemic. After graduation from medical school in 1794, Cutbush joined the Pennsylvania Militia in its campaign against the Whiskey Rebellion and became its surgeon general.

In 1799, joined the U.S. Navy and was assigned to the USS *United States*. He made his first voyage to Europe when that ship carried an American delegation to negotiate the agreement ending America's "quasi war" with France. As surgeon on the USS *Constitution*, Cutbush participated in the 1802–1803 blockade of the Barbary ports in North Africa.

On his return to the United States, Cutbush served on the first board to examine candidates for the U.S. Navy's medical service. He was an early proponent of smallpox vaccine, giving it to the entire crew of the *United States* in 1799, just a year after Edward Jenner's pamphlet describing the procedure was published. His 1808 *Observations on the Means of Preserving the Health of Sailors and Soldiers, with Remarks on Hospitals and Their Internal Administration* was the first book dealing with naval medicine by an American.

Cutbush left the navy in 1828 after the election of President Andrew Jackson, whom he opposed, and joined the faculty of Geneva College in New York. He was eventually named dean of the medical faculty and remained in Geneva until his death in 1843.

Jack McCallum

Further Reading

Luft, Eric. 2002. "Edward Cutbush, M.D. (1772–1843)." *Upstate Medical University Alumni Journal*, Spring.

Roddis, Louis. *A Short History of Nautical Medicine*. New York: Paul B. Hoeber, Inc., 1941.

Lovell, Joseph (1788–1836)

Joseph Lovell was born in Boston, Massachusetts to a politically prominent family. After graduating from Harvard College in 1807, he studied medicine and was

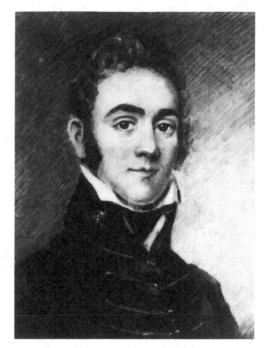

As commander of the Burlington Hospital during the War of 1812, Joseph Lovell made the facility a model of what a hospital should be. He subsequently became Surgeon General of the United States Army in recognition of his administrative skills. (National Library of Medicine)

among the first to receive the new M.D. degree from Harvard Medical School in 1811. In May 1812, Lovell entered the army as a major and surgeon in the 9th Infantry Regiment.

One of the formally trained physicians in the army, Lovell quickly made a name for himself with his superior surgical skills and organizational prowess. As U.S. troops campaigned along with U.S.-Canadian border, Lovell helped establish several hospitals there, including ones in Burlington, Vermont, and Williamsville, New York, which soon became models for how military hospitals were to be run. In June 1814 Lovell was elevated to the grade of full hospital surgeon.

In April 1818, Lovell was appointed surgeon general of the U.S. Army, a post he held without interruption until his death in 1836. He was the first person to serve in the post as a permanent, career officer. Lovell worked hard to enforce new medical regulations that had been passed by Congress, increase pay and benefits for career army doctors, and advocated for an overall increase in the number of medical personnel. Although not realized immediately, by the end of Lovell's tenure, all of these reforms had been instituted. During the 1820s, more organizational reforms occurred within the army's military branch, including the mandatory testing of all assistant surgeons and the creation of an apothecary general and related personnel.

Lovell died on October 17, 1836 in Washington, D.C., widely regarded as the father of the modern medical corps and a surgeon general who did much to advance and modernize the practice of military medicine.

Paul G. Pierpaoli, Jr.

Further Reading

Bayne-Jones, Stanhope. *The Evolution of Preventive Medicine in the United States Army, 1607–1939*. Washington, D.C.: Office of the Surgeon General, 1968.

Gillett, Mary C. *The Army Medical Department, 1775–1818*. Washington, D.C.: Center of Military History, 1981.

Tilton, James (1745–1822)

A surgeon general of the U.S. Army and one of the first graduates of the Philadelphia School of Medicine, James Tilton was born in the town of Kent, which was at that time part of Pennsylvania Colony but is now in Delaware. He joined the Continental Army as surgeon to the Delaware regiment in 1776 and was promoted to hospital surgeon in 1778. Tilton was present at the Yorktown surrender, after which he stayed behind to care for the sick and wounded. After the Revolutionary War, he served as state legislator and representative to Congress from Delaware while continuing to practice medicine.

He published his experience as a military surgeon in the *Economical Observations on Military Hospitals, and the Prevention and Cure of Diseases Incident to an Army*, which led to his appointment as physician and surgeon general of the Army in 1812, an office that had been created specifically for him. During the War of 1812, Tilton dedicated his efforts to reforming administration of the Army's medical system and improving military sanitation. Among his recommendations was the curious suggestion that the sick be kept in wood huts without chimneys so fireplace smoke would accumulate and presumably disinfect the surroundings. He also recommended that beds be placed around the hut's circumference with the patients' feet directed toward a fire at the center of the room.

Tilton remained in the army until cancer cost him a leg and forced his retirement. He died on his Delaware farm at the age of 76 in 1822.

Jack McCallum

Further Reading

Gillet, Mary. *The Army Medical Department, 1775–1818*. Washington, D.C.: Center of Military History, 1981.

Kelly, Howard, and Walter Burrage. *Dictionary of American Medical Biography: Lives of Eminent Physicians of the United States and Canada, from the Earliest Times*. Boston: Milford House, 1971.

Packard, Francis. *History of Medicine in the United States*. New York: Paul B. Hoeber, 1932.

DOCUMENT

In the years preceding the War of 1812, the U.S. naval establishment became aware of the inadequacies of medical care for seamen. There were too few naval surgeons to meet all the navy's requirements. In 1811, Congress voted to fund naval hospitals and set up a commission to draft governing regulations for the hospitals. Dr. Edward Cutbush, a Philadelphia naval surgeon, served as head of the commission. The secretary of the navy presented the commission's findings to Congress, but Congress failed to act. When the war began, Dr. Cutbush wrote to the new secretary of the navy, William Jones, of the problems caused by the lack of Congressional action.

In the communiqué Cutbush suggests that insufficient rank and pay deter American doctors from service in naval hospitals. He argues that army and civilian surgeons enjoy higher pay, and that the navies of France and Great Britain confer higher rank and greater respect on their surgeons. Based on his experience operating a small naval hospital at New Castle, Delaware, he also complains that some seamen refuse to submit to treatment, get drunk at every opportunity, and go rampaging around town. He argues that regulations are needed that would permit navy surgeons to impose discipline on the unruly convalescing seamen under their care.

Sir, A System of rules and regulations for the government of Naval Hospitals, drawn up by myself, and concurred in by Drs. Davis, Marshall and Ewell, were presented to Congress at the last session by Mr. Hamilton; they were examined by a Committee appointed for the purpose, and reported to the house with some amendments, July 11, 1812, but were not finally acted upon. Although there is *no law* authorizing the establishment of Naval Hospitals, yet as temporary buildings have been appropriated at different places, for the reception of the sick and wounded belonging to the Navy, I conceive that some rules and regulations for their government are necessary. The want of a system of rules, *authorized* by an act of Congress, was sensibly felt by me, during the last summer, in the small hospital at New Castle under my direction; I therefore beg leave to solicit your attention to the subject, for, without regulations, it is impossible to restrain the convalescents from acts injurious to themselves, to the service and to the inhabitants, who reside in the vicinity of those establishments. I likewise beg leave to state, that a certain number of Hospital Surgeons are appointed for the army, but none are authorized for the Navy!! With due deference, I conceive that the responsibility attached to those who *act* in that capacity in the Navy, not only entitles them to *the rank,* but to the *same pay and emoluments,* received by an Army Hospital Surgeon. Whilst engaged in attendance on the Hospital at New Castle,

I was only authorized to charge the *extra* expenses incurred in my visits, between the Navy Yard at Philadelphia and that place. Permit me, Sir, (as the subject of the rank of Officers has been brought before Congress) to solicit your attention to that of the surgeons of the Navy, when you take into consideration the relative rank of Officers. Although, it is apparently of little consequence, yet, I can assure you, that the description of a Naval Surgeon, by the pen of the celebrated Dr. Smollett in his Roderick Random, has prevented many men of professional abilities from entering our service, under an idea, that the surgeons and mates, were considered in the same *menial situation,* and I must add that the pay is not a sufficient inducement. There is scarcely a village in the US where a practitioner of medicine and surgery, does not receive a greater compensation than a Naval Surgeon. There is not a sufficient degree of respectability attached to the Surgeons of our Navy. In the British service, at present, the pay increases with the number of years that a surgeon serves, and the rate of the ship to which he is *advanced;* it is considered a promotion to be advanced from a sloop of war to a Frigate, and so on to a first rate; he likewise *ranks* with *Sea Lieutenants* and *Captains of the Army,* subject, however, to the orders of the Lieuts in the line of his duty as a surgeon. In the French service, I believe the rank has been made still more respectable. I hope, Sir, for the honor of our Navy and the profession of Medicine that, (although the army surgeon receives more pay) you will permit no invidious distinction in point of rank.

As to Naval Hospital Surgeons, I humbly conceive that they ought to rank with Hospital Surgeons of the army, and with the *same grade* of officers with whom they are ranked. I have the honor to remain your humble Servant, E. Cutbush

Source: Edward Cutbush, Letter on the Situation of Naval Surgeons, February 13, 1813. National Archives, Record Group 45, M148, Roll No. 11.

■ CHAPTER 3
Mexican-American War

___

INTRODUCTION

The Mexican-American War was the United States' first war with the overt goal of conquering foreign territory. As such, it imposed novel challenges for the U.S. military's medical corps. A long period of peace with all foreign powers preceded the war. During this time the army shrank, with a parallel reduction in the Medical Department. The nation's only military conflict between the end of the War of 1812 and the beginning of the Mexican-American War in 1845 involved border warfare with the Indians. During this time, the Medical Department, which had been established on a permanent peacetime basis in 1818, made some administrative improvements. It ended the schism between regimental and hospital surgeons. It established a clear command structure and devised a system for selecting and assigning personnel. However, there were few advances in medical science to match the improvements in bureaucratic oversight.

In 1844 came the election of President James K. Polk. Polk strongly supported the annexation of Texas, which at the time was an independent nation. However, Mexico refused to recognize Texas's right of independence. On March 1, 1845, Congress resolved to admit Texas into the Union. The Mexican government protested and broke off diplomatic relations. When Mexican forces crossed the Rio Grande and fought U.S. forces, the war began.

Major elements of the U.S. Army, supported by thousands of volunteers, concentrated along the Rio Grande to engage Mexican forces. The rapid American mobilization neglected the medical corps. Thereafter, the combination of difficult environment, poor preparation, and ineffective medical and surgical treatment made the Mexican-American War one of the least admirable episodes in United States military medical history. The U.S. Army experienced the highest death rate in its history, with the vast majority of fatalities due to diseases.

Between the war's preliminary maneuvers in 1845 and the war-ending Treaty of Guadalupe Hidalgo on February 2, 1848, 26,922 regular army troops and 73,260 volunteers served in the American military. Of those, 3,393 were wounded in action, 1,044 were killed in action, 505 died of wounds, and 10,196 died of disease. The seven to one ratio of death from disease to death from wounds compares to the American Civil War (1861–1865) ratio of approximately two to one.

Surgeon General Thomas Lawson had been unsuccessfully arguing for an enlarged Army Medical Department for years prior to 1845. Consequently, the service was woefully undermanned when the war started. It comprised a total of 1 surgeon general, 20 surgeons, and 50 assistant surgeons. When Congress authorized expansion of the regular army and creation of a volunteer force at the beginning of the war, they authorized one additional surgeon and one assistant surgeon for each volunteer regiment and an expansion of the Medical Department. By 1848, the service had grown to 50 regular army surgeons in Mexico, 2 in California, 2 in New Mexico, 1 in New Orleans, 1 in Baton Rouge, and a few scattered in various western posts. In addition, 50 medical officers were attached to the volunteers, none of whom had been required to take the rigorous examinations demanded of regular army surgeons. The majority of those who served in volunteer units were poorly educated and totally devoid of experience in treating either wounds or infectious disease. There were too few to handle adequately the workload.

The Medical Department's inadequacies became manifest well before the war actually started. When troops began mobilizing at Corpus Christi, Texas in 1845, poor sanitation and polluted water supplies created an epidemic of dysentery and other diarrheal diseases. As volunteers—many of whom came from rural areas—entered the camps, the problems multiplied. The farm boys had no experience with basic sanitation in crowded situations and were unwilling to learn. Most had not been exposed to epidemic childhood diseases and were thus vulnerable to outbreaks of measles and mumps, both of which might be minor in children but potentially fatal in adults. Many had not had smallpox vaccinations. The War Department greatly feared an epidemic outbreak of smallpox that fortunately never came.

Field and general hospitals accompanied the army's marches. While on the march, these hospitals relied upon tents for shelter. As the American army captured Mexican cities, the hospitals used local schools, churches, convents, and government buildings. American surgeons had some understanding that these facilities were unsuitable; "vermin-ridden" in the language of the day, referring to the host of rats, mice, fleas, and bedbugs that lived in the buildings. No one yet understood that pathogenic bacteria also thrived in such conditions. These bacteria caused wound infections and gangrene, producing an in-hospital mortality rate close to 20 percent. In fact, the death rate was not significantly different from that of large hospitals in the United States. But, the hospitals in Mexico acquired such a bad reputation among the American soldiers that they resisted entering them as long as possible. That behavior may have contributed to the mortality rate, since those admitted tended to be quite ill.

Additional factors produced poor hospital outcomes. Active duty soldiers provided the nursing staff. Those selected for nursing service were either convalescing from their own wounds or sickness, alcoholic, too weak, or too incompetent to participate in field campaigns. Supplies were a constant problem. Surgeon General Lawson insisted that linens, drugs, and equipment be purchased in New York, where prices were generally lower than places closer to the front. It took six weeks to ship those supplies to Mexico and as much as eight more weeks to move them overland to the field army. Thus, supplies arrived late and often spoiled by the long time spent in transit.

Medical techniques were little improved over those prevalent in the American Revolution. The only truly effective drugs were opium, which was useful for pain relief and for control of diarrhea, and quinine which was useful for malarial fevers (although it was regularly and inappropriately used for other fevers as well). A civilian surgeon brought ether and the equipment for administering it, but Lawson dismissed the innovation because the gas was too liable to explode and he deemed the equipment too fragile for military use. In addition, surgeons were skeptical about ether's use because they thought that pain was necessary to prevent shock during surgery. They also thought that muscle relaxation from ether encouraged bleeding, and that ether increased the risk of infection. Consequently, surgeons in the Mexican War performed most operations without anesthesia.

Amputation remained the most common operation. It was still performed in an unsterile environment with dirty instruments. Open fracture from a penetrating wound was considered an absolute indication for amputation to prevent osteomyelitis and likely fatality. Débridement, the removal of dead, contaminated, or adherent tissue from a wound, had been suggested as an alternative but was not widely adopted. Wounds of the head and chest could occasionally be managed successfully if infection did not intervene, but penetrating abdominal wounds were almost always fatal.

Mexico's tropical climate and poor sanitary facilities made infectious disease a great risk. The Medical Department's greatest worry was yellow fever because of its epidemic nature and high mortality. Malaria was a close second as a cause of concern, but both were dwarfed by the numbers suffering diarrheal disease from contaminated food and water. Scurvy, resulting from diets deficient in fruits and vegetables, was also widespread. Mandatory vaccination rendered smallpox a rare and sporadic occurrence.

Yellow fever never became the menace it was feared to be; a total of 402 cases with 109 deaths (a fairly typical 28 per cent death rate) were reported, but dysentery and malaria more than made up for that. Quinine was effective for malarial fever, but cupping, blistering, baths, mustard plasters, and mercury purges varied from ineffective to harmful. Of 6,466 of Scott's men hospitalized between April 1847 and March 1848, 775 died. The 12 percent death rate gave the hospitals a terrible reputation among the soldiers but was actually quite close to that of domestic hospitals in the United States. Venereal disease also became a problem for the Americans, with 46 cases of gonorrhea and 33 of primary syphilis reported by June of 1848.

Poor planning and organization and the attendant astronomical losses from largely preventable diseases made the Mexican War one of the darker chapters in the history of American military medicine.

Jack McCallum

ENTRIES

Casualties, United States

American losses in the Mexican-American War numbered 1,044 killed in action, 3,393 wounded in action, 505 mortally wounded, and 10,196 dead of disease.

The high mortality of American servicemen can largely be attributed to the poor state of medical care at the time. Any battlefield wound or non-combat accident could become life-threatening, especially those to the head or chest. The 12 percent death rate in army hospitals was, however, not that different from civilian facilities in the United States and far better than that of military hospitals of the belligerents in the Crimean War nearly a decade later.

Poor food, unsanitary practices, and lack of immunity to certain diseases carried off many men. Infection and disease were the largest killers of American soldiers. The connection between mosquitoes and diseases such as malaria and yellow fever was yet to be discovered. Yellow fever ("*vómito*"), in particular, frequently made its deadly round through American army camps. Furthermore, with American soldiers drinking often polluted river water and disregarding basic sanitary measures, not to mention the mixing of men from all parts of the country, other diseases took their toll as well. Measles, mumps, and smallpox, along with dysentery ("the bloody flux") and simple diarrhea ("the blues"), brought their own brand of misery and claimed the lives of many American soldiers.

American volunteer units tended to be less disciplined about field sanitation than regular army units. Thus, greater numbers of volunteers died from disease than did regulars. Disease epidemics often hit American soldiers from rural areas harder than they did their urban counterparts, likely because the city dwellers had developed proportionately more immunity to them.

Jack McCallum

Further Reading

Eisenhower, John S. D. *So Far From God: The U.S. War with Mexico, 1846–1848.* New York: Random House, 1989.

Henderson, Timothy J. *A Glorious Defeat: Mexico and Its War with the United States.* New York: Hill and Wang, 2007.

Wheelan, Joseph. *Invading Mexico: America's Continental Dream and the Mexican War, 1846–1848.* New York: Carroll and Graf Publishers, 2007.

Ether, First Use of

Ether, discovered in 1275 by Spanish chemist Raymundus Lullis, was first used as an anesthetic on the battlefields of North America during the Mexican-American War. Ether is an organic compound that contains an ether group, consisting of an oxygen atom attached to two alkyl or aryl groups. The type of ether used for anesthetic purposes is diethyl ether, which also acts as a highly flammable common solvent. It is the fumes from diethyl ether that are used as an anesthetic.

In the United States, Crawford W. Long, a Georgia doctor, was the first physician to use ether successfully in his private practice on March 30, 1842. The greater recognition, however, has gone to Dr. William Thomas Green Morton, a Boston dentist, who on October 16, 1846, at the Massachusetts General Hospital, publicly administered ether to relieve the pain of dental surgery. Dr. Edward Barton first used anesthetic ether in war during an amputation on March 29, 1847. Unlike alcohol, which was commonly used to moderate the pain of surgical procedures before the use of ether, ether was inhaled, not ingested, and therefore prevented asphyxiation during surgery.

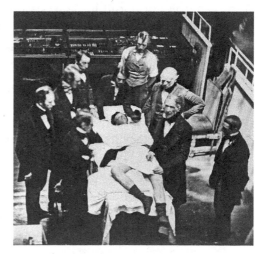

A public demonstration of ether anesthesia at Massachusetts General Hospital in 1846 led to this procedure becoming a surgical standard. (Wellcome Images, London)

Initially during the Mexican-American War, anesthetics such as ether were frowned upon as they were believed to detract from a soldier's masculinity. Despite such negative connotations, the use of anesthesia continued to grow. During the war, ether was administered as a vapor by an ether dome, which was placed over the patient's nose and mouth. Although ether gained more acceptance, other anesthetics, such as chloroform, became more popular because they were fast acting and easier to transport. Nevertheless, the use of anesthetics such as ether during surgical procedures led to less traumatic treatment of war-related injuries, and the widespread use of ether as a general anesthetic meant that doctors were able to perform major surgeries with fewer complications. Most surgeries during the war, however, continued to be performed without the benefit of ether or other anesthetic agents.

Lazarus O'Sako

Further Reading

Duncan, Louis C. "Medical History of General Scott's Campaign to the City of Mexico in 1847," *Military Surgeon*, 47 (1920), 436–470, 596–609.

Fenster, J. M. *Ether Day: The Strange Tale of America's Greatest Medical Discovery and the Haunted Men Who Made It*. New York: Harper Perennial, 2002.

Gillett, Mary. *The Army Medical Department: 1818–1865*. Washington, DC: Center of Military History, United States Army, 1987.

Moreno, Luis Gerardo Morales, et al., eds. *Echoes of the Mexican-American War*. Toronto, Canada: Groundwood Books, 2005.

Yellow Fever (Vómito)

Yellow fever is a deadly, painful viral disease, spread by the bite of the *Aedes aegypti* mosquito. It is also called yellow jack or *el vómito negro* (black vomit). Yellow fever is common in subtropical and tropical areas of the Americas and Africa, but is not found in Asia. Its prevalence in low-lying coastal areas of Mexico during the summer rainy season directly influenced Mexican and American strategy during the Mexican-American War. Victims, whose skin turns yellow as their livers are destroyed, suffer agonies ranging from fever, headache, constipation, nausea, diarrhea, and chills. Blood vessels in the skin often rupture and hemorrhage, creating black and blue patches, and the blood supply to the internal organs is cut off as hemorrhages filled the lungs. Victims literally drown in their own fluids, while vomiting coagulated blood.

Almost a third of those infected in the 19th century died from the disease. *El vómito* frightened the Americans more than it did the Mexicans because Mexicans had built up some immunity to the disease, which Americans lacked.

As 1846 drew to a close, President James K. Polk decided on an amphibious expedition against Veracruz, on Mexico's eastern coast, to be followed by a march on Mexico City. He appointed Major General Winfield Scott as commander-in-chief of the expeditionary force. As Scott meticulously planned the expedition, much of his concern was predicated upon seizing Veracruz before the end of January 1847, then marching his army rapidly into the Sierra Madres, beyond the "Yellow Fever Line," before *el vómito* took hold in mid-April. To counter Scott's plans, General Antonio López de Santa Anna, the Mexican commander, hoped to pin the American army on the coast so *el vómito* could ruin it.

In the event, Scott managed rapidly to move inland. Despite his haste, almost all his men subsequently contracted yellow fever to some degree. Death rates among serious cases in the army hospital at Veracruz averaged 28 percent. Doctors typically prescribed mercury, mustard, and camphor baths as treatments, but they were entirely ineffective and sometimes even harmful. Not until the 1890s did doctors and scientists isolate the cause of yellow fever. The first vaccines against the disease were administered in the 1930s.

Paul David Nelson

Further Reading

Duncan, Louis C. "Medical History of General Scott's Campaign to the City of Mexico in 1847," *Military Surgeon*, 47 (1920), 436–470, 596–609.

Eisenhower, John S. D. *Agent of Destiny: The Life and Times of General Winfield Scott.* New York: Free Press, 1997.

Gillett, Mary C. *The Army Medical Department, 1818–1865.* Washington: Center of Military History, U.S. Army, 1987.

Smith, George Winston, and Charles Judah, eds. *Chronicles of the Gringos: The U.S. Army in the Mexican War, 1846–1848.* Albuquerque: University of New Mexico Press, 1968.

DOCUMENTS

John Porter: Excerpt from Surgeon's Memoir (1847)

By modern standards, medical care during the Mexican-American War was primitive. Doctors and surgeons labored in ignorance of how infections and diseases were transmitted. They did know the cause of diseases, such as typhus (passed via contaminated water) or mosquito-borne diseases, such as malaria. They did not have access to effective drugs. Much of what they understood came from observations passed on through books and medical schools. The best medical practitioners sought to utilize these observations wisely. Others did not care. Regardless, medical practitioners had a very limited tool box. For example, the standard response to serious arm or leg injuries was amputation. Most soldiers understood that their best chance for recovery from disease or wounds was to stay out of the surgeon's hands. Still, conscientious surgeons did the best with whatever tools they possessed. Surgeon John B. Porter served with Zachary Taylor's army.

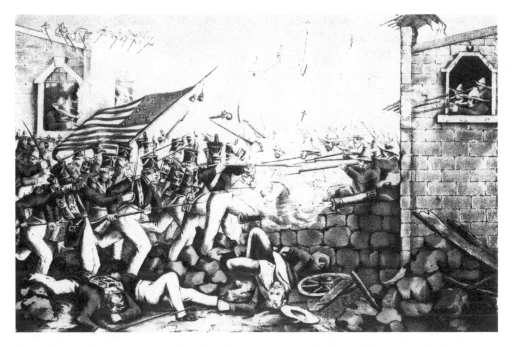

A Currier and Ives lithograph showing American forces fighting in Monterey in September 1846 during the Mexican-American War. (Bettmann/Corbis)

Porter was present on September 19, 1846, when General Zachary Taylor led his army to the Mexican city of Monterrey. The next day, the American attack began. A difficult, bloody combat ensued as the Americans advanced slowly in house-to-house fighting. Surgeon Porter tried to save some of the wounded. His account highlights the difficulties that medical men experienced during this era.

On the 19th of September we encamped within 4 miles of Monterey, in a grove of Peccan trees, called Walnut Grove; where we were abundantly supplied with clear and cold water, from a stream of considerable size, formed by the junction of numerous springs. The combination of wood and shade rendered the spot admirably fitted for an encampment. On the following day parties were employed in reconnoitering the enemy and in observation of the fortified position of the town. Toward evening my regiment, 3rd Infantry, with another, were advanced a mile toward the town, to cover a party of engineers, but returned to camp about 9 p.m.

On the morning of the 21st the whole division was thrown forward toward the city, with a view, as we supposed, of making a diversion while the 2nd Division, under General Worth, moved on the western side of the city by the Saltillo Road.... As soon as we emerged from cover the batteries opened their fire, completely sweeping the plain in a very direction and enfilading the advancing columns of our troops.

Now it was that my professional labors commenced; the nearest and only shelter that presented itself to me for the wounded, falling every moment, was a quarry pit, 4 or 5 deep and the same in breadth. Several of these were contiguous, and to them I directed the wounded to be carried. By stooping we were protected from the shots which became thicker every moment; as our troops had now advanced within range of the enemy's fire, and the moment they perceived a party of men bringing the wounded to us, they directed all their guns upon it. I already had performed one amputation and was preparing for a second, when three fugitives rushed into the pit, falling over the wounded that lay there crowded together, saying that a large body of lancers was approaching. So little credit did I attach to their report that I never raised my eyes to observe them: which circumstance doubtless saved us all. Had I been discovered all would have been massacred, as in their headlong fury they would neither have delayed to ascertain our character or profession, nor have paid much respect to our patients. Several soldiers who had sought an adjacent pit, with an officer, were slain. The lancers were soon after repulsed by a regiment of Ohio and Mississippi Volunteers....

The first wounds were received in crossing the plain and were inflicted by grape and cannon shot [solid shot]. These wounds were all low; generally at or just above the ankles. Of the first three men brought to me two had received wounds from 18-pound shot, just above the ankle, which had nearly severed the limbs, which were hanging only by a portion integuments. The other had his heel torn off by a 6-pound shot. Shortly after, our troops having advanced within reach and under fire of the Mexican infantry, numerous cases of wounds by musket and escopette consequently inflict a more severe and formidable wound. So numerous at this time because the wounded in our pit, and so constant and heavy the fire, as to compel us to remove our hospital several hundred yards further to the rear. We had not long been in our new position, when some covered wagons bringing the wounded attracted the attention of the enemy, who immediately reopened their fire, compelling us a second time to remove beyond the range of shot.

Among the numerous projectiles, occasioning severe and fatal wounds, were grape, canister, fragments of iron and copper shells and stones knocked by the balls from the corners of buildings and walls. Their shells were thrown with great accuracy, frequently into the midst of a body of troops, but fortunately killing and wounding but few.

Before speaking of any particular wounds, I will here take occasion to make some remarks reflecting the character they assumed, and the peculiar causes acting to prevent a favorable result, so far as regarded the healing of all, even the most slight. The first annoyance we experienced, and one which no doubt exerted an injurious effect, was one little anticipated at the time. The moment a limb was amputated numerous flies would alight on the stump, and must have deposited their eggs, for when it became necessary to dress the stump myriads of maggots were found buried in it, which could only be expelled with great difficulty; rendering it necessary in some instances to reopen the flap, for their complete extermination.

A much more formidable enemy made its appearance in an erysidelatous inflammation of the integuments covering the stump, which generally set in two or three days after the operation; and notwithstanding all the means made use of to arrest it, commonly ended in sloughing, and either proved fatal or rendered secondary amputation necessary. That some influence existed previously, external or internal, from causes connected with the state of the atmosphere, or habits of the men, arising from diet or water, was manifest. The slightest wound or scratch became in every case a tedious ulcer; in some cases proving a cause for serious alarm. Apparently the most trifling wounds required an unusual time for healing, and even those that had previously healed would break out again and present greater difficulty in their cure than in the first instance.

Source: Louis C. Duncan. "A Medical History of General Zachary Taylor's Army of Occupation in Texas and Mexico, 1845–1847." *The Military Surgeon* 48:1 (January 1921), 76–104. Excerpts on pp. 92–93.

Raphael Semmes: Book Excerpt Describing Yellow Fever

On March 2, 1847, General Winfield Scott's army landed near Vera Cruz in the largest amphibious operation in U.S. history up to that time. Among the sailors supporting that operation was Lieutenant Raphael Semmes. In this excerpt, Semmes showcases contemporary knowledge about "el vomito," which was the local name for yellow fever. The onset of yellow fever followed seasonal patterns. As Semmes observes, these patterns were well recognized as even trade into and out of Vera Cruz came to a standstill when the fever season struck. Semmes speculates intelligently about why the fever is so localized. He notes that aboard U.S. Navy ships operating offshore of Vera Cruz, no sailors fell ill from the fever. Semmes guesses that this is because of good hygienic practices. In fact, yellow fever was a mosquito borne disease, although this was not known at the time, and the mosquitoes did not venture offshore. General Scott also knew about yellow fever's seasonality. Consequently, he badly wanted to march his army inland, along the road Semmes describes, to the more healthy highlands before the weather warmed and the fevers set in.

When the norther has ceased to scour the coast in pursuit of victims, the vomito begins its more silent, but not less deadly, approaches. This scourge is not only the terror of the Americans and Europeans who trade with Vera Cruz, but is equally dreaded by the inhabitants of the interior of the country. When it prevails badly as an epidemic, almost all intercourse with the plateaus of the Cordilleras is suspended. Even the hardy arrieros, or mule-drivers, who are the common carriers of commerce, cease their regular visits to and from the infected city; when the whole interior of the country suffers more or less for want of its accustomed supplies. So pure and salubrious is the air of the upland regions, that an inhabitant of Puebla or Mexico, on descending to Vera Cruz, is more liable to take the disease than most foreigners. As Vera Cruz is the only seaport of any importance on the Mexican Gulf, and transacts three-fourths of the foreign business of the country, it is readily seen how pernicious an influence the prevalence of the vomito exercises on the pursuits of the mass of the population. Even the mines to which delay is death, in consequence of the vast amount of capital invested in them, not unfrequently suffer for want of quicksilver (used extensively for separating the precious metals, and almost all of which is imported from the mines of Almaden, in Spain), and the necessary machinery—none of which is manufactured in the country—for carrying on their operations. Indeed, so seriously have the inconveniences of this epidemic been felt, that, on more than one occasion, the question has been discussed, of razing the city to the ground, and abandoning it altogether.

These various discussions will give the reader an idea of the terror with which the vomito inspires the inhabitants of the mountain slopes, and elevated plains, Experience would seem to show, that extreme heat alone does not produce yellow fever. There are many islands in the West Indies, farther south than Vera Cruz—the Danish island of Santa Cruz, for instance—where the disease is unknown. But what is more remarkable, this scourge does not prevail on the western coast of Mexico. Even the unhealthy town of Acapulco, which, according to the observations of Humboldt, has a higher mean temperature throughout the, year, than Vera Cruz, is exempt from it. Malignant bilious and remittent fevers prevail here, but as yet there have been no well marked case of the vomito. Our squadron, which remained all the summer of 1846 in the vicinity of Vera Cruz—holding, of course, no intercourse with the shore—had no fever. The seamen were crowded in small spaces—there being as many as two hundred men on board a sloop-of-war of eight or nine hundred tons—were exposed to the same heat, somewhat tempered by tlie sea-breezes, slept in the open air on the decks, in their night watches, and were frequently drenched with rain, both and night; and yet they experienced no inconvenience. And the reason, no doubt, was, that under Commodore Conner's excellent system of discipline, the between decks were kept dry and well ventilated; and the men, every evening. At sunset quarters, were required to exchange their lighter duck-frocks and trowsers for woolen ones. Many valuable officers and men fell a sacrifice, in the following year; but we were then in possession of the enemy's ports and coasts; and it was necessary to maintain a constant communication with the shore, and even to garrison many points. It would seem to follow, from all these facts, that the vomito of Vera Cruz is local, and must, therefore, be produced by malaria arising somewhere in the vicinity of the town.

The vomito of Vera Cruz resembles, in all its essential futures, that of Havana and New Orleans. It is the same gastro-nervous disease, and is accompanied by the same yellowness of the skin, irritation of the stomach, intense headache, pain in the small of the back, and vomiting. It sometimes prostrates, so powerfully, the nervous system, as to kill the patient in five or six hours; but its more general course is from two to five days. Women are less subject to it than men, and very young children are rarely attacked by it. It is most to be feared at the commencement and end of the rainy season; and the reason assigned is, that there is more putrefaction of vegetable and animal matter going on at these periods, in consequence of the prevalence of alternate rain and sunshine, than when it is raining constantly; as constant humidity, like constant drowth, retards decomposition. There is, no doubt, a barometric cause also, hitherto unnoticed, which operates more powerfully upon the nervous system, while the atmosphere is undergoing these changes. It is remarkable that the natives of Vera Cruz do not suffer from this disease, and that those who have had it once need not fear it a second time. But n each particular place where it prevails, by local causes, more or less variant, and to require a new acclimation it is not a sufficient exemption for a stranger going to Vera Cruz, to have had il elsewhere. It seems to be modified in consequence. Thus we see that the eastern coast of Mexico has as powerful a defender in the vomito, as in the norther; and it is well known that the inhabitants of the interior plains, at the period of our invasion, relied greatly upon the chances of our being cut off by this disease. On the other hand, General Scott gave it due consideration in the formation of the plan of his campaign, and endeavored to avoid so great a calamity.

Source: Raphael Semmes. *Service Afloat and Ashore During the Mexican War.* Cincinnati: Wm. H. Moore & Co., 1851, pp. 112–16.

■ CHAPTER 4
American Civil War

INTRODUCTION

The Civil War in many ways represented an inflection point in the history of military practice and military medicine. When the war began in 1861, generals on both sides followed time-honored military tactics. One consequence was a horrific casualty rate. In the western theater at Shiloh (April 7–8, 1862), the combined loss total approached 25,000 men, marking Shiloh as the bloodiest battle fought in North America up to that time. In the eastern theater, the one-day Battle of Antietam, fought in Maryland on September 17, 1862, exceeded that total. The year 1863 featured even more costly engagements. Over 50,000 Americans were killed, wounded, missing, or prisoners at the July 1–3 Battle of Gettysburg. That autumn came the war's largest western engagement, the Battle of Chickamauga, Tennessee (September 18–20, 1863). Here another 34,000 Americans were casualties. By 1864, Civil War armies had perfected the art of entrenchment. The complex network of trenches, fortifications, and obstacles to impede an attacker provided a defender with tremendous tactical advantages and foreshadowed the bloody stalemate of trench warfare in World War I.

The Union Army lost 138,154 soldiers killed and mortally wounded and another 280,040 wounded. A total of 224,586 died from other causes, primarily disease, a figure nearly double the number who died in battle. The Confederate Army lost at least 94,000 soldiers killed or mortally wounded. An estimated 164,000 died from disease, including 30,000 who perished in northern prisons. The sheer number of battlefield casualties coupled with the high rate of death and sickness while in camp, overwhelmed both the Union and Confederate medical establishments.

On the eve of the Civil War, American medicine was beginning to question "heroic" practices such as purging, bleeding, and the liberal use of mercury and arsenic. However, the majority of practitioners had yet to admit that their standard remedies were actively harmful. Most physicians thought sanitation important, but, because microorganisms as a source of disease were as yet unknown, it was with the mistaken rationale that bad air (miasma) was responsible for most illnesses.

When the war began, the United States Army had only 16,000 troops and 115 physicians and medical assistants, almost all of whom were tied to specific regiments. After secession, eight of the surgeons and 29 assistant surgeons resigned and joined the Confederacy. The Union army grew to 109,000 in the first four months of the war and the Confederacy experienced a similar expansion. Most of the new volunteers joined geographically based regiments of around 1,200 men. The regimental commander was responsible for picking his own surgeon and assistant, and assigned a steward and 10 or 12 aides who were most often either members of the regimental band or physically unfit for combat. The physicians were generally from the regiment's home area. Although the local physicians had widely variable training and ability and almost never had experience treating major injuries, it was considered important for the new soldiers to be cared for by people they knew and trusted—a decision that had a generally detrimental effect on the quality of care.

In the war's first few battles, each regimental surgeon set up his own aid station in whatever protected area he could find within a few hundred yards of the front line and raised a red flag so the wounded or those tasked to carry them could find him. Although there were often better protected and better supplied hospitals farther to the rear, the regimental surgeons were reluctant to release their wounded and the men were reluctant to leave their friends. As a result, distribution of the wounded was erratic, leaving some aid stations overwhelmed with casualties while others lay idle.

In the July 21, 1861 Battle of Bull Run, the Union Army suffered 2,708 casualties. Appointed stretcher bearers fled, leaving the wounded abandoned on the field for days. Those who remained ambulatory and who were lucky enough not to be taken prisoner were forced to walk the 27 miles back to Washington before they could be treated. Those who made it to an aid station might have bullets removed, their skulls opened, or limbs amputated by men who had never seen operations, much less done them.

When the war commenced, Union Surgeon General Thomas Lawson was 72 years old and had neither the energy nor the ability to manage the demands on the medical corps. He was replaced by Clement A. Finley shortly after Fort Sumter's surrender, but Finley was 64 years old and, in spite of his 40-year army career, had no experience appropriate to his new job.

Recognizing the seriousness of the situation, a minister and three physicians (Henry Bellows, W. H. Van Buren, Elisha Harris, and Jacob Hansen) representing a variety of charitable and religious organizations, created the United States Sanitary Commission modeled after the similarly named British group. The commission successfully lobbied Congress for official status, and, under Executive

Secretary Frederick Law Olmstead, began furnishing food, clothing, and medical supplies to the Union troops and, over widespread objections from the medical corps, began supervising camp sanitation. The latter was especially important since typhoid, measles, and dysentery had become rife among groups of previously unexposed young men thrown into close quarters.

The commissioners also recognized Finley's shortcomings and pressed to have him replaced. In January 1862, 34-year-old William A. Hammond was named surgeon general. He cooperated in the commission efforts to sanitize camps, replaced the least qualified of his regimental surgeons, and removed some of the most dangerous drugs from the formulary. He went on to establish an army medical school, built a general hospital in Washington using the new pavilion design, created an army pathological museum that resulted in the monumental *Medical and Surgical History of the War of the Rebellion*, and the construction of a central laboratory for the army.

Perhaps Hammond's greatest contribution was in improved transport of the wounded. He insisted that ambulance transport be removed from line command and placed under the medical corps with designated bearers and drivers. Charles Tripler had been surgeon to the Army of the Potomac, but was unable to cope with the flood of injured and the explosion of disease in the malarial swamps of the March-August 1862 Peninsula Campaign. Hammond replaced him with Jonathan Letterman in July 1862. Letterman discarded Tripler's unwieldy 10-person ambulances in favor of smaller, better suspended wagons. He demanded and received one ambulance for every 150 soldiers and an additional two supply wagons for each regiment's medical supplies. He organized evacuation of the wounded so well that at Antietam on September 17, 1862, his stretcher bearers and ambulances had every one of the 9,420 Union wounded off the field before the day ended.

As a result of Hammond's challenges to the regimental medical system, his removal of treasured drugs from the formulary, his relative youth, and his frequent arguments with Secretary of War Simon Cameron, Hammond's career was in jeopardy. He was relieved as surgeon general and then, at his own insistence, was court martialed. He was relieved of duty in August 1864.

The Confederacy had a similarly talented surgeon general in Samuel Preston Moore. Although his government only allocated $50,000 for hospital construction and the additional liability of being chronically short of drugs and supplies, Moore created a creditable hospital system, devised ingenious substitutes for missing materials, and maintained a surprisingly high level of practice throughout the war.

From the beginning, field hospitals were most often in "walled tents" that could hold up to 20 patients or be strung together to hold twice that many. The earliest general hospitals were in whatever large buildings could be commandeered—hotels, houses, and warehouses being common solutions—and were under regimental control. Their inefficiency and poor sanitation led to their being replaced

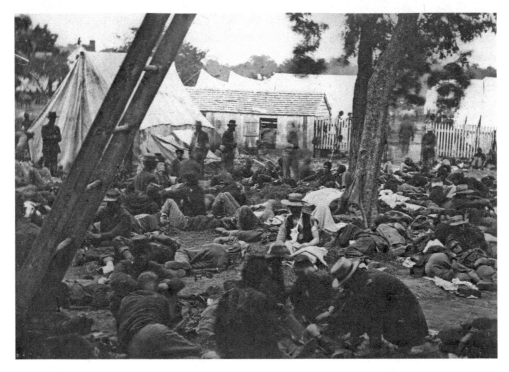

A Federal field hospital at Savage Station, outside of Richmond, Virginia, during the Seven Days Campaign in June 1862. (Library of Congress)

in the Union army by pavilion hospitals under the medical corps, especially after the numbers of sick and wounded went up in 1862.

By 1863, the United States Army Medical Corps had 151 hospitals and 58,716 beds, mostly well-ventilated and at least marginally clean. In 1864, Lieutenant General Ulysses S. Grant authorized a 6,000-bed hospital at City Point, Virginia, that ultimately expanded to 10,000 beds and had 18 trains continuously running between it and the front near Petersburg. The Union also created specialized hospitals for particular injuries and illnesses including Turner's Lane General Hospital in Philadelphia for nervous and neurologic problems, the DesMarres Hospital in Chicago for wounds and diseases of the eye, a hospital in Nashville for erysipelas, and another in New York City for the treatment of the severely mutilated. The Confederates also built a number of hospitals, although, with the exception of a few large facilities such as Chimborazo and Winder in Richmond, they tended to be dedicated to soldiers of particular states rather than to the army as a whole.

Throughout the war, most nursing care was done by men, but, particularly on the Union side, there were notable experiments with female nurses, beginning with Dorothea Dix, who was appointed the first superintendent of female nurses for the army, and including such women as Louisa May Alcott and Clara Barton.

By the war's end, 3,200 women had served as Union army nurses. After 1862, Confederate hospitals were assigned matrons responsible for "the domestic economy" of the institutions and for supervising the male nurses and African-Americans assigned to ward duty, but the South never matched the Union in its use of women caregivers.

The war's major advance in surgical care was the general use of anesthesia. Anesthesia had been used sparingly in the Mexican-American War and more widely in the Crimean War. Anesthesia became standard in the Civil War, although the potential benefits were tempered by the fact that Lord Joseph Lister would not apply emerging knowledge of bacterial infection and its control with antiseptics until the year after the war ended.

Chloroform as an anesthetic was not universally accepted when the war started. The gas could be prepared by distilling chloride of lime with alcohol in a copper still and was usually administered by soaking a sponge and placing it over a folded cloth cone covering the face. Depth of anesthesia was gauged by the noise and depth of breathing. If anesthesia was too deep, the patient was revived with fresh air, cold water on the face, or cold water enemas. Ether was used occasionally and was generally safer but harder to administer because of associated vomiting and a feeling of suffocation. In the end, about 80,000 operations were done under anesthesia by each side.

About 94 percent of Civil War wounds were caused by bullets, as compared to World War I in which 75 percent were caused by artillery. When a typical Civil War bullet struck human flesh, it carved out a large track and carried a high risk of vascular injury. Around 70 percent of projectile wounds involved the arms or legs. Amputation remained the surgical option of choice for serious injuries, particularly for extremity injuries that involved a joint, or that caused a compound fracture, removed chunks of bone, or became infected. Philadelphia surgeon William Williams Keen said it was seven times safer to have fought at the Battle of Gettysburg (July 1–3, 1863) than to have undergone a field amputation. Medical knowledge and practice was unable to deal with most head, chest, and abdomen injuries. Wounds requiring trephine (opening the skull) had 61 percent death rate, those penetrating the chest 62 percent, and those penetrating the abdomen 87 percent.

Even with those gruesome statistics, disease was a greater threat than battle injury on both sides. Overcrowded camps and poor camp sanitation promoted infectious diseases. Men from rural areas who had not developed immunities were particularly at risk for such diseases as measles, tonsillar abscesses, and upper respiratory infections. As conditions in camps deteriorated, sanitary shortcomings led to dysentery, typhoid, lice-borne typhus, erysipelas, and scabies. Venereal disease was a problem throughout the war. Soldiers serving in coastal regions suffered from malaria.

Ignorance of the mechanism of disease transmission made Civil War medical care resemble the care provided in earlier American wars. There were few clinical advances during the war. It was the first war in which the military recognized psychiatric casualties as a significant cost of war. In addition, there were some reforms and innovations that showed the way to an improved future, most notably in organizing transportation and care for mass casualties and the establishment of large-scale military hospitals and convalescent camps.

James R. Arnold

ENTRIES

Ambulance Corps

Prior to the establishment of a formal Ambulance Corps in 1862, medical evacuation in the Union army proceeded haphazardly. Insufficient vehicles, unreliable drivers and staff, and a lack of a unified command structure left thousands of wounded soldiers lying helplessly on the field sometimes for days after battles had ended. U.S. Army Surgeon (and Major) Jonathan Letterman endeavored to address this inadequacy.

Letterman became medical director of the Army of the Potomac near the end of the Peninsula Campaign (March–August 1862), and his most important innovation was the creation of an effective casualty evacuation system. On August 2, 1862, Letterman persuaded Major General George McClellan to sign Special Orders #147, which formally instituted the Ambulance Corps. This placed ambulances under the control of the Medical Corps (instead of the Quartermaster Corps). They also forbade the use of ambulances for anything except carrying the wounded and created a command structure of officers and men dedicated to retrieving the wounded from the field of battle, and, importantly, enjoined other soldiers from escorting maimed comrades to hospitals (this being a common means of avoiding combat). The orders provided for three ambulances per infantry regiment, each equipped with two stretchers.

The Ambulance Corps quickly proved its worth. By the First Battle of Fredericksburg (December 13, 1862), it was successfully evacuating all wounded to hospitals within 24 hours, garnering praise from line and medical officers alike. Through the remainder of the war, the Ambulance Corps provided timely and effective evacuation for Union wounded, although initially only in the Army of the Potomac. Other commanders quickly recognized its value, however. Major General Ulysses S. Grant mandated it for his Army of the Tennessee in March 1863, and by March 1864, pressure from line officers, uniformed and civilian physicians, and the public compelled Congress to pass the Ambulance Corps Act, which standardized the Ambulance Corps among all units in the Armies of the United States.

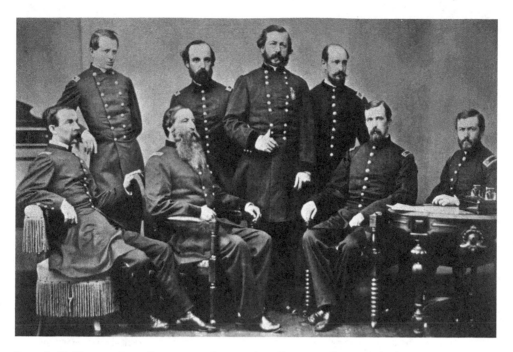

Joseph K. Barnes (standing, center) served as Surgeon General during the Civil War. Among his accomplishments was the expansion of the Army's Ambulance Corps. (National Library of Medicine)

The Confederate Army never developed an ambulance corps, relying throughout the war on whatever wagons were not otherwise occupied to move the wounded.

Letterman's creation and the subsequent army-wide implementation of the Ambulance Corps stand as one of the most important military-medical advances of the Civil War. Its fundamental structure remained largely unchanged in both American and European forces through World War I.

Justin Barr

Further Reading

Bollet, Alfred Jay. *Civil War Medicine: Challenges and Triumphs*. Tucson, AZ: Galen Press, Ltd., 2002.

Gillett, Marcy C. *The Army Medical Department 1818–1865*. Washington, D.C.: Center of Military History, 2000.

Barton, Clara (Clarissa) Harlowe (1821–1912)

Clara (Clarissa) Harlowe Barton was born in Oxford, Massachusetts, on December 25, 1821, into a middle-class family. She was educated at home, began teaching at age 15, and founded a free public school in Bordentown, New Jersey.

Prior to the Civil War, her only medical experience came while caring for a sickly brother for two years.

By 1861, Barton was living in Washington, D.C. Employed by the U.S. Patent Office, she decided to organize relief aid for soldiers of the 6th Massachusetts Regiment, who had been involved in the April 19, 1861, Baltimore Riots. Her efforts began an enduring commitment to humanitarian aid. Upon learning that many soldiers who fought in the First Battle of Bull Run (July 21, 1861) had died because of a lack of basic medical supplies, she took out an advertisement in the *Spy,* a Worcester, Massachusetts-based newspaper, to solicit donations for wounded Union soldiers. The response was nearly instantaneous and gratifying, and she was soon head of a highly successful relief organization.

In 1862 U.S. Surgeon General William Hammond gave Barton a travel pass so that she could accompany army ambulances to distribute aid and nurse ailing soldiers. Hammond's move was highly unusual for the time, as most women were barred from being on or near battlefields. For the following three years, Barton traveled extensively in Virginia and South Carolina, caring for wounded and dying soldiers and supervising relief and donation drives.

Barton carried out extensive nursing at hospitals in Fredericksburg, Virginia, as well as in field hospitals, where she cared for wounded soldiers in May 1864 both during the Battle of the Wilderness and at Bermuda Hundred, not far from Richmond. Her good work drew national attention and admiration on both sides of the conflict. In late 1864 and early 1865, Barton held her only official post during the Civil War when she served as Major General Benjamin Butler's superintendent of nurses. She also expanded her role and mission when she went to Camp Parole, Maryland, to establish a system for locating men listed as missing in action or captured. There she conducted extensive interviews with Union soldiers returning from captivity in Southern prisons and was many times capable of determining the status or whereabouts of men missing in action. She then passed the information along to families.

It is believed that Barton helped locate some 30,000 such soldiers. When the war was over, she traveled to Andersonville, Georgia, in an effort to identify and properly mark the graves of Union soldiers who had been buried there. Barton went to considerable lengths to locate missing servicemen, including the publication of lists of names in newspapers and direct communication with missing soldiers' families and friends.

In 1870, during a visit to Western Europe, Barton became active in the International Red Cross (founded in 1864), which led her to found the American Red Cross in 1881. Before long, Barton had broadened the scope of the Red Cross to include not only neutral aid in wartime but responses to other emergencies and natural disasters. She tried to go to Cuba during the Spanish-American War, but was prevented from doing so by U.S. military officials. Instead, she cared for Spanish prisoners of war and refugees in Key West, Florida. Her sometimes brusque demeanor and reluctance to delegate authority eventually led to her resignation in 1904, when she retired to her home outside Washington, D.C.

In addition to her humanitarian efforts Barton was active in the women's suffrage movement and the African-American fight for civil rights. She also authored several books, including a volume on the early history of the American Red Cross. Barton died in Glen Echo, Maryland, on April 12, 1912.

Paul G. Pierpaoli, Jr.

Further Reading

Hutchinson, John F. *Champions of Charity: War and the Rise of the Red Cross.* Boulder, CO: Westview Press, 1996.

Pryor, Elizabeth Brown. *Clara Barton, Professional Angel.* Philadelphia: University of Pennsylvania Press, 1987.

Bickerdyke, Mary Ann Ball (1817–1901)

Born on July 19, 1817 on a farm in Knox County, Ohio, Mary Ann Bickerdyke was the daughter of Hiram and Annie Ball. When she was 17 months old her mother died and she went to live with her maternal grandparents. Upon their deaths, she lived with her maternal uncle on a farm near Cincinnati, Ohio. Self-taught in the field of herbal medicine, she assisted doctors in Cincinnati during the cholera epidemic of 1837. Ball married Robert Bickerdyke, a widower with three boys, in 1847. The couple moved to Galesburg, Illinois, in 1856. After her husband's death in 1859, Bickerdyke supported herself and her children by practicing botanic medicine.

In 1861, after hearing of the deplorable conditions at the military hospital at Cairo, Illinois, the members of Bickerdyke's church collected $500 worth of supplies for the wounded soldiers, many of whom were from Galesburg. Church officials charged Bickerdyke with delivering the supplies to Cairo. Sensing a need for her services, she remained in Cairo and served as a volunteer nurse. Bickerdyke's energy and concern for Union troops made her wildly popular with wounded soldiers, who fondly called her "Mother Bickerdyke." Her ability to organize military hospitals, especially her concern for their sanitary conditions, was promptly brought to the attention of Brigadier General Ulysses S. Grant.

Shortly after capturing Fort Donelson in February 1862, Grant brought Bickerdyke and fellow nurse Mary Jane Stafford to the field hospital at Fort Donelson. Bickerdyke eventually worked on the hospital ships administered by the Western Sanitary Commission that transported wounded soldiers and supplies on the Mississippi River and its tributaries. By the beginning of 1863, Bickerdyke was the chief of nursing for Grant's troops. From April to July 1863, she accompanied Grant during the Second Vicksburg Campaign.

Bickerdyke routinely led campaigns to solicit supplies from the civilian population for wounded Union troops. Unfortunately, officers and surgeons frequently expropriated supplies designated for the wounded soldiers. Bickerdyke openly criticized Union officers and surgeons involved in this activity and reported their actions to Grant. Although many of Grant's staff officers complained about the outspoken Bickerdyke's disregard of military protocol, Grant consistently supported Bickerdyke. A highly resourceful and energetic nurse and administrator, Bickerdyke believed that it was her Christian duty to help the wounded soldiers as efficiently and quickly as possible.

As Grant's forces plunged deeper into the Confederacy, Bickerdyke followed the troops and established hospitals along the way. By the end of the war, Bickerdyke had aided the wounded on 19 battlefields, participated in the establishment of hundreds of field hospitals, and was instrumental in saving the lives of thousands of wounded soldiers, frequently searching battlefields at night with a lantern for wounded soldiers. Her popularity was so immense that soldiers frequently welcomed her with frenzied cheers rivaling those awarded to Grant. Bickerdyke's efforts even gained her accolades from Major General William Tecumseh Sherman, a man who routinely excluded women from his camp. Popular legend holds that Bickerdyke was the only woman that Sherman ever welcomed into his camp. At the conclusion of the war, Sherman insisted that Bickerdyke ride at the head of the XV Corps during the Grand Review of the Armies in Washington, D.C.

Once the war ended, Bickerdyke settled in Salina, Kansas, with her sons and opened a boarding house and dining hall for war veterans moving to Kansas. She also assisted war veterans and volunteer nurses in their quest for pensions from the federal government. Bickerdyke eventually helped more than 300 female volunteer nurses earn federal pensions. Although she was a volunteer for the duration of the Civil War, the U.S. Congress in 1886 awarded Bickerdyke a $25 annual pension. Bickerdyke died at Bunker Hill, Kansas, on November 8, 1901.

Michael R. Hall

Further Reading

Baker, Nina Brown. *Cyclone in Calico: The Story of Mary Ann Bickerdyke*. Boston: Little, Brown & Company, 1953.

De Leeuw, Adele. *Civil War Nurse Mary Ann Bickerdyke*. New York: Julian Messner, 1973.

Schultz, Jane E. "The Inhospitable Hospital: Gender and Professionalism in Civil War Medicine." *Signs* 17, 2 (Winter 1992): 363–392.

Billings, John Shaw (1838–1913)

John Shaw Billings was a surgeon, statistician, hospital architect, historian, bibliographer, and military physician for more than three decades. Billings was born on a frontier Indiana farm in 1838 and was noted early in his childhood to have an exceptional memory and facility for learning. He entered Miami University (Ohio) at age 14, graduated four years later, and enrolled in the Medical College of Ohio at Cincinnati in 1858. He graduated in two years and served briefly as a demonstrator in anatomy at the university before enlisting in the U.S. Army as a military surgeon in 1862.

Billings served in Washington and Philadelphia military hospitals until March 1863, when he was assigned to the Fifth Corps of the Army of the Potomac. He saw action at Chancellorsville, Gettysburg, the Wilderness, and Petersburg. His reputation for surgical skill brought to him many of the most difficult cases during this period, but he tired from overwork and was forced to spend six months recuperating in hospital before rejoining the Army of the Potomac, now under General Ulysses Grant, in March 1864. In August he was named medical director of the U.S. Army, and his reports formed a major part of the *Medical and Surgical History of the War of the Rebellion*.

In December 1864, Billings was transferred to the Surgeon General's office, where he spent the next 30 years. In 1869, his review of the Marine Hospital Service resulted in its reorganization into the Public Health Service. His ability to design hospitals was widely recognized, and he was responsible for plans of the first inpatient facility at Johns Hopkins University. He also chose William Welch, William Osler, William Halsted, and Walter Kelly to be the first medical staff.

Billings has been called the father of American medical statistics and was responsible for medical information being included for the first time in the 1880 U.S. census. He also suggested using an as-yet-uninvented mechanical counting device to tabulate the 1890 census, an idea translated by Herman Hollerith into the first computerized data processing machine. Billings created the Surgeon General's library, which became the National Library of Medicine, and supervised the publication of the *Index-Catalogue of the Library of the Office of the Surgeon General*, which has evolved into the *Index Medicus* and Medline.

He retired from the Army in 1895 to take the chair of hygiene at the University of Pennsylvania. In 1896 he left medicine to become director of the New York Public library and designed that institution's current building. He served there and as chair of the Carnegie Institution until his death after a brief illness on March 11, 1913. He is buried at Arlington National Cemetery.

Jack McCallum

Further Reading

Chapman, Carleton B. *Order out of Chaos: John Shaw Billings and America's Coming of Age*. Boston: Boston Medical library, 1994.

Garrison, Fielding. *John Shaw Billings: A Memoir*. New York: G. P. Putnam's Sons, 1915.

Gillet, Mary. *The Army Medical Department, 1865–1917*. Washington, D.C.: Center of Military History, 1995.

Lydenburg, Harry Miller. *John Shaw Billings: Creator of the National Medical Library and its Catalogue. First Director of the New York Public Library.* Chicago: American Library Association, 1924.

United States Surgeon General's Office, Joseph K. Barnes, Janvier Woodward, Charles Smart, George A. Otis, and David Lowe Huntington. *The Medical and Surgical History of the War of the Rebellion (1861–1865).* Washington, D.C.: Government Printing Office, 1870–1888.

Chimborazo Hospital

Richmond, Virginia's Chimborazo Hospital served the Confederate States of America during the American Civil War. It opened on October 11, 1861, and operated until April, 1865 when Union forces captured Richmond. Chimborazo was America's largest military hospital, with more than 8,000 beds at its peak. Established by order of Confederate Surgeon General Samuel Preston Moore, it was made an independent post under the command of Dr. James B. McGaw. McGaw, in turn, was a Medical College of Virginia faculty member and Richmond practitioner who had begun the war as a cavalry officer before being called back to run the hospital. The Medical College of Virginia was the only Southern medical school that remained open through the war. McGaw partially filled the education void by using Chimborazo to train more than 400 new physicians during the war.

The hospital occupied Chimborazo Heights above the James River outside Richmond on grounds that had originally been intended as winter quarters for the Army of Northern Virginia. It comprised 150 identical, one-story, wood-frame buildings measuring 100 feet long, 30 feet wide, and seven feet high with 10 windows in each structure. Each building housed from 40 to 60 patients, each of whom was intended to have 800 to 1,000 cubic feet of well-ventilated air space. In addition, eight to 10 convalescents occupied each of 100 Sibley tents pitched on the surrounding hillsides. The complex had five ice houses, Russian bathhouses, a bakery that produced 10,000 loaves of bread a day, a brewery that produced 400 kegs of beer at a time, and a farm with 200 cows and 3,500 goats. The hospital staff paid careful attention to sanitation and drainage from both hospital and farm facilities.

Chimborazo was divided into five administrative divisions of 30 buildings, each designated to care for men from specific states. Where possible, the men were housed with others from the same locality and cared for by physicians from as near their home counties as possible. Each division had a surgeon and a variable number of assistants with an average of 45 physicians assigned to the entire institution at any time. The divisions also had a matron and several assistants responsible for food preparation and laundry.

In spite of chronic shortages of medicine, supplies, and food, Chimborazo had an impressively low nine percent mortality rate for the war. Beyond that, detailed statistics are lacking since virtually all the hospital's records were lost in the Richmond fires of 1865. The hospital was formally surrendered when the city fell in 1865, and McGaw returned to practice and teaching, eventually becoming dean of the Medical College of Virginia in Richmond. His son, Walter Drew McGaw, served as chief surgeon of the American Expeditionary Force and established a number of hospitals in France during World War I.

Richmond was the Confederacy's center of medical care during the Civil War. In addition to the Medical College of Virginia, Richmond boasted 19 other large hospitals, the next largest being Winder with just under 5,000 beds.

Jack McCallum

Further Reading

Cunningham, H. H. *Doctors in Gray: The Confederate Medical Service*. Baton Rouge: Louisiana State University Press, 1958.

Hume, Edgar Erskine. 1934. "The Days Gone By: Chimborazo Hospital Confederate States Army; America's Largest Military Hospital." *Military Surgeon* 75 (September): 156–166.

Dix, Dorothea Lynde (1802–1887)

Dorothea Lynde Dix was born in Hampden, Maine (then part of Massachusetts), on April 4, 1802, and moved to Boston to live with her grandmother at the age of 12. Dix worked for a time as a teacher, then operated a finishing school for women in Boston, and authored several undistinguished books. In 1834, she traveled to Europe and visited numerous asylums for the mentally ill, hoping to bring reform to such facilities in the United States. Thus began a decades-long crusade to reform institutions for the mentally disabled and poor. Dix spent years lobbying Congress and local politicians to support her reforms. By the mid-1850s she had secured from Congress legislation that allotted thousands of acres of Federal land for the construction of modern—and humane—mental institutions. In the late 1850s Dix returned to Europe to study the management and physical layout of various hospitals, including military facilities.

In April 1861, when the Civil War began, Dix volunteered her services to the War Department. Appointed superintendent of all army nurses on June 10, 1861, Dix immediately began to recruit and appoint nurses and established efficient systems of management and medical delivery. During the war, she personally appointed more than 3,000 nurses. Dix also had charge of vast quantities of hospital supplies, which were distributed through her office in Washington, D.C. Dix maintained very stringent standards for nurse recruiting and training, which alienated some would-be nurses and which greatly annoyed some army doctors, who did not like to be beholden to a female nurse like Dix. Some nurses referred to her as "Dragon Dix," but most soon came to appreciate her exacting guidelines.

In October 1863, the surgeon general trimmed some of Dix's authority as a result of physicians' complaints. Order No. 351 empowered surgeons to appoint their own employees, including nurses. Dix was, however, undeterred and redoubled her efforts to provide the best nursing care possible among the employees she still controlled. She also tried to prevent her nurses from becoming victims of unwanted advances by male doctors, which infuriated some physicians all the more.

When supplies were short, Dix often raised private funds and purchased them herself. She toured many hospitals during the war and even operated a home where nurses could rest during leaves and furloughs. Dix accomplished all of this without receiving any pay from the government.

After the war, Dix continued her advocacy work on behalf of the mentally ill and indigent and founded a hospital in Trenton, New Jersey, where she died on July 17, 1887.

Paul G. Pierpaoli, Jr.

Further Reading

Brown, Thomas J. *Dorothea Dix: New England Reformer.* Cambridge, MA: Harvard University Press, 1998.

Muckenhoupt, Margaret. *Dorothea Dix: Advocate for Mental Health Care.* New York: Oxford University Press, 2004.

Hammond, William (1828–1900)

Responsible for the reorganization of the U.S. Army medical service during the Civil War before being court-martialed and dismissed as surgeon general of the Army, William Hammond was also a founder of American neurology.

William Hammond was born in Annapolis, Maryland, on August 28, 1828, the son of a physician. Both of Hammond's parents were descendants of prominent Maryland families. Hammond received his doctorate in medicine from the University of the City of New York in 1848 and enlisted as an assistant surgeon in the Army. He served in a variety of frontier posts during the Indian Wars before resigning in 1860 on account of ill-health.

When the Civil War began he reenlisted as an assistant surgeon, having lost both his rank and seniority. His superiors recognized his ability and experience and assigned him to inspect camps and hospitals in General William Rosecrans's army in West Virginia. The Union Army medical service was hopelessly inadequate at the beginning of the Civil War, and the civilian Sanitary Commission was appointed to evaluate and improve care, one result of which was the resignation of Surgeon General Clement Finley. The commission recommended that Hammond assume the post in spite of his youth and lack of rank, and he was appointed surgeon general on April 28, 1862, over a number of senior medical officers.

Almost all of the improvements in the Union Army's medical care came during Hammond's brief tenure. He started the Army Medical Museum, which became the Armed Forces Institute of Pathology; he adopted Jonathan Letterman's methods of patient transfer and his use of well-ventilated pavilion hospitals; and he instituted the data collection that resulted in the monumental *Medical and Surgical History of the War of the Rebellion*. In addition, he proposed formation of a permanent ambulance corps, an army medical school, a military medical laboratory, a permanent military research hospital in Washington, D.C., and a national library of medicine, all of which subsequently came to pass.

Hammond was a large, imposing man with an unhealthy measure of self-importance and arrogance. He got along poorly with Secretary of War Edwin Stanton, who finally removed him from Washington and stripped him of virtually all his powers. Hammond demanded a formal investigation or a court-martial to clear his name. He got the latter. The court found him innocent of charges that included fraud and corruption, but Stanton reversed that decision and directed a guilty verdict. Hammond was cashiered on August 18, 1864. In fairness to Stanton, Hammond had spent freely for drugs and supplies and had bought mostly from Philadelphia purveyors with whom he had a personal relationship. Although his behavior was so careless as to border on impropriety, no evidence exists that Hammond personally profited from his dealings. In fact, he was forced to borrow money to move his family to New York and restart his life after his dismissal.

In New York Hammond achieved both fame and fortune as a neurologist and "alienist" (psychiatrist), published a number of professional books and articles including the first American textbook of neurology. He was a founding member of both the New York and American neurological associations. Hammond's dogged efforts to clear his reputation culminated in 1878 in a congressional investigation that vindicated him and restored his rank of brigadier general.

Hammond retired from his New York practice in 1888 and moved to Washington, D.C., where he operated a private sanitarium for neurological disease until his death from cardiac failure on January 5, 1900. Hammond is recalled as the founder of American neurology.

Jack McCallum

Further Reading

Gillet, Mary. *The Army Medical Department, 1818–1865*. Washington, D.C.: Center of Military History, 1987.

Klawans, Harold. "The Court Martial of William A. Hammond." In *The Medicine of History from Paracelsus to Freud*. New York: Raven Press, 1982.

McHenry, L. C., Jr. 1963. "Surgeon General William Alexander Hammond." *Military Medicine*, 128.

Hoge, Jane Currie Blaikie (1811–1890)

Jane Hoge was born in Philadelphia on July 31, 1811. At the outset of the Civil War, she began providing relief supplies. She later became an associate manager of the northwestern branch of the United States Sanitary Commission in Chicago. In this position she came to see herself as a mother figure to the many men who fought for the Union.

Hoge shared her position at the Sanitary Commission with Mary A. Livermore. The two women worked smoothly together, imposing strict business standards on the Chicago branch and overseeing a massive supply effort. While the two women shared the office with two men, an accountant and a handyman, Hoge and Livermore represented the Commission to the hundreds of donors, family members, women, and soldiers who visited. They wrote thousands of letters, informing people at home about the needs at the front and facilitating correspondence between soldiers and their loved ones. In addition, they traveled extensively. For example, early in 1863 Hoge spent weeks on a ship that served as a supply depot and hospital in the Mississippi River in support of Union troops fighting to take Vicksburg. In an era when most women believed that speaking to mixed audiences was impolite, she learned to give moving and dynamic public speeches about the soldiers' experiences.

Hoge died in Evanston, Illinois on August 26, 1890.

Nancy Driscol Engle

Further Reading

Brockett, Linus P., and Marcy C. Vaughan. *Woman's Work in the Civil War*. Philadelphia: Zeigler, McCurdy & Co., 1867.

Hoge, Jane. *The Boys in Blue, or Heroes of the "Rank and File."* New York: E. B. Treat and Company, 1867.

Livermore, Mary A. *My Story of the War*. Hartford, CT: A. D. Worthington and Company, 1889.

Hospitals, Military

Before the Civil War, soldiers were treated in garrison hospitals or dispensaries located on the grounds of forts where they were stationed. These buildings were typically small and capable of holding some 18 patients. When the unit moved into the field, the regimental surgeon provided the medical care to the soldiers of his unit. The regimental surgeon had only two trained personnel, an assistant surgeon and an enlisted hospital steward, to assist him, but the regimental commander could detail additional soldiers to the surgeon as required.

The regimental surgeon was the primary focus of military health care in the early years of the Civil War. While the regiment prepared for battle, surgeons sent sick patients to general hospitals, usually converted hotels or warehouses or churches located in rear areas. During battle, the surgeon established a regimental hospital to treat the wounded. Regimental band members were responsible for carrying the wounded from the battlefield, while civilian teamsters drove the ambulances. Because the workload depended on whether the unit was engaged in battle or not, some regimental hospitals were overwhelmed with casualties while others were idle. After the battle, regimental hospitals consolidated the seriously wounded into depot hospitals, where they remained until they were well enough to be moved. Sometimes, regimental surgeons joined surgeons from the opposing army to treat all of the wounded from the battle. Some depot hospitals remained near the battlefield for almost a year.

Civil War battles produced enormous losses causing this system to collapse. Jonathon Letterman, medical director of the Army of the Potomac, recognized the need for a new system for taking care of the wounded. He proposed an ambulance corps of soldiers trained in the removal of the wounded under the control of medical officers. Each regiment was assigned an ambulance platoon under a noncommissioned officer. On August 2, 1862, Major General George B. McClellan signed the order implementing the ambulance corps within the Army of the Potomac. The organization was first employed during the Battle of Antietam on September 17, when the ambulance corps removed all 9,420 wounded, the heaviest casualties for a single day during the war, from the battlefield and had them under shelter by evening.

On October 30, 1862, General McClellan issued orders implementing Letterman's plan for consolidating regimental hospitals into division-level field hospitals. Regimental hospitals were transformed into dressing stations intended to stabilize patients before sending them to the newly established field hospitals. The new organization reduced the number of surgeons at the front and centralized medical staff far enough behind the lines to be accessible by all of the regiments while being close enough to ensure that the wounded would be treated in a timely manner. Letterman also established a supply system for the medical department separate from the quartermaster's corps.

Letterman's organization was in place when Major General Ambrose Burnside's Army of the Potomac attacked Fredericksburg on December 13, 1862. It was the first battle in which the surgeons had adequate supplies for treating the wounded. However, Letterman had planned to establish a depot in Falmouth, Virginia, and he failed to anticipate Burnside's eagerness to resume the offensive. When Burnside ordered the evacuation of all of the wounded to Washington, Letterman objected, arguing that not all of his patients could withstand a winter rail journey. Burnside was adamant and Letterman ordered the evacuation.

While the Fredericksburg campaign turned into a tactical debacle, the medical efforts were successful and became a model for handling wounded in the future.

The sudden order to remove wounded soldiers from Falmouth to make room for additional casualties from anticipated future combat became a common feature in future campaigns. Burnside's order had the unintended consequence of changing Letterman's army system into a national system for handling casualties, dovetailing into an evolving network of general hospitals and hospital trains.

The Medical Department was forced to begin building specially designed general or pavilion hospitals to accommodate large numbers of patients from the earlier Peninsula Campaign of March–August 1862. The designs emphasized sanitation and ventilation to minimize the miasmas that were believed to cause hospital infections. Each ward was in a single-story building, which ensured that there were no stairs to climb and impure vapors that patients on the second floor would have to inhale. By 1863, the Medical Department operated 151 hospitals accommodating 58,716 beds. Two years later there were more than 200 such hospitals.

Although most hospitals accommodated patients with virtually every kind of disease, some specialized hospitals began to emerge. Turner's Lane General Hospital in Philadelphia specialized in neurological and nervous disorders. A hospital for erysipelas cases was established in Nashville, Tennessee. Desmarres Hospital in Chicago focused on the treatment of wounds and diseases to the eye and a hospital for mutilated soldiers was located in New York City. The movement of patients away from the combat zone freed up beds in hospitals close to the battlefield for future casualties. On December 20, 1862, the War Department decreed that all wounded officers and enlisted be moved to a general hospital in their own state if they so requested.

The U.S. Navy had its own less elaborate system of hospitals. Sick and wounded sailors would be treated onboard the vessel, while those requiring definitive care were sent to shore-based hospitals located at major ports.

Hospitals were connected by a network of railroads and hospital trains that moved patients across the country. At first hospital trains used empty freight cars to move patients away from the battlefield. Straw or evergreen branches were laid on the floor of a flat car or a boxcar to accommodate the patients. In 1862, Dr. Elisha Harris designed a specialized hospital car that transported patients in stretchers hung from vertical posts with India rubber rings for shock absorbers. Four of these cars were placed in service on the rail lines connecting hospitals in Louisville, Kentucky, and Nashville, Tennessee, with the Army of the Tennessee, reducing travel time from Louisville to Nashville to 24 hours. The hospital trains were credited with preventing many cases of gangrene, common in the case of slower hospital ships. Many other hospital trains were also developed during the war. During the May 5–September 2, 1864, Atlanta campaign, 25,184 wounded men made the 12-hour journey to the general hospitals in Nashville or on to Louisville.

The hospital system during the Civil War was not exclusively a military venture. Civilians, horrified at the carnage of the war, organized to help the sick and wounded soldiers. The most influential of these organizations was the U.S. Sanitary Commission led by Frederick Law Olmstead, which was given semi-official status by President Abraham Lincoln in 1861. The Commission demonstrated its political clout by ensuring that their candidate, William H. Hammond, was appointed surgeon general of the U.S. Army in 1862. The Commission solicited donations and raised money by holding Sanitary Fairs in several major cities to fund the construction of hospital trains, purchase medical supplies, and garner support for 25 soldiers' homes. Other organizations, such as the Christian Commission and the Young Men's Christian Association, also provided supplies and relief to the sick and wounded.

The nursing profession received a major boost from this system of hospitals. Regimental surgeons, at the beginning of the war, were authorized one enlisted assistant, whose duties included nursing. Ambulatory sick or wounded soldiers also performed nursing duties for their less fortunate comrades. Dorothea Dix and Elizabeth Blackwell, the first woman medical doctor, trained 3,214 women to serve as nurses for the U.S. Army, most of whom served at general hospitals in cities. However, that was only a fraction of the more than 18,000 women paid by the U.S. Army and 2,000 unpaid volunteers who took care of the sick and wounded at hospitals within the combat zone. These women were sent by organizations or just showed up and started working. At the beginning of the war, doctors and nurses had a testy relationship that evolved into a grudging mutual appreciation and respect. After the war, physicians' support of nurses led to the demand for nursing programs at medical colleges and hospitals.

Although the Confederate Medical Service suffered from a chronic shortage of supplies and personnel and never matched Letterman's success in evacuation of the wounded, it did have a few impressively designed hospitals, the largest of which was Chimborazo in Richmond, Virginia. This facility opened October 11, 1861 and operated until the fall of Richmond in 1865. It was America's largest military hospital with more than 8,000 beds at its peak. The staff at Chimborazo demonstrated an enlightened attitude toward sanitation that contributed to the hospital's impressively low nine percent mortality rate for the war. Richmond was the Confederacy's medical center, and there were 19 other large hospitals in the city, the next largest being Winder with just less than 5,000 beds.

Medical care for Federal forces during the Civil War evolved from a group of individual regimental surgeons into a national network to tend to the sick and wounded. It influenced the medical profession to begin seeing health care as system rather than as the work of individual doctors. In the network of hospitals developed during the war, the outlines of how health care would be organized in the 20th century became visible.

Alan J. Hawk

Further Reading

Robertson, James I., ed. *Medical and Surgical History of the Civil War.* Wilmington, NC: Broadfoot Publishing Company, 1991.

Schultz, Jane E. *Women at the Front: Hospital Workers in Civil War America.* Chapel Hill: The University of North Carolina Press, 2007.

Hospital Trains

Initially used in 1854 to evacuate wounded during the Crimean War, hospital trains remained a major means of medical transportation through World War I. When the American Civil War started, the United States had 31,000 miles of railroads (21,000 of which were in Union states), and President Abraham Lincoln put them under federal management and appointed Colonel Daniel McCallum superintendent of the U.S. Military Railroad in January 1862. The intent was primarily to use railcars to move food, forage, ammunition, and some medical supplies with no real thought of using railroads to move the wounded.

The first time railroads were used for that purpose in the United States was in August 1861 when Assistant Surgeon S. H. Melcher used boxcars to move Union

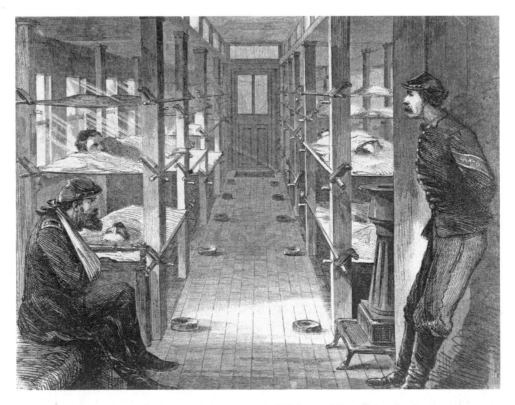

Specially designed hospital cars carried wounded Union soldiers from the front to rear area hospital facilities. (Corbis)

wounded from Rolla, Missouri, to the general hospital at St. Louis after the Union's defeat at the Battle of Wilson's Creek. Empty cars returning from the front became a preferred method of evacuating the wounded for both the Union and the Confederacy in spite of the fact that the men often had to lie on straw, leaves, or bare boards in cars that were either open entirely or closed boxes without ventilation. When stretchers were available, they were usually either hung by ropes from the ceiling or rested on stanchions bolted to the walls of the car. In either case, they left the men subject to the rocking and jerking of a moving train.

As part of Jonathan Letterman's reform of medical transport beginning in 1862, evacuation trains from the front to rear-area hospitals became standard in the Army of the Potomac. In October 1862, Dr. Elisha Harris of the U.S. Sanitary Commission designed a car in which stretchers were suspended by their handles with rubber-ring shock absorbers to ease suffering during evacuation of the wounded. The Philadelphia, Wilmington, and Baltimore Railroad subsequently built 15 of the Harris cars.

After the Battle of Antietam, Letterman was able to move more than 9,000 wounded to the general hospital in Frederick, Maryland, in less than three days. After the Battle of Gettysburg, 11,425 men were transported by rail to hospitals in Baltimore; York, Virginia; and New York City. The wounded at Gettysburg were initially taken to a field hospital, and those able to be moved were then transferred to Sanitary Commission tents that had been erected at the railhead. The large numbers of wounded led to a bottleneck at the railhead, but, as trains became available, movement farther to the rear was generally smooth.

By 1864 J. McCricket, assistant superintendent of Union military railroads, had designed hospital cars that could hold up to 60 wounded on permanently mounted stretchers. Eighteen trains a day ran the 20 miles from the front at Petersburg to the 6,000-bed Union hospital at City Point, Virginia, in June of that year. Although these were primarily boxcars in the beginning, by January 1865 they had all been replaced by dedicated hospital cars. In contrast, the Confederates never got beyond using back-loaded freight cars and commandeered passenger cars and never had an organized program of rail evacuation.

Combined Franco-British "ambulance trains" not only transported wounded from the front during World War I but also acted as mobile medical and surgical wards and kitchen and supply cars. In spite of those advances, men continued to be transported on straw palettes in empty boxcars on return journeys from the line. Trains were again used to move casualties within France after D-Day in World War II and during the Burma Campaign. Various sorts of rail transport were also used during the Korean Conflict. More recently, rail transport has largely been supplanted by road or air evacuation.

Jack McCallum

Further Reading

Haller, John S. *Farmcarts to Fords: A History of the Military Ambulance, 1790–1925*. Carbondale: Southern Illinois University Press, 1992.

Hawk, Alan. 2002. "An Ambulating Hospital: Or, How the Hospital Train Transformed Army Medicine." *Civil War History* 48: 197–219.

Plumridge, John H. *Hospital Ships and Ambulance Trains*. London: Seeley, Service & Co., 1975.

Letterman, Jonathan (1824–1872)

Jonathan Letterman was born in Cannonsburg, Pennsylvania, on December 11, 1824, the son of a surgeon. He graduated from Jefferson Medical College in 1849 and enlisted in the Army as an assistant surgeon. For the next 12 years, Letterman served in a variety of Army posts and in a number of Indian campaigns. On July 1, 1862, Surgeon General William Hammond appointed him to succeed Major Charles Tripler as chief surgeon in Major General George McClellan's Army of the Potomac.

From that position, Letterman instituted the changes that became standard practice in Army medical services through World War I. Realizing that wounded men were being left in the field for as much as a week, Letterman first instituted an organized system of evacuation. He arranged for rapid construction of carts and two-and four-wheeled horse-drawn vehicles to evacuate the wounded. He utilized French practice to create a permanent group of stretcher bearers and ambulance drivers. The litter bearers were taken from line regiments but were organized by division and placed under the corps medical officer. The ambulance vehicles were restricted to transporting the sick and wounded rather than doubling as carriers of ammunition and supplies. By the Battle of Antietam on September 7, 1862, Letterman had 200 new ambulances (roughly one for every 175 combat soldiers) and was able to remove all wounded from the field in less than 48 hours.

Letterman adapted lessons learned in the Crimean War to completely reorganize the Union hospital system. He replaced converted public buildings and warehouses that had previously served as fixed hospitals with well-ventilated, modular pavilions organized on a divisional rather than a regimental level that became the model for Type A and B hospitals of the American Expeditionary Force in France during World War I. He established a sequential evacuation that started with tented hospitals near the front from which patients were moved to field hospitals and then to general hospitals in rear-area cities. This step-wise evacuation was subsequently adopted by all the powers in World War I.

Letterman resigned from the Army in 1864 after Hammond's court-martial. He unsuccessfully tried business in Southern California before moving to San Francisco, where he went into private practice and briefly served as city coroner. He died at age 47 on March 15, 1872.

Jack McCallum

Further Reading

Ashburn, P. M. *A History of the Medical Department of the United States Army.* Boston: Houghton Mifflin Co., 1929.

Gillet, Mary. *The Army Medical Department, 1818–1865.* Washington, D.C.: Center of Military History, 1987.

Haller, John S. *Farmcarts to Fords: A History of the Military Ambulance, 1790–1925.* Carbondale: Southern Illinois University Press, 1992.

Packard, Francis. *History of Medicine in the United States.* New York: Paul B. Hoeber, Inc., 1931.

Livermore, Mary Ashton Rice (1820–1905)

Born in Boston on September 19, 1820, Mary Ashton Rice graduated from an all-female seminary in Charlestown, Massachusetts, in 1836. From 1839 to 1842 she was a tutor on a Virginia plantation, an experience that caused her to become an abolitionist. She then was the head of a private school in Duxbury, Massachusetts, for three years. In 1845 she married Universalist minister Daniel P. Livermore, and in 1847 they moved to Chicago.

Before and during the Civil War, she rose through the ranks of Chicago's voluntary associations, including the U.S. Sanitary Commission, the Chicago branch of which she help to organize. Livermore held the office of associate director along with two men and Jane Hoge, a friend who shared with Livermore the great workload and inspired her with confidence. To countless visitors, the two women became the faces of the commission. Many times each day they convinced skeptical would-be donors of the agency's merits. In addition, they oversaw the sorting of tons of donated goods, packing and sealing boxes to be sent to the front lines. They recruited nurses to serve at army posts and handled a voluminous correspondence. Finally, they planned and led two huge sanitary fairs in Chicago that raised considerable funds. Eventually they disbursed more than one million dollars in relief.

Besides office responsibilities, Livermore's war-time activities involved a fair amount of travel, during which she met both President Abraham Lincoln and Lieutenant General Ulysses S. Grant. Following an early 1863 visit to the armies camped outside Vicksburg, Livermore helped prevent an outbreak of scurvy there by collecting and shipping more than 1,000 bushels of vegetables to the troops. Finally, in an era when women who spoke to mixed audiences were considered inappropriate, Livermore learned to give compelling speeches before large mixed groups of men and women.

Livermore's wartime work made her aware of the restrictions that society imposed on women. In 1863, a builder refused to sign a contract with Livermore and Hoge because they were women, even though they were agents of the Sanitary Commission and had in their possession both the money and the lumber necessary to construct the building. In the decade following the war, women's rights became one of Livermore's most important causes. She wrote articles for various magazines and helped organize the Illinois Woman Suffrage Association.

Still in print today, Livermore's *My Story of the War* (1889) sold approximately 60,000 copies in its first decade. It offers a woman's perspective on the Civil War, gives details about military hospitals and relief work, describes her encounters with prominent Union officials, and provides glimpses into the operations of the Sanitary Commission. Livermore was a nationally known figure by the time of her death in Melrose, Massachusetts, on May 23, 1905.

Nancy Driscol Engle

Further Reading

Livermore, Mary A. *My Story of the War*. Hartford, CT: A. D. Worthington and Company, 1889.

Venet, Wendy Hamand. *A Strong-Minded Woman: The Life of Mary Livermore*. Amherst: University of Massachusetts Press, 2005.

Medical Department, Confederate

Southern efforts to organize and operate a Medical Department confronted difficult obstacles because the Confederacy lacked sufficient numbers of doctors, hospitals, medicine, and medical supplies for a long war.

Surgeon General Samuel P. Moore modeled the Confederate Medical Department on its Union counterpart, although his government allocated only $50,000 for hospital construction and supply. As a result, Moore's administrative staff in Richmond was relatively small, although it oversaw an extensive field network. Three categories of Confederate military medical personnel directly treated patients. Surgeons and assistant surgeons were military officers and qualified physicians. They served as doctors and staff officers in units and at hospitals. Stewards were enlisted soldiers who performed nursing and administrative services for the army. The Confederacy also had a support force of medical purveyors and storekeepers, including pharmacists who specialized in buying or making medicines, and medical inspectors, who reported to the surgeon general on the efficiency of the system. Qualified medical personnel were always in short supply; although, as with the Union army, the Confederate department used short-term volunteers to supplement the regular military personnel.

The department provided medical services in three types of hospitals. The largest, called general hospitals, were permanent facilities located in buildings in major cities in the South. Smaller than general hospitals and less permanent were depot hospitals. One could find these in combinations of tents and temporarily commandeered buildings at the major Confederate supply depots (hence the name). The third category of hospital was the field hospital, which directly

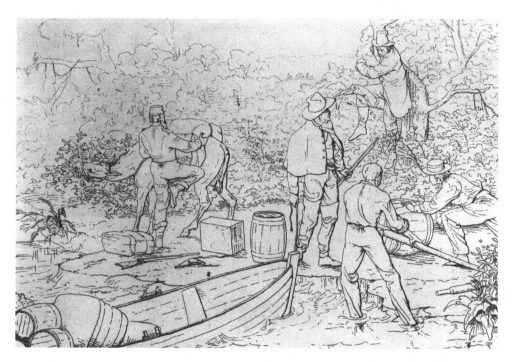

Because of the cessation of trade and the imposition of the Federal blockade, the South was cut off from its traditional sources of medicine. Smugglers brought medicines into the South to alleviate the drug shortage. (Bettmann/Corbis)

supported the fighting units and were the nearest to the front lines. At the beginning of the war, the law only assigned medical personnel to the regiments, so field hospitals started as regimental hospitals. However, regimental hospitals were too small to be efficient. The field hospitals gradually consolidated into informal brigade, division, and even corps hospitals.

Evacuation of wounded soldiers from the battlefield to hospitals was haphazard at best. Confederate President Jefferson Davis vetoed the bill that would have established an ambulance corps of specially trained and equipped soldiers to move the wounded, so the Southern armies made do with informal ambulance arrangements.

The Confederate Medical Department suffered under a significant disability in that there was no major producer of pharmaceuticals in the South and the surgeons were forced to rely on pre-war stockpiles, drugs that could be imported through the Union blockade from Europe, and herbals harvested from local sources. A significant exception was the anesthetic chloral hydrate which could be distilled from chloride of lime and alcohol and which was more widely used by the Southerners than by their Northern counterparts, especially early in the war. Ether was also used by both sides, and, by war's end, each had carried out approximately 80,000 operations under anesthesia.

Southern military surgeons labored under other significant disadvantages. The Confederacy did not have a unified civilian support agency such as the U.S. Sanitary Commission to help the Medical Department. Although state and local aid societies provided important assistance, the effort was never coordinated. In a similar vein, the Richmond Ambulance Company, a civilian volunteer organization, participated in all the major eastern campaigns, but there was no similar organization in the western theater.

Because the Confederacy had no formal system of medical record keeping analogous to that created by United States Surgeon General William Hammond, and because most Confederate military medical records were burned in Richmond at the end of the war, statistics are incomplete. It is estimated that the Confederacy lost about 94,000 men in battle and 164,000 to disease of the approximately 1.3 million who served, compared to 138,154 who died in battle and 224,586 who died of disease of the 2,893,304 who served in the Union army.

J. Boone Bartholomees

Further Reading

Cunningham, H. H. *Doctors in Gray: The Confederate Medical Service*. Baton Rouge: Louisiana State University Press, 1958.

Freemon, Frank R. *Gangrene and Glory: Medical Care During the American Civil War*. Madison, NJ: Farleigh Dickinson University Press, 1998.

U.S. Surgeon General's Office. *The Medical and Surgical History of the War of the Rebellion (1861–1865), Prepared in Accordance with the Acts of Congress, under the Direction of Surgeon General Joseph K. Barnes, United States Army*. 2 vols. in 6 serials. Washington, D.C.: U.S. Government Printing Office, 1870–1888.

Medical Department, U.S.

The U.S. Army Medical Department was entirely unprepared for the Civil War. In April 1861, there were only 115 doctors in the Medical Department, including one surgeon general, 30 surgeons, and 84 assistant surgeons. Eight surgeons and 29 assistant surgeons left the army when the southern states seceded. The head of the Medical Department was the conservative 72-year-old Surgeon General Thomas Lawson. After his death in May 1861, he was succeeded by the equally conservative Dr. Clement Finley.

The small, tradition-bound medical bureau fared poorly at the outset of the conflict. There were no plans in place for supply and evacuation on the scale produced by the war, nor were there plans for a hospital system to care for the mass of sick and wounded. Representatives of charitable and religious organizations responded to the situation by creating the United States Sanitary Commission modeled after the similarly named British group. The commission successfully lobbied Congress for official status. Led by Executive Secretary Frederick Law Olmstead, it began providing food, clothing, and medical supplies to the Union troops. In spite of strenuous objections from the medical corps, the commission also began supervising camp sanitation. This was especially important since measles and dysentery had become rife among groups of previously unexposed young men sharing close quarters.

During the 37th Congress (1861–1863), Senator Henry Wilson of Massachusetts introduced a bill proposing a complete reorganization of the Medical Department; this went into effect on April 16, 1862. At the urging of the U.S. Sanitary Commission, Secretary of War Edwin Stanton removed Finley from his post and on April 25, 1862 appointed in his stead the 33-year-old William A. Hammond as surgeon general.

The Medical Department now underwent a vigorous reorganization. Its structure was modified and new positions were created: the surgeon general enjoyed the rank and pay of a brigadier general, and the assistant surgeon general, inspector general of hospitals, and eight at-large medical inspectors had the same privileges and pay as cavalry colonels. Improvements included the creation of a corps of medical cadets to assist in hospitals and as ambulance attendants and the employment of female nurses in general hospitals. Physicians were organized into seven categories: surgeons and assistant surgeons of the regular army; surgeons and assistant surgeons of U.S Volunteers; regimental surgeons and assistant surgeons commissioned by state governors; acting assistant surgeons, U.S. Army (civilian physicians employed by the Union army as part-time or full-time surgeons under contract); medical officers of the Veterans Corps; acting staff surgeons; and surgeons and assistant surgeons of U.S. Colored Troops. Each regiment was authorized a surgeon and two assistant surgeons, and individual armies had brigade, division, corps, and army medical directors who were responsible for supervising the medical officers of that particular army unit.

Large general hospitals were established for the overflow of patients from post and regimental hospitals. These had one surgeon in charge of administrative matters, another in charge of hospital staff, and assistant surgeons and medical cadets responsible for one to two wards of 70 to one 100 patients each. The hospitals also had a chaplain and hospital stewards who supervised clothing, hygiene, cooking, and the dispensing of medicines. Convalescent soldiers were responsible for nursing and cleaning each individual ward. Larger hospitals also had blacksmiths, attendants for the dead, washerwomen, and female nurses. Also, the Medical Department constructed laboratories to formulate and compound medicines, and employed medical purveyors to distribute medicines and hospital supplies. Between 1861 and 1865, the Union constructed 204 hospitals with an aggregate capacity of 137,000 beds, an impressive feat by any measure.

In early 1863, Dr. Hammond appointed Jonathan Letterman to succeed Charles Tripler as medical director of the Army of the Potomac. Together they created a new ambulance and field relief system, and control of the ambulance system was moved from the Quartermaster Department to the Medical Department. In late 1863, Congress implemented the Letterman system throughout the Union army.

From the beginning, field hospitals were most often in "walled tents" that could hold up to 20 patients or strung together to hold twice that many. The earliest general hospitals were in whatever large buildings could be commandeered—hotels, large houses, and warehouses being common solutions—and were under regimental control. Their inefficiency and poor sanitation led to their being replaced by pavilion hospitals under the medical corps, especially after the numbers of sick and wounded went up in 1862. By 1863, the United States Army Medical Corps had 151 hospitals and 58,716 beds, mostly well ventilated and at least marginally clean. In 1864, Lieutenant General Ulysses S. Grant authorized a 6,000 bed hospital at City Point, Virginia, that ultimately expanded to 10,000 beds and had eighteen trains continuously running between it and the front near Petersburg. The Union also created specialized hospitals for particular injuries and illnesses such as Turner's Lane General Hospital in Philadelphia for nervous and neurologic problems, the DesMarres Hospital in Chicago for wounds and diseases of the eye, a hospital in Nashville for erysipelas, and another in New York City for treatment of the severely mutilated.

Shauna Devine

Further Reading

Gillett, Mary. *The Army Medical Department, 1818–1865*. Washington, D.C.: Government Printing Office, 1987.

Wintermute, Bobby. *Public Health and the U.S. Military: A History of the Army Medical Department, 1818–1917*. New York: Routledge, 2011.

Mitchell, Silas Weir (1829–1914)

Silas Mitchell was the foremost practitioner of both clinical and experimental neurology during the American Civil War. Mitchell was born February 15, 1829, in Philadelphia, the son of a well-to-do physician and professor at the Jefferson Medical College, from which Mitchell himself graduated in 1850. He went on to study with Claude Bernard in Paris before returning to Philadelphia and entering private practice. While in practice he became friends with William Hammond, who later became surgeon general of the Union Army, and the two coauthored several papers.

Mitchell enlisted in the U.S. Army in October 1862 as a contract surgeon and was assigned to the hospital at the old Armory building at 16th and Fulton streets in Philadelphia where he began his studies of nerve injury. On May 5, 1863, Hammond ordered the establishment of the U.S. Army Hospital for Diseases of the Nervous System at Christian Street, also in Philadelphia. That facility was overwhelmed with casualties from the Battle of Gettysburg and moved to a larger building at Turner Lane, where Mitchell joined with George R. Morehouse and William Williams Keen in directing what had become America's first large hospital devoted to injuries of the nervous system. The three collaborated on the groundbreaking *Gunshot Wounds and Other Injuries of Nerves* (1864), which Mitchell expanded to *Injuries of Nerves*, published in 1872. That volume became a standard that, in its English and French versions, remained in use through World War I. Mitchell also wrote *Reflex Paralysis* (1864), in which he coined the term "causalgia" (intractable pain and skin changes caused by partial nerve injury) and described shock caused by the brain's reaction to bodily injury.

After the war Mitchell became America's foremost clinical neurologist. He was elected the first president of the American Neurological Association by acclamation but declined to serve. Mitchell died January 4, 1914.

Jack McCallum

Further Reading

Burr, A. R. *Weir Mitchell, His Life and Letters.* New York: Duffield and Co., 1929.

Earnest, E. S. *Weir Mitchell, Novelist and Physician.* Philadelphia: University of Pennsylvania Press, 1950.

Walter, R. D. S. *Weir Mitchell, M.D., Neurologist.* Springfield, IL: Charles C. Thomas, 1970.

Moore, Samuel Preston (1813–1889)

Born on September 16, 1813 in Charleston, South Carolina, Samuel Preston Moore graduated from the Medical College of South Carolina at the age of 21. After several years of private practice in Little Rock, Arkansas, Moore applied for a commission as an assistant surgeon in the United States Army, which he received in March 1835. He served as a medical officer in the army for more than 26 years. While tending wounded soldiers in the Mexican-American War, Moore met and became friends with Colonel Jefferson Davis, later president of the Confederacy. In February 1861, shortly after his native state joined the Confederacy, Moore resigned his U.S. Army commission.

On July 30, 1861, President Davis selected Moore to serve as the surgeon general for the Confederacy, a post he held for the duration of the Civil War. His decades of prior service provided him with the experience necessary to lead the medical department, but his strict, abrasive, martinet management style won him few friends. Nevertheless, fellow officers believed that Moore was one of the ablest Confederate administrators. Despite chronic shortages of both medical supplies and qualified doctors, Moore built from scratch a Medical Corps of some 3,000 personnel by 1865 that credibly supported the Confederate war effort.

Moore's insistence on examination boards to assess the competency of incoming physicians, his strong support for modern pavilion hospitals, and his recognition of the importance of dentistry stand out among his many achievements in military medicine. In September 1861, Moore became the first surgeon general in American history to grant a commission to a woman: Captain Sally Louisa Tomkins.

After the war, Moore retired from medical practice. He held a variety of civic and government posts, including a seat on the Richmond School Board, and served as the first president of the Association of Medical Officers of the Army and Navy of the Confederacy. Moore died on May 31, 1889 in Richmond, Virginia.

Justin Barr

Further Reading

Chancellor, Charles W. "A Memoir of the Late Samuel Preston Moore, M.D., Surgeon General of the Confederate States Army." *Southern Practitioner* XLII (1903): 275–284.

Cunningham, H. H. *Doctors in Gray: The Confederate Medical Service*. Baton Rouge: Louisiana State University Press, 1958.

Farr, Warner D. "Samuel Preston Moore: Confederate Surgeon General." *Civil War History* XLI, 1 (1995): 41–56.

Morphine

Morphine is an alkaloid and is the chief active ingredient in opium. It is extracted from immature seed capsules of the *Papaver somniferum* plant. The opium poppy is native to southeastern Europe and western Asia but is currently cultivated in Europe, India, Canada, South and Central America, and much of central Asia. Heroin, codeine, meperidine (Demerol), oxycodone, and fentanyl are all semi-synthetic derivatives of morphine. Morphine's pain-relieving properties were known to the Sumerians as early as 4000 B.C. and to the Egyptians two millennia later. In his 1517 *Fieldbook of Wound Surgery*, Hans von Gersdorff described performing battlefield amputations after having the patient inhale from a "sleeping sponge" soaked in opium, mandrake root, henbane, hemlock, and lettuce. By the late 17th century, a typical military surgeon's field chest contained his instruments; a variety of folk remedies such as sandalwood, dog fat, and mummy dust; and a handful of useful drugs such as aloe and, especially, opium.

Rosengarten and Company of Philadelphia (the predecessor to modern pharmaceutical company Merck, Sharpe and Dohme) began manufacturing morphine salts in 1832, and, by the beginning of the American Civil War in 1861, a variety of opioid preparations were available, including Laudanum (tincture of opium), paregoric (tincture of camphorated opium), powdered opium (which contained 9–12 percent morphine), opium gum, Dover's powders (10 percent opium and 10 percent ipecac), and an assortment of narcotic-containing patent medicines and elixirs.

Medicinal use of morphine underwent a dramatic change during the Civil War with the introduction of the hypodermic syringe. Injected morphine proved such an effective pain reliever that it went from prescribed use in field and general hospitals to self-administration by soldiers with chronic pain who were supplied with both the drug and syringes for self-administration. Paregoric was also routinely used to manage diarrhea from the ubiquitous dysentery, and various morphine powders were standard therapy for malarial fevers.

During World War I, the U.S. Army had the Mulford Company of Baltimore devise "hypo units" containing morphine that a soldier could administer to himself with one hand, and several hundred thousand of the syringes were produced. In 1938, the Army and the Navy asked Squibb to improve on the Mulford unit, and, ultimately, 75 million of the improved syrettes were produced during World War II.

Jack McCallum

Further Reading

Albin, Maurice. " 'Opium Eaters' and 'Morphinists'—Narcotic Addiction and the Civil War: Did It All Start There?" *Anesthesiology* 2002: A1162.

Newsom, Ella King (1838–1919)

Ella King Newsome was born in June 1838 in Brandon, Mississippi. In 1854, she married William Frank Newsom, a wealthy doctor and landowner, and the couple moved to Winchester, Tennessee. He died a short time later. When the Civil War began, Newsom pursued nursing training and instruction from Dr. James Keller, a Memphis City Hospital physician, and the Roman Catholic Sisters of Mercy. Her nursing career began in December 1861 at Bowling Green, Kentucky. She was soon promoted to superintendent of the Bowling Green hospitals. The Confederate evacuation of Bowling Green and surrender of Forts Henry (February 6) and Donelson (February 16, 1862) forced her to re-establish a hospital in the Howard High School buildings in Nashville.

After the fall of Nashville, Newsom moved patients to Winchester, Tennessee, and organized another hospital, which acquired the nickname "The Soldiers' Paradise" because of its excellent care. Following the Battle of Shiloh on April 6–7, 1862, Newsom was summoned to the Corinth House and the Tishomingo House Hospitals in Corinth, Mississippi.

Other hospitals with which Newsom was associated were the Crutchfield House at Chattanooga, Tennessee; hospitals at Okolona, Columbus, and Meridian, Mississippi; the Emory and Henry College hospital in Abingdon, Virginia; and hospitals in Marietta and Atlanta, Georgia. Among hospital administrators, soldiers and friends, Newsom was known as "The Florence Nightingale of the southern army."

After the war, Newsom married a former Confederate officer, but upon his death in 1885, her financial status declined. In 1908, Dr. Samuel E. Lewis and the

Association of Medical Officers of the Army and Navy of the Confederacy established the Newsom Home Fund to help Newsome financially. She eventually moved to Washington, D.C. and worked in the Patent, Pension, and General Land Offices until her retirement in 1916. She died in Washington on January 20, 1919.

M. Lynn Barnes

Further Reading

Massey, Mary Elizabeth. *Women in the Civil War.* Lincoln: University of Nebraska Press, 1994.

Richard, J. Fraise. *The Florence Nightingale of the Southern Army: Experiences of Mrs. Ella K. Newsom, Confederate Nurse in the Great War of 1861–65.* New York: Broadway Publishing Co., 1914.

Nurses

Prior to the Civil War, most nursing was done by men or was conducted in private homes because it was considered socially inappropriate for women to have contact in public areas with men who were not family members. During wartime, many nursing duties had been performed by recuperating soldiers prior to their full recovery and return to military service.

American nursing was in its infancy when the Civil War began, and nursing schools, diplomas, and credentials did not exist. Early on the U.S. government recognized the great need for skilled nursing and the lack of available male nurses. In 1861 the government sought the expertise of Florence Nightingale, a pioneering nurse during the 1853–1856 Crimean War. When the Union decided to accept women into the nursing profession, thousands, from all levels of society, sought available appointments. Documents show that at least 21,000 women served as nurses on the government payroll during the war.

The majority of nurses were assigned to general hospitals, medical transports, and regimental aid stations, with few actually posted on battlefields. As a general rule, one nurse was assigned to a single hospital division, with duties including organization of wards, direction of subordinates, supervision of special diets, and distribution of food and medical supplies. Other nursing duties included dressing wounds, assisting with amputations, cleaning wards, bathing soldiers, cooking, laundering, and mending uniforms. Literate nurses often read to and wrote letters for soldiers. Most importantly, women nurses cared for the emotional and spiritual needs of wounded and ill soldiers. The Civil War marked the first time in American history that women played a significant role in a war effort.

Critical to the advancement of American nursing was the formation of The United States Sanitary Commission on June 18, 1861. Dorothea Lynde Dix was appointed superintendent of the nursing program administered by the Commission, and in this

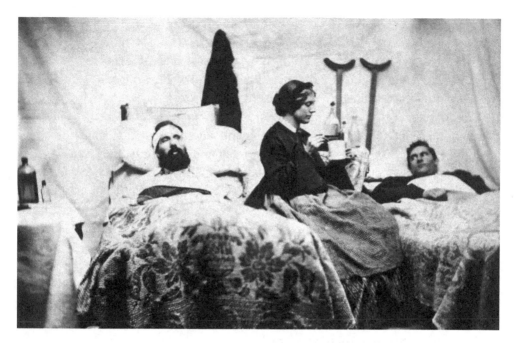

Two wounded Federal soldiers are cared for by Anne Bell, a nurse during the American Civil War. (Corbis)

capacity supervised more than 3,000 women nurses for the Union army. She required all female nursing recruits to be 35 to 50 years old, "plain looking," and have recommendations from two people attesting to their morality, integrity, seriousness, and capacity for care of the sick.

Women nurses committed to serve at least three months and were paid $12.00 per month. Because uniforms were not supplied by the army, their dress code included a brown, gray or black dress with no bows. Nurses were not permitted to have hair curls, jewelry, or hoop-skirts. The nurses recruited by Dix were found in every Union hospital and virtually all battlefields of the war.

Clarissa "Clara" Harlowe Barton was another significant influence on the American nursing profession. After the July 21, 1861 Battle of Bull Run, Barton, who was working as a clerk for the U.S. Patent Office, encountered wounded Union troops who were housed in the U.S. Senate chamber. Supplying food, comfort, and aid to these soldiers, she realized that her greatest contributions did not lie as a patent clerk. Shortly afterward, she founded a civilian agency that gathered and distributed medical supplies to the wounded and sick soldiers. She supported other relief organizations and was one of the few women nurses during the Civil War who actually worked on battlefields. Labeled the "Angel of the Battlefield," she nursed Union soldiers during and after many battles. In 1863, President Abraham Lincoln appointed Barton supervisor of the Missing Soldiers Office.

Her most lasting legacy was the establishment after the war of the American National Red Cross on May 21, 1881. She served as its president for 22 years.

Other notable Union nurses include Mary A. R. Livermore, Margaret Breckinridge, Helen Louise Gilson, Katherine Wormeley, the Woolsey Sisters, Annie Wittenmyer, and Mary Ann Bickerdyke.

The first nurses on the Confederate side had also been recuperating male soldiers. In the South, there were no government-sanctioned standard qualifications or formal training for nurses. Prior to the war, nursing of family members was considered a woman's duty; therefore Southern women were already accustomed to caring for ill patients. Throughout the war, most women depended on past experience and natural talent to care for the wounded soldiers. Confederate hospitals were generally established in any available buildings such as private homes, churches, donated structures, and even barns. Unlike the requirements imposed on Union nurses by Dix, there were no age restrictions for Southern nurses. Duties were much the same as for Union nurses, however, although supplies and medicines in sufficient quantities were often lacking. In addition, when fighting drew near a medical facility, nurses often evacuated patients to safer locations and frequently became frontline nurses.

Notable Confederate nurses were Fanny Beers, Kate Cumming, Ella K. Newsom, and Sally Louisa Tompkins. Tompkins equipped her Richmond home as a 22-bed infirmary and was the only woman to hold a commission as a captain in the Confederate cavalry.

Orders of Catholic Sisters also participated in caring for sick and wounded soldiers on both sides during Civil War. At the outbreak of the war, the Catholic sisters were among the few organized and trained nurses. By the end of the war, more than 280 sisters had nursed both Union and Confederate soldiers in 28 established hospitals, aboard steamships, and on battlefields. Called the "black caps" by the soldiers, they worked on the battlefields in full habits. Nine sisters are known to have died in service during the Civil War.

By the end of the Civil War, more than 20,000 women and 30,000 men had been involved with nursing and relief aid.

M. Lynn Barnes

Further Reading

Eggleston, Larry G. *Women in the Civil War.* Jefferson, NC: McFarland & Company, Inc., Publishers, 2003.

Garrison, Webb. *Amazing Women of the Civil War.* Nashville, TN: Rutledge Hill Press, 1999.

Oates, Louise. "Civil War Nurses." *The American Journal of Nursing* 28, 3 (March, 1928): 207–212.

Sanitary Commission, U.S.

The United States Sanitary Commission was the outgrowth of a meeting of representatives of various relief organizations and concerned citizens in New York City in April 1861. The meeting resulted in a petition to the U.S. government to establish a Sanitary Commission patterned on the British example for the aid of soldiers in the field. The U.S. War Department issued, and President Abraham Lincoln signed in June 1861, an official warrant establishing the U.S. Sanitary Commission, which quickly became the overarching organization that coordinated Union civilian relief efforts nationwide. Often considered a "women's organization," the commission was actually headed by men. Most prominent were its president, Reverend Henry W. Bellows, and general secretary, Frederick Law Olmsted.

The commission classified its activities in three categories and organized itself along those same lines. The first was preventive services. These entailed inspections of camps and hospitals for sanitary and health problems and the publication of pamphlets and tracts on medical and field sanitation issues. Because the civilian inspectors usually knew little about military medicine or field sanitation, the commission developed and published extensive checklists to guide inspections. Especially early in the war when officers, soldiers, and military doctors were learning their trades, such inspections produced significant results.

The commission considered its largest function to be general relief. This comprised collecting and distributing food, clothing, blankets, medicines, and other medical supplies for sick and wounded soldiers in both field hospitals near the armies and general hospitals in major Union cities. The commission gathered and sorted supplies from more than 1,000 chapters nationwide and shipped them to agents assigned to geographical districts that corresponded roughly with the Union armies.

The third category was special relief, the term for care provided soldiers outside the normal control of the army. This included assistance to soldiers going on or returning from leave or moving from facility to facility in the medical system. The commission operated soldiers' homes and lodges to provide these men food and shelter as they traveled. Additionally, the commission outfitted and ran special hospital ships and railroad cars for the transportation of sick and wounded.

Initially, the Sanitary Commission collected and distributed food and material primarily donated by individuals and families. However, as the war progressed and the need grew, the commission sought funds to purchase supplies. It instituted large and very popular fairs in major cities in the North to raise money. Direct contributions from businesses such as free or reduced train fares or discount printing costs made contributions go farther.

The Sanitary Commission dominated relief organizations in the North. It was also able to quash occasional efforts by subordinate relief groups trying to target their efforts exclusively on units from their home states. Only in the western theater where the U.S. Christian Commission had a considerable presence, did the Sanitary Commission have significant competition. The Christian Commission eventually limited its activities in the east to matters concerning the soldiers' religious well-being.

J. Boone Bartholomees

Further Reading

Newberry, J. S. *The U. S. Sanitary Commission in the Valley of the Mississippi, During the War of the Rebellion, 1861–1866.* Cleveland: Fairbanks, Benedict, 1871.

Wormeley, Katherine Prescott. *The Other Side of the War with the Army of the Potomac: Letters from the Headquarters of the United States Sanitary Commission During the Peninsular Campaign in Virginia in 1862.* Boston: Ticknor, 1889.

Sanitary Fairs

From the fall of 1863 through the spring of 1865, cities throughout the North experienced outpourings of patriotic fervor that led to a host of Sanitary Fairs to supplement the diminishing finances of the United States Sanitary Commission (USSC). The USSC had the mandate to care for wounded and sick soldiers. Volunteers organized Sanitary Fairs to help finance the Sanitary Commission.

The brainchild of Chicagoans Mary Livermore and Jane Hoge, the first fundraising fair opened in their city on October 27, 1863 to widespread popular support. Aided by the region's various women's groups, businessmen, teachers, clergy, politicians, and farmers, the Chicago Sanitary Fair raised almost $100,000 in two weeks. Its success inspired other Northern women to organize similar events, beginning with the Western Sanitary Fair in Cincinnati, which raised triple the amount of the Chicago Fair.

Despite the enormous success of the sanitary fair movement, USSC leaders became alarmed at some of the unintended consequences of the mania. Some female branch leaders in New York and New England, for example, became concerned that many patriotic women were devoting their spare time to planning fairs while neglecting the more critical but mundane tasks of sewing shirts, knitting socks, and preparing jams and jellies for the troops. Their concerns became manifest as the USSC had to use sanitary fair proceeds to purchase clothing and supplies to replenish diminished stocks in their central supply depots. In addition, the extravagant publicity surrounding the sanitary fairs created an illusion among many women that an enriched USSC had no compelling need for their continued exertions for the troops. The USSC commissioners, all of whom were men, made an effort to exert some measure of control over the sanitary fair phenomenon. They threw their support behind the 1864 male-organized Metropolitan Fair in New York City, which proved to be the most successful fund-raiser of the war, netting more than one million dollars.

Despite the USSC's frequent misgivings about the sanitary fairs, they marked an important watershed in the history of women's involvement in national affairs. By organizing fairs on their own, women, rather than men, made the decisions about the nature of their contribution to the war effort, moving beyond the traditional domestic realm. The sanitary fairs for which records were kept netted a total of $4,393,980, an impressive sum for the middle of the nineteenth century.

Errol MacGregor Clauss

Further Reading

Attie, Jeanie. *Patriotic Toil: Northern Women and the American Civil War.* Ithaca, NY: Cornell University Press, 1998.

Giesberg, Judith. *Civil War Sisterhood: The U.S. Sanitary Commission and Women's Politics in Transition.* Boston: Northeastern University Press, 2006.

Tompkins, Sally Louisa (1833–1916)

Born on November 9, 1833, in Matthews County, Virginia, Sally Louisa Tompkins from an early age showed interest in nursing and aiding the sick. With the help of 10 surgeons and two cooks, she cared for more 1,300 sick and wounded soldiers from July 31, 1861 to June 13, 1865 at Richmond's Robertson Hospital. Tompkins's hospital was so successful that she obtained an honorary commission as a captain in the Confederate army from Confederate President Jefferson Davis. The president's action allowed Tompkins to keep her hospital open until war's end, long after other private hospitals had been taken over by the Confederate government. Of the 1,333 men treated at Robertson Hospital, only 73 died, a success rate of 94.5 percent, and a figure unequaled in any other Confederate hospital.

Tompkins never married, and after the war she depleted her remaining financial resources with various charitable works for Confederate veterans. She died in Richmond, Virginia on July 25, 1916.

E. Susan Barber

Further Reading

Holtzman, Robert S. "Sally Tompkins, Captain, Confederate Army." *American Mercury*: 127–130.

Massey, Mary Elizabeth. *Women in the Civil War.* Lincoln: University of Nebraska Press, 1994.

Western Sanitary Commission

Numerous charitable and relief organizations arose in both North and South during the war. These charities came about as civilians sought to care for soldiers and as the dramatic expansion of the size of the military outstripped the government's attempts to provide adequate supplies and medical care. While the United States

Sanitary Commission (USSC) was organized in the East in June 1861, the need for a corresponding organization in the West was met by the Western Sanitary Commission (WSC). The WSC supplemented military efforts by providing food, supplies, and medical care to soldiers.

The WSC was formally established on September 10, 1861 by Major General John C. Frémont's Special Order No. 159 in response to a request by Reverend William Greenleaf Eliot. The organization was headquartered in St. Louis. James E. Yeatman served as its president and, together with Reverend Eliot and three other members comprised its executive committee.

The WSC provided soldiers with food, clothing, and other essentials that supplemented what they had received from the army. It also provided medical supplies, established and managed hospitals, and appointed nurses. The WSC raised money to provide these supplies and services through individual donations and charity events. It also solicited civilians to become volunteer workers. The WSC developed floating hospitals to serve on the Mississippi River and secured government permission to transport supplies by river and by rail, which allowed it to operate in a wide area. The WSC also maintained careful records of patients and of places of burial, allowing family members a better chance of locating the soldiers they sought.

While its primary mission was caring for Union soldiers, the WSC was also active in aiding former slaves and even sought to improve conditions for Confederate prisoners of war. The work of the WSC was thoroughly appreciated by soldiers and commended by many notable Union commanders in the western theater. However, its relationship with the USSC was acrimonious. The USSC had sought jurisdiction over the WSC, but this effort failed and the two agencies continued to function independently in their respective theaters for the duration of the war.

Joshua Michael

Further Reading

Forman, Jacob Gilbert. *The Western Sanitary Commission: A Sketch*. St. Louis, MO: R. P. Studley, 1864.

Parrish, William E. "The Western Sanitary Commission." *Civil War History* 36 (1990): 17–35.

Wittenmyer, Annie Turner (1827–1900)

Sarah Ann Turner was born on August 26, 1827, in Sandy Springs, Ohio. In 1847, she married merchant William Wittenmyer and three years later moved to Keokuk, Iowa. In March 1853, Wittenmyer began her life of charitable work, founding the first tuition-free school for underprivileged children. William died in 1860, leaving Annie a single mother.

When the Civil War began, Wittenmyer joined the Union war effort as a nurse. The unsanitary conditions, inadequate food, and psychological turmoil the soldiers suffered horrified her. In 1861 the Keokuk Ladies' Soldiers' Aid Society (KLSAS) elected Wittenmyer its corresponding secretary. In that capacity she visited the hospitals in her region to determine their needs, gathered and distributed supplies, secured transportation for the wounded, and helped organize a coalition of women's groups.

Wittenmyer's work was often impeded by the Iowa branch of the United States Sanitary Commission (USSC), run by local men with connections to state politicians. To circumvent these problems, Wittenmyer eventually accepted a salaried position as one of the Iowa State sanitary agents. Once the state legislature approved her position in September 1862, she and the KLSAS gained official status. As a sanitary agent, she continued collecting and distributing food, medicine, bandages, clothing, and beds.

Wittenmyer gained nationwide fame through her establishment of more than 100 Special Diet Kitchens in Union army hospitals. She worked to reorganize kitchens so that each patient would receive individualized doctor-prescribed menus, suitable for that patient's condition. Wittenmyer's model helped save countless lives as the wounded and ill began receiving healthier, more nutritious, and better tasting food. At her request, the United States Christian Commission agreed to help fund and organize these kitchens. Wittenmyer hired the staff, appointed managers, and supervised the 200 paid women working in the kitchens.

Wittenmyer had other concerns as well. She began organizing orphanages in Iowa for Union soldiers' children in the fall of 1863, with the first one opening in 1864. In 1865 she applied to Congress for barracks in Davenport, Iowa, where the Iowa Soldiers' Orphans' Home was built later that year.

Wittenmyer is perhaps best known as the founder and first president of the Women's Christian Temperance Union, organized in 1874. In 1889 she moved to Pennsylvania and was elected president of the Woman's Relief Work of the Grand Army of the Republic, a national organization dedicated to helping former Union hospital workers obtain homes and pensions. She helped ensure the passage of the Army Nurses Pension Law in 1892.

Wittenmyer died on February 2, 1900 in Sanatoga, Pennsylvania.

Paula Katherine Hinton

Further Reading

Holland, Mary Gardner. *Our Army Nurses: Stories from Women in the Civil War.* Roseville, MN: Edinborough Press, 1998.

Schultz, Jane E. *Women at the Front: Hospital Workers in Civil War America.* Chapel Hill: University of North Carolina Press, 2004.

DOCUMENTS

Mary Loughborough: Letter about Visiting Casualties of the Battle of Shiloh

Mary Ann Webster Loughborough, the 27-year-old wife of Confederate Major James M. Loughborough, and her two-year-old daughter had left their home in St. Louis to follow her husband's army, eventually coming to Vicksburg, Mississippi. There she endured the 1863 Union siege and life in one of the hastily-dug caves where civilians took refuge from the continuous shelling. She kept a diary of her experiences under siege, which she published in 1864 as My Cave Life in Vicksburg. *Appended to her account are her contemporary letters. This letter, written after the Confederate army had retreated following its defeat at the Battle of Shiloh (April 6–7, 1862) to Corinth, Mississippi, details her hospital visits. It emphasizes the grievous wounds and illnesses endured by the combatants. The Confederate army suffered terribly in Corinth as thousands of soldiers camped in a confined area and suffered from poor sanitation that led to the rapid spread of diseases such as dysentery.*

The expected battle has not yet come off, and I am still awaiting the result; busying myself about many things, visiting and returning visits from my old friends; dividing my time between the world and the hospital, the lights and shades of life. Ah, the shades! My dear J——, you can little imagine how much suffering I have witnessed in the last few weeks—how much, that acts or kind words have no power to mitigate. There have been many wounded brought in from Corinth, many who have died since their arrival, many who will die; but, saddest of all, a young boy, too young to be a soldier, yet possessing all a soldier's spirit. I walked into a ward, one morning, that I had visited the evening before—a ward of very sick patients— and saw an old man sitting by a new cot, fanning a young boy, who lay with flushed face, and burning eyes fixed on the ceiling. As I advanced toward them, the weather- bronzed man stood stiffly erect, making me a quaint, half-awkward, military salute, saying, as he did so, "My boy, ma'am!" "Is he wounded?" I asked. He threw back the sheet that covered him, pointed to the stump of a limb amputated near the thigh: "He has gained the cross," he said, while his head grew more erect, as he held back the sheet with the fan, and his eye shot out the grim ghost of a smile.

A proud, iron soldier the man was, I could see. The boy was delirious; so I shall tell you of the man. Refusing to be seated as long as a lady remained standing in the room, he stood stiffly upright at the head of the cot, keeping each fly from the face of the boy with the tenderness of a mother. A limp brown hat was on the side of his head, shading his eyes, that followed me in all parts of the room. A red cord and tassel hung from one side of his hat, and gave him a jaunty air that was quite out of keeping with the quaint stiffness of his manner. After speaking to the sick and wounded soldiers around, asking after their wounds and wants, I returned to the young boy's cot, and heard the old man's story. Don't be weary if I give it to you; he had so much pride in his boy, let that be my extenuation.

"We belong to the Texas Rangers, ma'am, the boy and me; he could ride as well as the rest of them, ma'am, a year ago. When the war broke out, and we practised regularly like, he was the best rider in the company—could pick anything he wanted off the ground as he was going. He's only fourteen, ma'am—a fine-grown lad, indeed. His mother was the likeliest woman I ever seed," with a deprecating bow to me; "he's got her eyes—the finest eyes God ever made, she had, ma'am. She died when quite young like, leaving him to me, a little shaver, and he's been by me ever since. The boys and me tried to overpersuade him out of the army; 'peared like he was too young for such business; but he wouldn't hear to it, not he, ma'am, and here he is," passing his sleeve across his eyes.

"Well, ma'am, so he staid with us; and when we got to Corinth, General Beauregard offered a cross of honor to the ones that showed themselves the best soldiers. So our boys talked a heap about who'd get it; but this boy says nothing. Well, one day we were ordered out to scout, and we came up with the Yankees, and we fit 'em a half hour or so, when I seed this youngster by my side kind adrooping by a tree, but standing his ground. Well, we routed them at last, when I found the boy's leg was all shattered, and he'd kept up like nothing wan't the matter. So when we went back to Corinth, it got noised about like from the soldiers to the officers—how he'd held out. And, more'n all, the time when his leg was being cut off, we couldn't get any chloroform, morphine, or the like: he just sit up like a brave lad, and off it went, without a word out of him. So the doctors they talked of that; and he's been notified that he'll get the first cross, and the boys'll be monstrous fond of him, and feel most like they'd got it themselves. If he'd get rid of his fever and pick up like, I'd be a happy man," he said anxiously. Pardon me do I tire you; but let me take you to visit the sick prisoners. The old man that we pass in the hall, with his arm and leg in a frame, will never recover; yet he does not know it, and frequently asks me if I think he will get a pension when he is well, if he loses his leg and arm. He persists in keeping his face covered with a handkerchief, raising it up and peeping out, if he hears my voice, each day, with his usual salutation: "You've come, have ye?" If I bring any little article of food that I think the patients will relish, this old man must be fed by me, and I am frequently amused at the directions he gives me, for he is extremely practical and particular: "Now, if you will turn the spoon a little to one side, I will turn my mouth in this direction, and the custard will pass safely in." Poor man, without a friend, both arms badly wounded, and leg shattered, dying by degrees, yet to the last the handkerchief would be raised, and the cheery welcome greet me, "Ye're come, have ye?"

I think I can see you looking around in this ward to learn which are the prisoners, for all seem cheerful and talkative. In this cot by the door, with a wounded limb in a frame—like a huge lion—lies a man, large whiskered, large bodied, and long limbed, yet with a pleasant smile of greeting as we enter and make our inquiries after his wound. He is "better this morning, thank you," or, "I am obliged to you, not quite so well." A little picture on the table by his side, of a child three years of age, is never closed. A little child, blue eyed, with bare white neck, and plump round arms, showing the mother's wish that the picture should be fair and lovely to the father's eye. The Federal flag is on the cover. The man, a captain, is of an Illinois company. The child and mother, with tearful eyes and wistful hearts, look over the wide expanse of land and water that separates, over the cruel bounds that man has set—still faithful in their love. Still watching, and hoping, for the time when liberty will be his, and he, constant and true, will return to them. He tells me the name of the little one, with a sorrowful look at me with his dark eye. If he is free, if he ever sees these words, he will remember how the little one was gazed on by a lady in deep mourning, to whose heart a child of three years brought a sad and tearful memory. Come to the next cot with me; do not shrink from this blackened brow. Yesterday this was a noble-faced, gray-haired, old Confederate soldier, with the plaintive, lovely smile of perfect resignation. He suffers much from a wound in his body; seldom talks, yet always smiles gratefully for the slightest attention. This morning I find the erysipelas has broken out, spreading over his forehead and a part of his face. He cautions me, with the same pleasant, resigned smile, about coming near him, lest I take the disease. The blackened skin is from the effect of iodine to stay its progress. He will not live: dear, patient old man, my heart aches for him, yet I can give him nothing but kind words.

This morning I brought the men in this ward toast. The old man slept, and I gave to each his portion. Engaged in talking to a prisoner in another part of the room, I heard the Illinoisian say: "Let me divide this toast with you; I do not need it all." I turned, and heard the old man reply: "Oh, no; you keep it." I procured his toast and brought it to him, laughingly telling the prisoner I believed I saw the dawn of the millennium.

Do you not wish, dear J——, that the dawning was indeed with us; that brave and noble men should no more suffer, bleed, and die, but live; and in their lives grow more thankful and worthy of the Divine blood that has been shed for the removal of the fearful suffering and warfare that is all around us?

Pardon me for the length of time I have detained you, and remember me as ever, dear J——,

Yours.

Source: Mary Ann Webster Loughborough, *My Cave Life in Vicksburg*. Little Rock: Kellog Printing, 1882, pp. 159–165.

Charles A. Humphreys: *Field, Camp, Hospital and Prison in the Civil War, 1863–1865*

Charles Alfred Humphreys was born in Massachusetts in 1838. After completing his bachelor's degree he went on to the Harvard Divinity College and was ordained on July 14, 1863. He then applied for and was accepted as chaplain of the newly formed Second Massachusetts Cavalry. Part of a chaplain's duty was to visit the sick and wounded. In 1864, Humphreys resolved to perform a more onerous service by driving from camp in northern Virginia to the battlefields in a thickly wooded area of Virginia known as the Wilderness. Beginning on May 5, 1864, the Union Army of the Potomac had fought a series of intense and costly battles in and around the Wilderness. During the three-day Battle of the Wilderness the army suffered about 18,000 casualties. Because the Union army continued to advance after this battle and engage in new, and even bloodier actions, it left in its wake uncounted numbers of hurt soldiers. In the following excerpt, Humphreys relates his experiences as he tries to locate wounded soldiers and transport them to the hospital.

We had entered that region of gloom to carry away any of our own wounded whom it might be possible to move. Word had reached Washington through some of our men, who had so far recovered as to be able to walk to our lines, that there were three hundred of our wounded men in a field hospital at Locust Grove in the Wilderness, and Colonel Lowell was ordered to take seven hundred men and fifty four-horse ambulances, and try to bring them away.

I was delighted to be able to assure this one of Bartlett's brave followers, now wounded beyond cure and still lying on the field of the Wilderness, that his loved commander was doing well. I took the names of all these patients, and such messages as they wished to send to their homes, and with unutterable regret that we could not transport them to Washington, we left them to the kindly though unskilled nursing that the place afforded.

While we were halting thus at Parker's Store, a detachment had pushed on six or eight miles further to Locust Grove, but found that most of the wounded had been removed to Orange Court House three days before. At this we were greatly disappointed, for we could easily have brought off two hundred. Still, as there were some left. Colonel Lowell took ten ambulances — sending the rest for safety back over the ford — and we found at Locust Grove forty-six of our men who, we thought, could safely be moved. Their wounds were all very bad, and the ride was to be very long — more than fifty miles, — yet they were all ready to take the risk and perfectly delighted at the prospect of getting among friends. There were two who were dying, and whom, of course, we would not move; yet even they longed to go, that at least they might close their eyes for the last time among friends. One of these, before he had been told that he could not go, although he was already so weak that he could not turn on his couch, asked me to take his haversack from under his pillow, that he might have some provision for the journey. But he had no need of food on the journey that his soul would speedily take, nor would he taste again the bread of earth till it was transformed into the bread of the immortal life. We hastily loaded the rest into the ambulances, all except three for whom there was no room. But their prayers to be taken along were so piteous that I begged Colonel Lowell to let me see that they were carried on stretchers to the ford where were the rest of the ambulances. He gave me a detail of forty-eight men, and I had twenty-four dismount at a time, the others leading the riderless horses, and I put eight at each stretcher, four to carry and four to rest alternately. In this way we carried them twelve miles between five and eleven o'clock. It was very hard work, as the road was exceedingly rough. I took hold myself a part of the time; and though I was very much exhausted, with lack of food and sleep, and with the peculiarly trying labors of the day, in the excitement of the occasion I felt very strong, and often carried alone one end of a stretcher with its precious but heavy load of suffering loyalty. To add to the difficulties of our weary tramp, towards evening it began to rain, and by nine o'clock it was so dark we could not see a yard before us, and we stumbled over every slightest obstacle. We reached the ford and the rest of the ambulances a little after eleven; but it was not safe to cross in the darkness, so we lay down on the wet ground till half-past three o'clock, when we fed horses and started again. This crossing of the Rappahannock was the hardest place in the whole journey for the wounded. All were now provided with room enough in the ambulances; but in descending the steep bank to the river, one ambulance was upset, throwing out three wounded men and breaking again the limbs which had first been broken by bullets. Like true soldiers these sufferers looked upon the bright side even of this calamity, and found some comfort in thinking that their limbs had been poorly set and would in any event have had to be broken again.

Then the crossing of the river was very rough. It seemed at times as if the large round stones in the bed of the river would upset the wagons into the water. In one of the ambulances a horse had given out, and we had supplied his place with a mule, but as the team entered the water the two animals — from incompatibility of temper — refused to pull together. The mule especially sulked, and seemed disposed to shift the burden upon his more aristocratic companion. So, procuring a long pole and putting a little pointed persuasion into the end of it, I managed by persistent punching, to induce the mule to draw at least his half, and at last we were out of the water. But in climbing the bank, the wheels got stuck in the mud, and then the horse refused to pull — showing how catching is depravity. In this complication I had ten men dismount, and what with pulling at the tongue and pushing at the back and tugging at the wheels and lashing the horse and punching the mule, the ambulance was finally drawn up the bank. But the sufferings of the wounded during these wrenchings and joltings of the wagon were simply indescribable.

We found a camping-ground about four miles from the river and halted for breakfast. We had concentrated beef-tea for the sick, and heated three large iron kettles full of it, and thickened it with soft bread. The patients had had nothing to eat for twenty-four hours, and it was a great refreshment to them.

I will not stop to give in detail the rest of the journey. Suffice it to say that only one of the wounded men succumbed to the dreadful fatigues. The rest reached Washington in safety. As we approached our camp late on the second night of our journey, I galloped ahead of the column, and waked up the band, and had them play a "welcome home" for the command as it came in. The joy of the wounded captives whom we had rescued may be imagined but cannot be described when they heard once more the inspiring strains of "The Star Spangled Banner" and "Hail, Columbia." For were they not also heroes who "fought and bled in freedom's cause," and did they not deserve the trumpet's "All Hail!" and do they not still deserve a nation's grateful remembrance.

Source: Charles A. Humphreys. *Field, Camp, Hospital and Prison in the Civil War, 1863–1865.* Boston: George H. Ellis Co., 1918, pp. 51, 54–58.

Inspection Report on Fort Delaware

About 195,000 Union soldiers entered Southern prisons. Over 30,000 died while in captivity, a mortality rate of 15.5 percent. In contrast, some 215,000 Confederates entered Union captivity. Almost 26,000 died in prison, a mortality rate of about 12 percent. This death rate stemmed from overcrowded conditions that triggered the outbreak of diseases. Fort Delaware Prison was one of the worst northern prisons. The prison commander, General Albin Schoepf, was a brutal man known among the inmates as "General Terror." The fort was located on low, marshy ground making sewage disposal difficult. The prison featured numerous outbreaks of communicable diseases. An estimated 4,000 men died while being held at Fort Delaware. The Gettysburg Campaign yielded thousands of additional Confederate prisoners. Overcrowded conditions at Fort Delaware grew worse. On August 26, 1863, the Federal officer in charge of prisoners ordered Surgeon Charles H. Crane to embark on a round of inspections of northern prisons. Crane's mandate was to examine the condition of the sick and wounded and to assess whether medical officers were adhering to regulations when caring for the prisoners. His grim findings are presented in the following excerpt.

Col. WILLIAM HOFFMAN,

Commissary. General of Prisoners, Washington, D.C.:

There are 8,000 prisoners of war at this point, and they have been much crowded together, sick and well, in the same barracks, which it has been impossible to keep clean. The opening of a new hospital at this post which contains 600 beds will improve the condition of affairs very much, and the separation of the sick will improve their sanitary condition immensely. . . . I do not consider Fort Delaware a desirable location, in a sanitary point of view, for a large depot of prisoners. The ground is wet and marshy and the locality favorable for the development of malarious diseases. There have been many deaths at this place from typhoid fever, the result of their being crowded together in large numbers in a confined space.

C. H. CRANE.

Source: U.S. War Department, *War of the Rebellion: A Compilation of the Official Records of the Union and Confederate Armies,* Ser. II, Vol. VI.

■ CHAPTER 5

Indian Wars and the Spanish-American War

INTRODUCTION

The end of the Civil War brought a rapid demobilization of the U.S. military. Accordingly, the Army Medical Department went from 204 general hospitals in 1865 to none in 1866. In 1865 there were 12,343 medical officers; at the lowest point in 1866, there were just 213. For American military surgeons, the medical care of large numbers of men engaged in organized campaigns changed to looking after small groups engaged in guerrilla warfare against Indians. The Medical Department under William Hammond and Jonathan Letterman had made huge improvements by the end of the Civil War. Their organized system of ambulance transport, triage, and stepwise movement of the sick and wounded through field, general, and specialty hospitals had made it possible to manage large numbers of casualties and had measurably improved outcomes. That system, however, was not at all suited to an army of 25,000 scattered among 134 posts, the largest of which had 700 men, with more than one-third of the posts having fewer than 60 men. Skills necessary to treat casualties from set-piece battles fought by thousands of men using rifles and artillery were not helpful in treating frostbite, malnutrition, and the occasional arrow wound seen on the western frontier.

Living conditions for soldiers stationed on the western frontier were generally abysmal. Most forts were either adobe or simple wooden structures with dirt floors and no plumbing or heat. Water was brought in barrels from the nearest stream or well, and there was virtually none available for bathing. During the winter when bathing in streams became impractical, the odor of bunk rooms was usually overwhelming. Privies were so-called earth closets, and the incidence of fecally transmitted disease was a major factor in a sick rate that regularly exceeded ten percent. Vermin were a constant problem until washable sheets, wire spring mattresses, and bed frames became available in the 1880s. Facilities for providing medical care were little better than the barracks.

The rate of venereal disease in the army hovered around 70 per 1,000, although some posts were much worse. Admissions for alcoholism were around 30 per 1,000. Malaria remained a significant problem. Three grains of quinine along with an ounce of whiskey were a standard addition to reveille each morning. In the 1870s, sanitation was the responsibility of camp commanders, who generally had little knowledge of and less interest in the subject. By the mid-1880s a new understanding of infectious disease and its transmission pushed responsibility for camp sanitation more into the hands of the medical officers, and regular post sanitary reports were required after 1885. A report that year emphasizing the importance of contaminated water in typhoid transmission resulted in a 50 percent decrease in the incidence of typhoid in the camps.

The Indian Wars effectively ended at Wounded Knee on December 29, 1890. The period between 1865, the end of the Civil War, and 1890 witnessed tremendous advances in both general and military medicine. Military medicine went from a practice dominated by toxic drugs (compounds containing mercury and arsenic in particular) and amputation to an understanding of the nature and cause of infection and application of that understanding to the practice of surgery and sanitation.

A key development came in 1871, the year Lord Joseph Lister published his experience using phenol as an antiseptic during surgical procedures. Robert Koch in his 1878 *Study of the Etiology of Wound Infection* described six different microorganisms that could cause specific types of infection. By the 1880s some American military surgeons were operating under clouds of phenol, although many of their more traditional colleagues refused to change. In 1885 the antiseptic method was used in 42 of 170 American military operations; the following year the percentage increased to 60 of 108. Understanding and acceptance of the importance of infection in American military medicine and surgery culminated in the 1893 appointment of bacteriologist George Sternberg as Surgeon General. Although sanitation would again be a problem with the widespread mobilization incident to the Spanish-American War, the U.S. Army Medical Department was poised to assume a role at the forefront of research and management of infectious disease.

In spite of intellectual advances, the U.S. Army Medical Department was unprepared when the Spanish-American War began in 1898. Just four years earlier, Congress had stripped 15 commissioned surgeons and the entire allotment of contract surgeons from a corps that had consistently and justifiably complained that it was incapable of meeting even peacetime requirements. The Medical Department's organizational structure was antiquated. Each regiment had its own surgeons and each division its own hospital. All were under a corps-level chief surgeon. Physicians had an advisory role only over matters directly pertaining to medical care of patients. Hospital administration and evacuation of the wounded

were the province of line officers. Even worse, line officers selected camp locations and arrangement with little regard to camp sanitation.

The Medical Department was led by Surgeon General George Sternberg, an
internationally renowned bacteriologist with almost no administrative experience.
Besides a severe shortage of physicians, he had no nurses, which left hospital care
to an undermanned, untrained, and largely unmotivated collection of stewards
assigned to the Hospital Corps. The Medical Department had no transportation resources of its own, being entirely dependent on the Quartermaster Corps. Although
war was a near certainty after the February 15, 1898, sinking of the U.S. battleship
Maine at Havana, Sternberg was legally barred from spending any more money to
stockpile supplies than had already been budgeted for 1898. He had barely sufficient equipment, hospital supplies, and medicines on hand to take care of the
27,000-man prewar force. The March 9, 1898, Fifty Million Dollar Bill intended
to fund the war allocated only $20,000 to the Medical Department. Even when
purchases were authorized after the declaration of war in April, supplies and drugs
were almost entirely unavailable on such short notice.

After Congress authorized purchases, supply depots were established at Lytle,
Georgia, and at Tampa, Florida. But because of the difficulty in buying what was
needed and transporting it, nothing arrived in either place for more than a month.
When the trains finally started coming in, the system was overwhelmed. Freight
was seldom labeled, and one complete field hospital was found only after the
war had ended. Still, to their great credit, Sternberg and his staff found and distributed 272,000 first-aid packets, 7,500,000 quinine pills, 18,185 cots, 23,950 blankets, and 2,259 litters in 1898.

The rapid expansion of the military brought thousands of regulars and volunteers to training camps in the southern United States to acclimate the men to a
hot, damp climate. Typhoid soon afflicted the crowded camps, striking particularly
hard at the volunteer units whose men routinely ignored basic sanitation practices.
More than 90 percent of the volunteer regiments had typhoid within eight weeks of
arriving in camp, and not a single regiment escaped the disease. In the end, far
more men died in camp than in battle, and 80 percent of those succumbed to what
was likely typhoid, although the disease was often confused with malaria. The
Medical Corps had initially planned for one percent of the volunteer force to
require hospitalization while in camp. Once reality set in, a network of military
hospitals had to be created.

When the war began, nursing care was provided by the 791 noncommissioned
officers and privates of the Hospital Corps since the Medical Corps had no female
nurses. It proved much more difficult to get volunteers for the Hospital Corps than
for line regiments, a deficit that was often made up by forced transfer of unwilling
soldiers. To help alleviate the problem, Congress authorized the hiring of female
nurses on contract. In August 1898, the Army Nurse Corps Division of the

Surgeon General's Office was formed and placed under Dr. Anita Newcombe McGee, who was made an acting assistant surgeon. A total of 1,563 women were hired, with a maximum of 1,158 serving at any one time, but since the first American nursing school had only been founded 25 years earlier, the supply of trained nurses was quite limited.

American forces invaded Cuba on June 22, 1898. As American troops moved inland, a series combats occurred that taxed the medical service. A field hospital at Siboney treated the wounded from the battles on the San Juan Heights and El Caney. That facility had an adequate supply of surgical instruments and dressings and was able to keep six operating tables working around the clock. Soldiers in the field had a good supply of first-aid packs and splints, and most of the men—who were transported to Siboney on a short-haul railroad pressed into service for that purpose—were well splinted and well dressed. A combination of antisepsis, anesthesia, and relatively clean wounds from the high-velocity Spanish Mauser rifles resulted in cleaner injuries and better surgical results than in prior wars. Of the 1,142 men wounded in the Battle of San Juan Hill and the Battle of El Caney, the War Department reported a mortality of less than 1 percent. The Surgeon General's Report for 1898, however, said that 1,457 men were injured by guns that year, with a mortality rate of 6 percent. Regardless, the death rate from gunshot wounds was strikingly lower than in prior wars.

Although the number of battle injuries was relatively low and the complications less frequent than in earlier wars, disease was a major problem. By mid-July, an army corps at the forefront of the fighting reported 1,500 men sick with fever, and 10 percent of those had yellow fever. The death rate from disease peaked at 6.14 per 1,000 in August 1898, with malaria being the most common problem and yellow fever the most feared.

As many as 75 percent of the American force in Cuba may have ultimately suffered from malaria, with typhoid, dysentery, and other diarrheal diseases also common. Overall, in 1898, there were 217,072 cases of disease or injury among the men serving in the U.S. Army. The rate of men reporting for sick call was an astounding. On average, each soldier reported sick more than twice each year. Battle wounds were numerically almost insignificant. In fact, significantly more men were disabled by rupture (the contemporary term for cases of inguinal hernia) than by gunshot wounds. Disease, however, became such a problem that in late July the city of Siboney was burned to the ground as a sanitary measure.

One immediate effect of the outbreak of disease was the Round-Robin Letter in which senior American officers demanded the immediate return of the American force to the United States. Because there was a widespread fear that returning soldiers would bring yellow fever with them, the decision had been made to build what was in essence a quarantine facility at Camp Wikoff on eastern Long Island. The Round-Robin Letter led to a hurried transfer of troops to Camp

Wikoff in spite of the fact that transport ships were disastrously underequipped and the camp not nearly finished.

There were a handful of military medical innovations attributable to the Spanish-American War. Difficulty in identifying dead and seriously wounded men led to the use of metal identification tags subsequently worn by all soldiers. X-rays were used both in hospitals in the United States and on hospital ships to locate metallic foreign bodies and to visualize fractures. But the biggest changes came as a result of the postwar investigation of shortcomings in medical care led by Major General Grenville Dodge. The Dodge Commission's report recommended a major increase in the number of commissioned medical officers, the establishment of a volunteer hospital corps, and a permanent corps of trained nurses. It also recommended maintenance of a stockpile of medical stores sufficient to supply an army four times as large as that maintained in peacetime and a separate transport service dedicated to medical needs. Virtually all of the commission's recommendations were adopted, and the changes in the Medical Department formed the basis of its preparation for the larger wars to come.

The Spanish-American War is generally recognized as one of the last conflicts involving modern Western armies in which casualties from sickness and disease outnumbered those related to accidents and combat. Mortality from battle wounds in Cuba was 4.1 percent of those wounded as compared to 17.5 percent in the Civil War. Much of that improvement came from the use of aseptic surgical techniques and the fact that unlike in the earlier conflict, the vast majority of extremity injuries were treated without amputation.

The rate of death and disability from disease was a more dismal story. The ratio of death from disease to that from battle-related wounds in the Cuban phase of the Spanish-American War was 7.4:1 as compared to 2:1 in the Civil War. The majority of the disease-related deaths occurred in training camps before the men were ever deployed. Most of the disease in the camps was related to inadequate sanitation.

In sum, medical care during the Spanish-American represents a transition from a deeply ignorant tradition-based approach toward a more scientific approach. Doctors better understood the pathology of wounds and developed new procedures for antiseptic surgery.

Jack McCallum

ENTRIES

American National Red Cross

The American National Red Cross was founded on May 21, 1881, by Clara Barton. Its goal was to offer humanitarian assistance in the event of war or natural disasters. Organized into state chapters with numerous subchapters, the American

National Red Cross (ANRC) offered relief to the victims of floods, hurricanes, tornadoes, and rail disasters across the United States prior to the Spanish-American War.

During her 23-year stewardship of the organization, Barton exercised a tight grip on the ANRC's activities, frequently alienating its middle-class and wealthy patrons who sought greater roles in its administration. Exercising full right of veto over all requests for assistance, which she reviewed personally, Barton often left the national headquarters in Washington to direct relief efforts on-site, frequently acting at cross-purposes to the actual need and local capabilities. Hence, the ANRC was occasionally criticized as being poorly run and subject to the whims of its founder.

Even before the Spanish-American War, the ANRC was active in Cuban relief efforts, with Barton herself visiting Havana in 1897 and again in early 1898. There, beginning on February 9, 1898, she personally oversaw relief for victims of the Spanish regime's policies in Cuba. She also took an active role in revealing the extent of Spanish abuses, accompanying numerous American visitors on tours of the bleak and squalid *reconcentrado* (reconcentration) camps. These visits served a dual purpose: they highlighted Spanish indifference to the plight of civilians and the charitable impulse of Americans toward the war's unfortunate victims.

In late March 1898, Barton returned to the United States, where on April 1 she chartered a freighter, the *State of Texas*, in Key West, Florida. As war appeared imminent, she hurriedly arranged for 1,400 tons of food, clothing, and supplies to be loaded on the ship for one final delivery of humanitarian supplies to Cuba before war broke out. Events overtook her efforts, however. The *State of Texas* was ordered by the U.S. Navy to remain in port, as Rear Admiral William T. Sampson's North Atlantic Squadron instituted the blockade of Cuba on April 22, 1898.

With the official outbreak of hostilities between the United States and Spain on April 21, 1898, the flaws in Barton's personal administration style became readily apparent. ANRC efforts to mount a wartime relief program were hamstrung by its leader's absence and the overall lack of structure in the organization. While Barton remained with the *State of Texas* in Key West, ANRC representatives in Washington were struggling to gain recognition and permission from the War Department to work in the military volunteer camps scattered throughout the United States. Accordingly, and without clear direction at its head, the ANRC's response drifted aimlessly, with individual members and chapters taking the initiative and acting without coordination. Across the country, local relief committees raised money, gathered supplies, and provided support to volunteer militia and National Guard units as they departed for their mustering camps. The range of support from local ANRC chapters was varied and included collecting reading material and tobacco products, outfitting special-diet kitchens and laundry facilities for regimental and brigade hospitals, and purchasing field surgical kits for volunteer regiments.

Compounding the problems of disorganization was the appropriation of the ANRC's name and insignia by various independent and temporary relief groups. Many of these organizations ultimately competed with the ANRC for support from local philanthropists and volunteers. Without strong leadership at the helm in Washington, the ANRC was helpless to act against its competitors. As a result, the general public came to see the ANRC's response to the war as fragmented and chaotic.

The chief obstacle to direct coordination between the ANRC and the U.S. War Department was Surgeon General George Miller Sternberg. Mindful of Barton's tendency toward meddling and interfering with army physicians during the Civil War, Sternberg was willing to accept any supplies and material support donated by the group. He was far less charitable toward the prospect of ANRC volunteers in camp hospitals, however, where he believed that they would cause more harm than good.

The typhoid fever epidemic forced Sternberg to revise this position. Following a July 16 interview with representatives of the ANRC Committee on Maintenance of Trained Nurses, he agreed to allow ANRC female nurses to serve in general hospitals in the United States, Cuba, and the Philippines. ANRC nurses, however, never gained the full access that Sternberg had accorded to the volunteer nurses under the direction of Anita Newcomb McGee.

Meanwhile, on June 25, 1898, the *State of Texas* finally departed Key West for the V Corps beachheads at Daiquirí and Siboney, Cuba. In fact, Barton and her supplies arrived in the immediate aftermath of the Battle of Las Guásimas. On July 1, after the battles at El Caney and San Juan Heights, V Corps commander Major General William Shafter sent a request to Barton for all essential medical supplies. Barton then commandeered two army wagons, loaded them with supplies, and personally delivered the material to the front. After two weeks in hospitals caring for American and Spanish wounded, Barton and her delegation traveled throughout V Corps offering supplies and assistance to sick soldiers as needed. After the August truce, she turned her attention toward civilian-relief, offering clothing and food to the poor and opening several relief hospitals in Havana.

Despite, or perhaps because of, Barton's efforts in Cuba away from the ANRC's headquarters in Washington, several members began to agitate for her retirement after the war. During the next four years, a group opposed to Barton's stewardship coalesced around the efforts of Cleveland socialite Mabel L. Boardman. The struggle for leadership continued until 1904, when Barton finally resigned in the face of growing opposition. A year later the ANRC was reorganized, and a new charter was granted to the organization by the U.S. Congress.

Bob Wintermute

Further Reading

Barton, Clara. *The American National Red Cross*. Washington, D.C.: American National Red Cross, 1898.

Dulles, Foster Rhea. *The American Red Cross: A History*. New York: Harper and Brothers, 1950.

Gillett, Mary C. *The Army Medical Department, 1865–1917*. Washington, D.C.: Center of Military History, United States Army, 1995.

Dodge Commission

The Dodge Commission was named after its chairman, former U.S. Army major general and former Republican congressman from Iowa Grenville Mellen Dodge. First convened on September 26, 1898, the Dodge Commission ended its assignment on February 9, 1899. Its findings were published in an eight-volume report.

At the conclusion of hostilities with Spain, President William McKinley called upon Dodge to head a commission to investigate charges of mismanagement and incompetence leveled against the U.S. Army and Secretary of War Russell A. Alger. Dodge, a loyal and influential Republican, organized a committee composed of 12 members, all of whom were Civil War veterans.

During its inquiry, the Dodge Commission requested comprehensive reports from the U.S. Army's adjutant general, quartermaster general, commissary general, surgeon general, chief of engineers, and chief of ordnance. It investigated 10 specific areas. Among these were the amount and kind of camp and garrison equipment on hand at the start of the war; the arming and equipping of the volunteer regiments in the various camps; the quantity, quality, and kind of food furnished; the number of tents, beds, linens, medicines, and other necessaries for hospitals; the efficiency of the medical staff; and the conditions and operations of both the Engineer Department and the Ordnance Department.

The Dodge Commission's most important investigative focus was directed at hygiene and public health in the army camps. Of the 274,000 officers and men who served in the war, 5,462 had died in theaters of operation and camps in the United States. Yet, only 379 of those deaths were battle-related. The commission heard testimony from 495 witnesses and visited most of the encampments. It also conducted interviews with soldiers and officers in several locales around the country. Based on a report submitted by Majors Walter Reed, Edward Shakespeare, and Victor C. Vaughan, who examined the incidence of typhoid fever in army encampments, the commission found that the Army Medical Department was understaffed and not properly organized to meet the demands of a modern war. It also pointed out that the Medical Department had failed to investigate the sanitation conditions in the camps, had too few nurses available and discounted their valuable service, and had to rely on an ineffective Quartermaster Corps for the distribution of medical supplies and equipment.

The Dodge Commission's findings produced numerous recommendations that included an increase in the number of medical officers, the establishment of a nursing reserve component, and the securing of a sufficient amount of medical supplies equivalent to the army four times its present strength. The commission also recommended that the Medical Department take charge of the delivery of supplies.

Despite some criticism that the Commission was a rubber stamp and partisan cover-up for the shortcomings of the McKinley administration, it examined every aspect of the U.S. Army's and War Department's actions. No formal charges were brought against either, although McKinley did request Alger's resignation in 1899. Many of the Dodge Commission's recommendations regarding military hygiene and medical treatment were implemented within a few years. Military officer training manuals were also rewritten to ensure that line officers developed a sense of responsibility for the overall health of their command. Also, curriculum in hygiene and public health was implemented at the United States Military Academy at West Point and other military training schools. Thus, the Dodge Commission is credited with establishing new policies governing hygiene and medicine within the U.S. military.

By far the most controversial topic with which the committee dealt was the Embalmed Beef Scandal. During his testimony to the Dodge Commission, Major General Nelson A. Miles, commanding general of the army, pointedly accused Brigadier General Charles Patrick Eagan, who was the commissary general during the war, of providing U.S. troops with substandard canned beef that most soldiers despised because of its poor taste. Miles also accused the commissary general and U.S. meatpacking companies of experimenting with unknown chemical preservatives that had resulted in sickness among many who had consumed the beef. Eagan denied the allegations and lashed out at Miles publicly, an action that brought a court-martial, conviction, and reduction in rank. In the end, the Dodge Commission concluded that while much of the meat fed to U.S. soldiers may indeed have tasted terrible, it was not defective and had not caused the widespread sickness claimed by Miles and others.

Charles F. Howlett

Further Reading

Bollet, Alfred J. "Military Medicine in the Spanish-American War." *Perspectives in Biology and Medicine* 48(2) (Spring 2005): 293–300.

Cirillo, Vincent J. *Bullets and Bacilli: The Spanish-American War and Military Medicine.* New Brunswick, NJ: Rutgers University Press, 2004.

Cosmas, Graham A. *An Army for Empire: The United States Army in the Spanish-American War.* College Station: Texas A&M University Press, 1994.

Hirshon, Stanley P. *Grenville M. Dodge: Soldier, Politician, Railroad Pioneer.* Bloomington: University of Indiana Press, 1967.

Dysentery

Dysentery is an inflammatory disease of the bowel characterized by fever, abdominal pain, and bloody or purulent diarrhea and most often caused by *Escherichia coli (E. coli)*, *Shigella*, *Salmonella*, or *Campylobacter* species. Because these organisms are usually transmitted by water or food contaminated with human feces as a result of poor sanitation, dysentery regularly marches with armies.

During the American Civil War, dysentery and other diarrheal diseases were the most common causes of hospitalization, accounting for 1,585,236 admissions and 44,448 deaths in the Union Army alone. By comparison, the North lost 110,070 to battle injuries, a situation that led directly to formation of the U.S. Sanitary Commission.

Dysentery was once again a prominent factor in the Spanish-American War, where the death rate in training camps in the United States significantly exceeded the death rate on Cuban battlefields.

In the 1894 Sino-Japanese War, Japan suffered 12,052 cases of dysentery and almost 50,000 other cases of infectious disease in an army of 200,000. The impact on military effectiveness precipitated drastic reform of the Imperial Army Medical Corps so that, in the Russo-Japanese War a decade later, out of a total force of 600,000 only 10,565 infectious illnesses occurred, and the death rate was only 1.2 percent. This was the first time a major military force had so effectively lowered disease rate with an organized sanitary program, and it served as a model for armies for the rest of the 20th century.

In 1910, U.S. Army Major Carl Rogers Darnall showed that water could be purified by anhydrous chlorine. Five years later, Major William Lyster developed the "Lyster bag," which effectively chlorinated water with sodium hypochlorite contained in cloth. In World War I, Sir Almroth Wright's typhoid vaccine finally controlled that disease but did nothing to prevent the other forms of dysentery. Dysentery became easier to control after World War II due to the development of broad-spectrum antibiotics generally effective against diarrhea-causing bacteria.

Recently, antibiotic-resistant strains of *E. coli*, Shigella, nontyphoid Salmonella, and Campylobacter have emerged among U.S. troops in Southeast Asia. During Operation Desert Shield, 57 percent of American troops stationed in Saudi Arabia had suffered at least one bout of diarrhea within two months of deployment, and the majority of organisms isolated from those patients were strains of *E. coli* and Shigella that were resistant to available antibiotics.

Jack McCallum

Further Reading

Bayne-Jones, S. *The Evolution of Preventive Medicine in the Unites States Army: 1607–1939*. Washington, D.C.: Office of the Surgeon General, Department of the Army, 1968.

Hyams, K. C., A. I. Bargeris, and B. R. Merrill. 1991. "Diarrheal Diseases during Operation Desert Storm." *New England Journal of Medicine* 325 (May 16): 1423–1428.

Lim, M. L., G. S. Murphy, M. Calloway, and D. Tribble. 2005. "History of U.S. Military Contributions to the Study of Diarrheal Diseases." *Military Medicine* 170: 30–38.

Lim, Matthew, and M. R. Wallace. 2004. "Infectious Diarrhea in History." *Infectious Disease Clinics of North America* 18: 261–274.

Embalmed Beef Scandal

An acrimonious U.S. Army procurement scandal arose from the Spanish-American War of 1898 in which hundreds of tons of meat sent to feed U.S. troops were thought to have been tainted. Major General Nelson A. Miles touched off the Embalmed Beef Scandal during his testimony to the presidential-appointed Dodge Commission on December 21, 1898. While defending his military decisions in Puerto Rico, Miles attacked the Commissary Department and, indirectly, the William McKinley administration with accusations that chemically tainted meat had been deliberately issued to the troops and that this had resulted in many illnesses and deaths. Miles's accusations centered on 337 tons of refrigerated beef and 198,508 pounds of canned beef sent to Cuba and Puerto Rico during the war. He contended that the refrigerated rations were so unpalatable that the men refused to eat them. He also claimed that the canned beef was not much better. To meet the low prices of competitive bidding, contractors often used waste and offal from other packing processes for the army rations. Miles claimed that when this meat was consumed, often disguised in stews, the results were diarrhea, dysentery, and even death. Many believed that the Commissary Department and its civilian contractors were experimenting with chemical preservatives, including boric acid, salicylic acid, and nitrate potash, which gave the refrigerated meat an embalmed smell and appearance.

Many important military and political leaders responded to these charges, which quickly became a national sensation. Major General Wesley Merritt, who commanded the Philippines expedition, denied any incidence of bad beef under his authority. Not surprisingly, the meatpacking industry also denied any wrongdoing. Retired army major general Grenville Dodge, head of the presidential commission, found no concrete evidence of chemical tainting and concluded that Miles was attacking McKinley in an effort to become the next Democratic Party presidential nominee.

Commissary General Charles P. Eagan attacked Miles with considerable vehemence, accusing him of lying, deceit, and political chicanery. So harsh were Eagan's condemnations, in fact, that a military court later found him guilty of conduct unbecoming of an officer. Secretary of War Russell A. Alger, himself the object of scrutiny during the scandal, attempted to bring charges against Miles

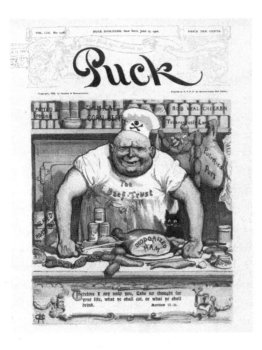

The Embalmed Beef Scandal provoked a number of satirical cartoons. This cartoon shows a butcher labeled "The Beef Trust" standing behind a counter in a butcher shop, surrounded by meat products labeled Potted Poison, Chemical Corn Beef, Bob Veal Chicken, Tuberculosis Lard, Decayed Roast Beef, Deodorized Ham, Embalmed Sausages, and Putrefied Pork. A verse from the Bible appears below the counter: "Therefore I say unto you, Take no thought for your life, what ye shall eat, or what ye shall drink." Matthew VI:25. (Library of Congress)

for issuing unauthorized press releases. Almost all the participants in this scandal suffered significant damage to their reputations and careers.

In the end, neither the Dodge Commission nor the Miles Court of Inquiry could prove that the refrigerated beef was tainted, but they did conclude that the canned beef was of inferior quality. Congress released the two-volume *Record of Court of Inquiry* on March 30, 1900. But the political infighting and issues of dishonesty haunted the scandal's primary participants for much longer. Elihu Root ultimately replaced Alger as secretary of war, and Miles entered into a lengthy battle about military reform with the new secretary. The dissension over military reform eventually damaged both the army organization and Miles, who retired in disgrace.

For its part, the meatpacking industry suffered even more scrutiny, and writer-journalist Upton Sinclair mentioned the Embalmed Beef Scandal in his muckraking exposé *The Jungle*, published in 1906. Sinclair's book revived the charges of unhealthy and unsanitary conditions in America's meatpacking industry (which was centered principally in Chicago) and prodded the Roosevelt administration into action. Indeed, Roosevelt, who had read Sinclair's book and was still convinced that the meat rations during the war had been tainted, pushed Congress into passing legislation to regulate more closely meatpacking and other food industries. The result was the Pure Food and Drug Act of 1906 and the Meat Inspection Act of 1906, two of the first significant pieces of legislation of the incipient Progressive era. Their passage is often attributed, at least in part, to the president's experiences with Spanish-American War meat rations.

Dawn Ottevaere

Further Reading

Grivetti, Louis. "Food in American History, Part 6—Beef: Reconstruction and Growth into the Twentieth Century." *Nutrition Today* 39 (May–June 2004): 128–138.

Keuchel, Edward. "Chemicals and Meat: The Embalmed Beef Scandal." *Bulletin of the History of Medicine* 98 (Summer 1974): 65–89.

Miller, Everett B. "Veterinary Medical Service of the Army in the Spanish-American War, 1898 (with Notes on the 'Embalmed Beef' Scandal)." Paper presented in part before American Veterinary History Association, July 20, 1987. Reprinted in Veterinary Heritage (February 1988): 14–38.

Roosevelt, Theodore. *The Letters of Theodore Roosevelt. Edited by Elting E. Morison.* 8 vols. Cambridge: Harvard University Press, 1951.

Sinclair, Upton. *The Jungle.* 1906; reprint, New York: Longman, 1998.

Wooster, Robert. *Nelson A. Miles and the Twilight of the Frontier Army.* Lincoln: University of Nebraska Press, 1993.

Gorgas, William Crawford

Born on October 3, 1854, in Mobile, Alabama, William Crawford Gorgas was the son of the former Confederate chief of ordnance and grandson of a former governor of Alabama. He was raised on the family plantation near Mobile and, unable to obtain an appointment to West Point, decided to join the Army Medical Corps after obtaining a medical degree from Bellevue Medical College in New York. In the 1880s, while stationed at Fort Brown, Texas, he met Marie Doughty, his future wife, while they were both recovering from yellow fever. Because he was subsequently immune to the disease, Gorgas spent much of the next two decades in posts where yellow fever was common. In 1898, during the Spanish-American War, he was sent to Cuba to be the director of sanitation.

Working under Brigadier General Leonard Wood, who was both a physician and Cuba's military governor, Gorgas applied the research done by Walter Reed's Yellow Fever Commission into a coordinated effort to rid Cuba of mosquitoes. The resultant mosquito control program, which included draconian punishments for leaving standing water, virtually eradicated yellow fever and dramatically reduced the incidence of malaria within less than three years. Since the legs of hospital beds were placed in flat dishes filled with water to keep crawling bugs from getting onto patients, Gorgas treated the water and placed screens around patients to keep the disease from spreading.

In 1904, the United States acquired the rights to the Panamanian isthmus and bought the equipment left by the French after their failed effort to dig a canal. Realizing that the death rate among workers from yellow fever and malaria had been a major factor in the French failure, the army sent Gorgas to take charge of sanitation in the Canal Zone. Unfortunately, the Canal Commission and Colonel George Goethals were unwilling to spend any money on improving sanitary conditions and controlling mosquito breeding. An outbreak of yellow fever in late 1904, however, convinced the Canal Commission to fund Gorgas's attempts at mosquito control. Because of insufficient funding, it was not until late 1905 that yellow fever and malaria were eradicated in the Panama Canal Zone. Following President Theodore Roosevelt's visit to the Panama Canal Zone, Gorgas was made a member of the Canal Commission. Determined to see the completion of the Panama Canal, he refused an offer in 1911 to become president of the University of Alabama. He was the only U.S. official who remained on the canal project from the beginning to end.

In 1914, Gorgas was promoted to brigadier general and named surgeon general of the United States, an office he held through World War I. He is credited with having made the medical corps more efficient and with standardizing medical evaluation of new recruits.

Retiring from the army in 1918, Gorgas accepted an offer from the Rockefeller Foundation to travel to South America to advise on the eradication of yellow fever and malaria. He also served as president of the American Medical Association and the American Society of Tropical Disease. Gorgas died in London on July 4, 1920, shortly after suffering a stroke. Following a large funeral in St. Paul's Cathedral, his body was returned to the United States and buried in Arlington National Cemetery.

Michael R. Hall and Jack McCallum

Further Reading

Gibson, John M. *Physician to the World: The Life of General William C. Gorgas*. Durham, NC: Duke University Press, 1989.

Gorgas, Marie Cook. *William Crawford Gorgas: His Life and Work*. Garden City, NY: Doubleday, 1935.

Gorgas, William Crawford. *Conquest of Malaria: The Views of Surgeon-General Gorgas*. N.p.: Argus, 1914.

Hospital Corps

Because the first women's nursing school in the United States was not established until 1873, there was no supply of female hospital nurses, and in 1898, the corps was entirely male. The Hospital Corps was divided into three classes; steward, acting steward, and private. In time of war, the Hospital Corps was charged with providing patient care in military hospitals and with operating the military ambulance service.

Each regiment had four litter bearers. After serving for a year and passing an examination, these men could be promoted into the Hospital Corps. A private in the Hospital Corps, after serving a year and passing another examination, could be promoted to acting steward. Initial rules called for another year of service and yet another examination for promotion to steward. However, personnel shortages during the Spanish-American War led to a reduction in the service requirement to three months. The minimal pay differential between the Hospital Corps and line regiments coupled with physically demanding work and the risk of infection led to the corps being quite unpopular and chronically understaffed.

As of May 1, 1898, the Hospital Corps comprised 99 hospital stewards, 100 acting stewards, and 592 privates, but these men served in the regular army and thus did not address the needs of the rapid volunteer expansion. The April, 1898 act of Congress that established the volunteer force authorized 1 steward for each regular army battalion, 25 hospital privates for each regiment, and an additional 50 privates for each division. These men were, however, attached to the line units, and no formal Hospital Corps was authorized for the new volunteer units. Even those National Guard units that already had Hospital Corps were forced to disband them. As a result, regimental nursing was regularly done by men who had neither training nor enthusiasm for their jobs. Most had been assigned to hospital duty because they were either poor soldiers or were physically unable to function as combat soldiers.

The obvious deficiency led to a change in the law allowing transfer of 25 men from each regiment and an additional 50 men from each division to a hospital corps. In spite of the change, the hospital nursing in the volunteer units remained inadequate. Line commanders often simply refused to give up men to the Hospital Corps. Those who did get posted were of wildly variable ability. At the top end were men who had been pharmacists, medical students, and even practicing physicians in civilian life. At the bottom were otherwise worthless men who had been detailed from units that did not want them. A course in hospital nursing had been developed at Washington Barracks, but the rapid expansion of the volunteer force left no time for training new corpsmen. Most were simply given the *Handbook for the Hospital Corps* and trained on the job.

By June, the Hospital Corps numbered 133 stewards, 172 acting stewards, and 2,940 privates, and by November, the Corps had grown to more than 6,000. However, the greatest improvement in hospital care came as a result of Surgeon General George Sternberg's authorization to contract with 1,700 female nurses. After the war, the Dodge Commission recommended retention of a permanent Hospital Corps for volunteer units to be supplemented by a reserve corps of trained female nurses.

Jack McCallum

Further Reading

Ashburn, P. M. *A History of the Medical Department of the United States Army.* Boston: Houghton Mifflin, 1929.

Gillett, Mary C. *The Army Medical Department, 1865–1917.* Washington, D.C.: Center of Military History, United States Army, 1995.

Maass, Clara Louise

Born in East Orange, New Jersey, on June 28, 1876, Clara Louise Maass was the oldest of 10 children in a devout Lutheran German immigrant family. She helped in an orphanage during her high school years and at the age of 17 entered the newly established Christina Trefz Training School for Nurses at Newark's German Hospital. She graduated in 1895, and her competence earned her a promotion to head nurse only two years later.

On the outbreak of the Spanish-American War in April 1898, Maass volunteered to serve as a contract nurse for the U.S. Army. From October 1898 to February 1899, she served with VII Corps in Jacksonville, Florida; Savannah, Georgia; and Santiago, Cuba. After her discharge, she joined VIII Corps in the Philippines, which was battling Filipino insurgents in the Philippine-American War (1899–1902). She remained in the Philippines until mid-1900, when she was sent home after having contracted dengue fever, a serious disease of the tropics transmitted by infected mosquitoes.

The wars in which she had served had given Maass considerable expertise in fighting malaria, yellow fever, and other tropical diseases. In October 1900, she returned to the Las Animas Hospital in Havana, Cuba, at the request of Major William Gorgas, chief sanitation officer, and Dr. John Guitares. The U.S. Army's Yellow Fever Board (also known as the Reed Commission), headed by Major Walter Reed, an army physician, had been established in Cuba after the war to find out the means of transmission for this tropical fever and develop effective immunization against it.

In order to determine whether yellow fever was caused by contaminated filth, person-to-person transmission, or the bite of a mosquito, the commission recruited volunteers to test their theories. They were paid $100 for risking their lives, with an offer of an additional $100 if they became ill. In March 1901, experiments revealed that men living in filth without exposure to mosquitoes were not infected with yellow fever. Next, seven volunteers offered themselves to be bitten by infected mosquitoes. One of them was Maass, who contracted a mild case of the fever and recovered quickly; however, two men who volunteered died. Because the other volunteers remained healthy, however, researchers were not sure whether the mosquitoes were truly the carriers of the disease.

On August 14, 1901, Maass volunteered for a second mosquito bite, hoping to prove that her earlier case of yellow fever had immunized her against the disease. This time, however, she became severely ill. She died of yellow fever on August 24, 1901, at the age of 25 and was buried in Colón Cemetery in Havana with full military honors. Her death confirmed the theory of transmission by mosquitoes, but public protest put an end to further experiments on humans. Maass's death also seemed to prove that the body did not produce sufficient antibodies to ward off further infections of yellow fever. In fact, the original illness was almost certainly not yellow fever, and Maass was not immune. Several years later, vaccines would be developed to build the body's defenses against infection.

In 1952, Newark's German Hospital was renamed Clara Maass Memorial Hospital (now located in Belleville, New Jersey) in her honor, and she was inducted into the American Nursing Association's Nursing Hall of Fame in 1976.

Katja Wuestenbecker

Further Reading

Cunningham, John T. *Clara Maass: A Nurse, a Hospital, a Spirit.* Belleville, NJ: Rae, 1968.

Herrmann, E. K. "Clara Louise Maass: Heroine or Martyr of Public Health?" *Public Health Nursing* 2(1) (1985): 51–57.

Samson, J. "A Nurse Who Gave Her Life So That Others Could Live." *Imprint* 37 (1990): 81–89.

Tengbom, Mildred. *No Greater Love: The Gripping Story of Nurse Clara Maass.* St. Louis, MO: Concordia, 1978.

Native American Medicine

Native American medicine was (and continues to be) a system of professional practices based on the native concept of health and wellness. Health is seen as a proper balance among the physical, psychological, and spiritual states of the individual as well as personal harmony with the surrounding natural environment. This system predates and is quite similar to the concept of homeostasis that is currently gaining popularity in modern medicine. Native Americans see the natural world as having a significant spiritual nature, and the medicine of Native American culture reflects this concept.

As in Western medicine, Indian medical practice is based on observations of the progression of illness and is strongly rooted in cause and effect. The profession was and still is practiced by specialists who are trained in their medical system of specialized procedures, particular (natural) medicines, and specific rituals. The practitioners fulfill this specialized role in their culture after extensive training and internship with an established healer.

In Native American culture, good health is the result of an individual maintaining a proper balance of his or her own physical, psychological, and spiritual natures. The belief is that a deficiency in any of these aspects can cause illness to the individual. The goal of the medical professional is to restore the person to a proper balance. Therefore, the healer must treat the physical problems as well as perform procedures to address the emotional and spiritual imbalances observed in the patient. It is important to note that the spiritual aspect often involves the group as well as the individual. Thus, medical procedures will often include members of the patient's extended family, acquaintances, and even the entire band or

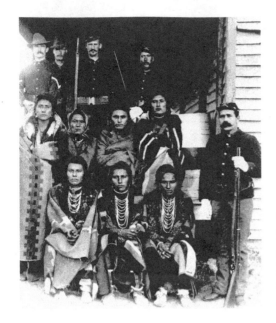

Compared to the more urbanized east, there was a shortage of medical services and facilities on the western frontier. Eight Crow prisoners under guard at the Crow agency in Montana in 1887. (National Archives)

tribe. When balance within the individual is restored, the patient becomes well again.

A Native American healer has knowledge of medical procedures, medicines, and ceremonies. He or she is trained in the use of specific physical procedures to remove objects and toxins from the body, reset bones, relieve stress, and realign muscles and other biological systems. The healer collects, prepares, and administers a large number of naturally occurring plant, fungi, and animal substances (medicines). These medicines are believed to be effective in treating the specific physical symptoms presented by the patient.

Most Native Americans believe that the natural world is directly influenced by spirits of both beneficence and harm; therefore, the effects of these spirits are important in their cultures' practice of medicine. The healers are trained in specific ceremonies that are designed to enhance the effect of beneficial spirits as well as to mitigate the actions of harmful spirits. The healer observes the patient, diagnoses the particular problem, and treats the illness with a particular combination of procedures, medicines, and ceremonies specific to the patient's illness. The healers believe that they are part of a continuum of healing forces in the harmony of nature. Their actions perform a coordinating role in balancing the significant physical, emotional, and spiritual aspects within the patient.

Over the centuries, Native American medicine has been shown to be quite effective in the treatment of numerous illnesses. Western medicine has observed Native American practices over time and has often concluded that many procedures and medicines are useful, and Native American and Western healers continue to exchange knowledge to the benefit of both systems. This was particularly true during the 18th and 19th centuries. Today Native American healers are frequently important partners with Western doctors, particularly in areas with significant Native American populations.

Lawrence E. Swesey

Further Reading

Bonvillain, Nancy. *Native American Medicine.* Philadelphia: Chelsea House, 1997.

Kavasch, Barrie, and Karen Baar. *American Indian Healing Arts: Herbs, Rituals and Remedies for Every Season of Life.* New York: Bantam Books, 1999.

Reed, Walter

Walter Reed was born on September 13, 1851, in Belroi, Virginia. His father, a Methodist minister, encouraged him to enroll at the University of Virginia, where he earned an MD degree in 1869. At the time, he was the youngest person to earn such a degree at the university. He earned a second medical degree from Bellevue Hospital Medical College in 1870. On June 26, 1875, he was appointed as an assistant surgeon in the U.S. Army Medical Corps with the rank of first lieutenant. His first assignment was Fort Lowell, Arizona. In 1880, after serving at various posts in the West, he was promoted to captain and transferred to Fort McHenry, Maryland. During the early 1880s, he attended lectures at Johns Hopkins University in Baltimore. He also studied bacteriology and pathology under the guidance of William Henry Welch, the foremost bacteriologist in the United States. In 1893, after being promoted to major, Reed was appointed professor of bacteriology at the U.S. Army Medical School.

Alarmed by the number of U.S. deaths caused by yellow fever during the Spanish-American War, in May 1900 the U.S. Army appointed Reed to head the Yellow Fever Board in Cuba. Reed and his team, which included James Carroll in charge of bacteriology, Jesse Lazear in charge of experimental mosquitoes, and Aristides Agramonte in charge of pathology, arrived in Havana on June 25, 1900. Volunteers were infected with yellow fever, which allowed Reed to prove the hypothesis that mosquitoes caused the disease. He made his conclusions by October of that year. His tests were based on a theory first postulated by Cuban physician Carlos Juan Finlay in 1881 that identified mosquitoes as the carriers of yellow fever. Until Reed had verified Finlay's hypothesis, it had been commonly held that yellow fever was contracted by contact with clothing and bedding soiled by the excrement and body fluids of yellow fever victims. Reed also conducted experiments to determine if survivors were immune to the disease from subsequent mosquito bites. These generated a great deal of controversy when nurse Clara Maass died of yellow fever on August 24, 1901.

As a result of Reed's efforts, Colonel William Crawford Gorgas, the U.S. Army's chief sanitary officer in Cuba, was able to virtually eliminate yellow fever from Cuba by destroying the mosquitoes' breeding grounds. In 1901, Reed returned to Washington, D.C., to resume his duties at the U.S. Army Medical School and George Washington University. Following an appendectomy, he died of peritonitis on November 23, 1902.

Reed's pioneering research stymied the mortality rates caused by yellow fever and facilitated the construction of the Panama Canal from 1904 to 1914. Although there is still no cure for the disease, a vaccine to protect against yellow fever was eventually developed in 1937. Opened in 1909, the Walter Reed General Hospital (Walter Reed Army Medical Center) in Washington, D.C., is named in his honor.

Michael R. Hall

Further Reading

Bean, William. *Walter Reed: A Biography.* Charlottesville: University of Virginia Press, 1982.

Pierce, John R., and James V. Writer. *Yellow Jack: How Yellow Fever Ravaged America and Walter Reed Discovered Its Deadly Secrets.* New York: Wiley, 2005.

Sternberg, George Miller

Born on June 8, 1838, at Hartwick Seminary in Orange County, New York, George Miller Sternberg graduated from the Columbia College of Physicians and Surgeons in 1860 and entered the Army Medical Department in 1861. He then held appointments as a battlefield and post surgeon and engaged in path-breaking medical research. He conducted exhaustive research into the pathology of yellow fever, a very serious public health threat at the time. He lectured extensively on his research and by the 1880s was recognized as one of the world's top bacteriologists. In consequence, he was appointed over several more-senior officers to the post of surgeon general on May 30, 1893, and was advanced in rank from lieutenant colonel to brigadier general.

Sternberg strongly advocated the new medicine rooted firmly in science. Over the years, he had witnessed firsthand the scourge of hospital gangrene, erysipelas (a potentially deadly communicable skin disease), and typhoid fever among soldiers at war and peace. Following early work on disinfectants, in 1880 he was the first researcher to identify the *pneumococcus* microbe that causes pneumonia and related diseases. Upon taking charge of the Army Medical Department in 1893, he opened the Army Medical School, one of the nation's first postgraduate medical schools, with a dual emphasis on military sanitation and hygiene and microbiology.

From the onset of the Spanish-American War, Sternberg sought to impose some order on the rapid mobilization of volunteers and the political rush for a speedy decision in Cuba. Both Sternberg and commanding General of the Army, Major General Nelson A. Miles, opposed an early invasion of Cuba, preferring to wait for the passing of the rainy season (April to September). Their reservations were overcome by the testimony of Cuban physician Juan M. Guiteras, who opined that careful sanitation preparation by an invading army would keep yellow fever and malaria infections at a minimum. Sternberg next pressed for careful sanitary guidelines with special regard to garbage, latrines, drinking water, and cleanliness in camps.

Despite his efforts to promote higher standards and readiness in the Medical Department, Sternberg remained stubbornly defiant on several issues, particularly on the subject of female nurses and physicians in military service. He outright refused to appoint female physicians as contract surgeons. Before the camp fever crisis exploded in September 1898, he also resisted calls to allow female nurses into the camps. Female nurses, he believed, would present a needless distraction in camp hospitals and were only capable of providing menial support. The typhoid epidemic caused him to reassess this view, and he then took a personal interest in building up a cadre of trained and uniformed female nurses to assist in the camps. Ultimately, 1,563 women were selected as contract nurses. Sternberg later gave full support to the permanent establishment of the female Army Nurse Corps on February 2, 1901.

The war revealed that Sternberg's chief failing as a department head came in organization. Reluctant to delegate authority, he spent long hours micromanaging supply shortages, interviewing volunteers for new positions, and making personal recommendations on the conduct of troops in the tropics. As reports of growing chaos reached his office, he issued new circulars to his medical officers. Pleading overwork, he failed to conduct personal inspections of the camps as the crisis unfolded, instead dispatching subordinates who had limited authority to intervene. By September 1898, Sternberg was moved to quick action in authorizing new hospital camps and routing supplies, food, and personnel where needed, but by then the worst was over.

Nevertheless, Sternberg claimed that the overall experience in the war was a triumph for his model of scientific-based medicine, despite the typhoid fever outbreaks. Comparing death rates from disease in the recent conflict with the first year of the American Civil War in 1861, he concluded that the mortality rate from disease during the war (May 1, 1898–April 30, 1899) was half than that of the first year of the earlier conflict. However credible Sternberg's efforts were to point out the successes of his department, the fact remained that in the midst of the much-heralded new scientific revolution in medicine, more than five times as many men died of disease than wounds.

In defending his Medical Department, Sternberg garnered criticism for shifting the blame to the volunteer establishment. Civilian physicians in volunteer service frequently owed their appointments to political favors rather than military necessity, he complained, and generally had little if any instruction in hygiene and sanitation. He also noted that the overwhelming preponderance of National Guard and volunteer militia officers had little respect for regimental surgeons. Hence, all essential hygiene recommendations—including those elaborated upon in three different circulars issued by his own office—were generally ignored.

Sternberg's influence on the postwar Medical Department, which he would direct until 1902, was greater than the sum of the criticism against him. His use of scientific medicine and leadership by example also dramatically affected the overall progress of medicine. In the midst of the camp fever crisis, he convened the Typhoid Fever Board, under the leadership of Majors Walter Reed, Edward Shakespeare, and Victor Vaughan. In 1900, Sternberg authorized the formation of the now-famous Yellow Fever Board under Reed's direction. Both boards brought about significant advances in the state of disease etiology and prevention by establishing beyond question the significance of mosquitoes as the vector of yellow fever and the presence of healthy carriers in typhoid fever and disproving once and for all the fomite theory of disease transmission in yellow fever.

Sternberg continued as surgeon general until he retired in June 1902. After his retirement, he lent his name to numerous humanitarian causes. Sternberg died in Washington, D.C., on November 3, 1915.

Bob A. Wintermute

Further Reading

Gillett, Mary C. *The Army Medical Department, 1865–1917*. Washington, D.C.: Center of Military History, United States Army, 1995.

Sternberg, George M. *Sanitary Lessons of the War and Other Papers*. New York: Arno, 1977.

Typhoid Board

The Typhoid Board was created by Surgeon General George Sternberg on August 18, 1898, to investigate the typhoid epidemic ravaging military training camps and recommend sanitary measures to alleviate the crisis. The commission comprised Major Walter Reed of the Army Medical Corps and Majors Victor C. Vaughan and Edward O. Shakespeare, both surgeons in the U.S. Volunteers.

The Department of the Army and the American public had been shocked at the morbidity and mortality from fevers in training camps late in the summer of 1898. Losses from febrile disease were greater even than those in the first year of the American Civil War, even though the fact that typhoid was bacterial in origin and that the exact organism responsible for the disease had recently become known.

Reed had been professor of bacteriology and clinical microscopy at the Army Medical School and was a recognized authority on typhoid. Shakespeare had studied the 1885 typhoid epidemic in Plymouth, Pennsylvania, and Vaughan was the founder of formal bacteriologic training in the United States. Between August 20 and September 30, 1898, the three visited every major military training camp in the United States and all of the secondary camps to which men had been moved to escape the disease. They then personally reviewed the sick reports of 107,973 officers and men who had become ill prior to leaving the United States. By the time the work was finished in June of 1900, Shakespeare had died, and Reed had been transferred to Havana, where he was in charge of the Yellow Fever Board.

The Typhoid Board suspected that the disease could be transmitted by asymptomatic carriers, although this would not be definitively demonstrated until 1907. They believed that the disease was transmitted by contaminated water and suspected (incorrectly) that flies played a major role in that spread. They decried the common diagnosis of typho-malarial fever since the serological Widal test could identify typhoid with certainty and since microscopic examination of the blood could do the same for malaria. The board insisted that every camp have a laboratory capable of making the differentiation. They also placed the blame for the epidemic squarely at the feet of line officers who refused to follow the sanitary recommendations of their medical officers. The board's two-volume *Report on the Origin and Spread of Typhoid Fever in U.S. Military Camps during the Spanish War of 1898* is still regarded as the most complete study of epidemic typhoid ever published.

Jack McCallum

Further Reading

Cirillo, Vincent J. *Bullets and Bacilli: The Spanish-American War and Military Medicine.* New Brunswick, NJ: Rutgers University Press, 2004.

Typhoid Fever

Typhoid fever is an enteric fever caused by *Salmonella typhi* (formerly *Bacillus typhosus*). The disease is characterized by fever, headache, abdominal pain, diarrhea, and a rose-colored rash sometimes followed by delirium, vascular collapse, and death. There are still 21 million cases of typhoid and 200,000 deaths each year, mostly in developing countries in Africa, Asia, and Latin America. Typhoid was one of the earliest diseases shown to be caused by a specific microorganism, having been cultured by Georg Gaff in 1884 only two years after his mentor Robert Koch elucidated his four postulates for proving infectious causation of an illness. In 1896, Felix Widal demonstrated that serum from a typhoid patient would cause clumping in broth cultures of the causative organism, giving physicians a reliable way to differentiate typhoid from other febrile illnesses. By the beginning of the Spanish-American War, military physicians had access to enough information about the disease that they should have been able to diagnose it accurately and should probably have been able to deploy effective means of prevention. They did neither, and typhoid was by far the major cause of death during the Spanish-American War.

The majority of typhoid cases occurred in training camps among volunteers who never left the United States and was the direct result of abysmal sanitation practices. Sixty thousand men—the number assigned to Camp George H. Thomas in Chickamauga Park, Georgia—produce 21,000 gallons of urine and 9.4 tons of feces a day. The dense clay around Camp Thomas could not begin to absorb that volume of waste. The sinks (latrines) quickly overflowed and emanated a nauseating stink. In addition, many of the recruits had come from cities and had no experience with outdoor sanitation. They deposited their waste directly on open ground and ignored pleas from medical officers to bury it. A person could not walk anywhere in the surrounding woods without tramping through piles of feces. With the arrival of heavy rains in July and August, the mess spread and was washed into streams that supplied the camp's water.

Camp Alger in Virginia had most of the same problems and, by early September 1898, the entire camp had to be abandoned and the men moved to Camp Meade in Pennsylvania. Camp Cuba Libre in Jacksonville had better soil but no better sanitation and a high water table, and it ultimately had to be abandoned as well.

Because typhoid was endemic in the late 19th-century United States, because the disease can reside in asymptomatic carriers, and because the War Department had opted to congregate its new volunteer regiments in a few camps, an outbreak was virtually inevitable. Typhoid in the camps was not a problem as long as the inhabitants had been members of the regular army, but the story changed when the volunteers came. Within three weeks of their arrival, 82 percent of the volunteer regiments had typhoid, and that number reached 90 percent after eight weeks. Eventually, the total number of cases reached 20,738, of whom 1,590 died (a 7.7 percent mortality rate). In retrospect, 86.8 percent of all deaths from disease during the Spanish-American War were probably from typhoid.

Responsibility for those deaths lies with both line officers and the medical corps. The regimental surgeons had no operational authority outside direct treatment of the sick and wounded. To the extent that they made recommendations on camp sanitation, those suggestions were generally ignored by officers who had little interest in and less understanding of infectious disease. The line officers almost universally viewed sanitary measures as a waste of time. The physicians, however, also contributed to the problem. Because many of them were ancillary to the volunteer regiments, their training and ability were far from uniform. Many had only a sketchy idea of how infectious diseases were transmitted, and a number of them were still unable to differentiate among various febrile illnesses, with the most obvious result being the widespread use of the diagnosis typho-malarial fever even though William Osler had discredited that diagnosis in 1896 and laboratory tests were readily available to separate the two. Thermometers had been available in the United States since 1866, but many physicians continued to diagnose fever by feeling the patient and had yet to make the connection between febrile illness and body temperature, much less the connection between the amount of temperature elevation and the severity of the disease and the risk of death.

Even the best of physicians in 1898 did not fully understand that typhoid was generally transmitted by contaminating food and water with infected feces. The least educated thought that the disease was transmitted by bad air. The better educated thought that it was primarily waterborne. Even the postwar Typhoid Board persisted in the belief that flies were the main culprit. In fact, most disease came from camp kitchens but not—as line officers and men suspected—from deteriorated food. The disease really came from cooks who failed to wash their hands, and it would be almost a decade before physicians learned that asymptomatic carriers were a primary source of typhoid epidemics.

If diagnosis was bad, treatment was nearly nonexistent. Calomel, strychnine, alcohol, and sedatives were all tried, but none were actually of any use. It was somewhat helpful to treat the fever since the rate of death approached 100 percent in those whose temperature surpassed 107 degrees. Aspirin and cold baths were used to that end but had minimal impact on overall mortality. Fortunately, the disease ran its course as the camps emptied. The incidence peaked in September and was virtually gone by December.

Distress over the unnecessary loss of life was, however, not gone by the end of 1898. Surgeon General George Sternberg had created a special commission—the Typhoid Board chaired by Major Walter Reed—in August 1898. The board personally inspected the camps and reviewed records of those who had suffered from the disease. Its work culminated in a two-volume report released in June 1900. Although the report mistakenly attributed typhoid's spread to flies, it firmly placed responsibility for the debacle on poor sanitation. The report placed the blame for the epidemic squarely at the feet of line officers who refused to follow the sanitary recommendations of their medical officers. The Spanish-American War was the last American conflict in which the loss of life from disease outweighed that from trauma.

Jack McCallum

Further Reading

Ashburn, Percy M. *A History of the Medical Department of the United States Army.* Boston: Houghton Mifflin, 1929.

Cirillo, Vincent J. *Bullets and Bacilli: The Spanish-American War and Military Medicine*. New Brunswick, NJ: Rutgers University Press, 2004.

Gillett, Mary C. *The Army Medical Department, 1865–1917*. Washington, D.C.: Center of Military History, United States Army, 1995.

Wood, Leonard

Born on October 9, 1860, in Winchester, New Hampshire, the son of a marginally trained and generally unsuccessful family doctor who died before his children reached adulthood, Leonard Wood was forced by finances to earn a living. Opting for medicine, he earned a degree from Harvard in 1884. He was accepted as an intern at Boston City Hospital but was fired for generally insubordinate behavior before completing his internship.

Wood joined the army as a contract surgeon in 1885 and participated in a protracted pursuit of Apache leader Geronimo through the mountains of southern Arizona and northern Mexico, for which he ultimately received the Medal of Honor. In 1890, Wood married Louise Conditt-Smith, ward of Supreme Court justice Stephen Field. Wood subsequently parlayed his wife's social connections to become a force in Washington politics.

Wood, along with his friend Theodore Roosevelt, encouraged President William McKinley to support war with Spain in 1898. Subsequently, the two friends recruited the 1st Volunteer Cavalry Regiment. Wood was colonel and commander, and Roosevelt was lieutenant colonel and second-in-command.

During the fighting in Cuba Wood rose to the rank of brigadier general. Shortly after the Spanish surrendered Santiago, he was made first military governor of the city and then of the province. He used his medical training to bring disease and starvation under control and proved an exceptional and exceptionally stern administrator. His success in Cuba coupled with his Washington ties and a talent for political machinations led to him being named military governor of Cuba in December 1899. As governor, he made notable strides in education, public health, and prison reform and established a fiscally responsible republican government. Perhaps his most notable accomplishment was his sponsorship of and acceptance of responsibility for Walter Reed's yellow fever experiments. Immediately after Reed demonstrated the mosquito's role as a vector for the disease, Wood used his autocratic power to authorize draconian insect control measures carried out by his chief surgeon, Major William Gorgas. The campaign transformed Havana from one of the most dangerous cities in the world to one of the healthiest.

Wood subsequently had a long and controversial military career culminating in promotion to chief of staff of the army in 1910. He died in Boston on August 7, 1927, during surgery to remove a benign brain tumor.

Jack McCallum

Further Reading

Hagedorn, Hermann. *Leonard Wood: A Biography.* 2 vols. New York: Harper and Brothers, 1931.

Lane, Jack. *Armed Progressive: General Leonard Wood.* San Rafael, CA: Presidio, 1978.

McCallum, Jack, *Leonard Wood: Rough Rider, Surgeon, and Architect of American Imperialism.* New York: New York University Press, 2006.

Yellow Fever

Yellow fever is a lethal systemic disease caused by a *Flavivirus* and transmitted by the bite of the female *Aedes aegyptii* mosquito. Yellow fever begins with a flulike illness and may progress to necrosis of the liver with subsequent diffuse internal and external bleeding, kidney failure, coma, and death. Mortality is still approximately 20 percent, and there is no effective treatment.

The *Aedes* mosquito is not native to the Western Hemisphere and was first introduced to Barbados in 1647 and to Cuba and the Yucatan in 1648 by ships carrying slaves from West Africa, where the disease is endemic. Although the mosquito requires ambient temperatures above the low 70s, yellow fever could be transmitted

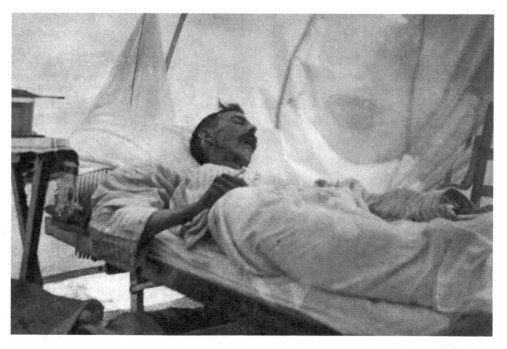

During the Spanish American War, diseases killed far more soldiers than Spanish bullets. Here a victim of yellow fever in hospital at Siboney, Cuba, July 1898. (National Library of Medicine)

to northern cities during the summer months, and epidemics were a recurrent event in American seaports. Yellow fever caused more than 100,000 deaths in the United States between 1793 and 1901, and the threat was so serious that Thomas Jefferson was of the opinion that the United States would never be able to support major cities.

Fear of a yellow fever epidemic among American soldiers sent to Cuba during the Spanish-American War, and the worry that they would bring the disease home with them, played a major role in both the planning and execution of the 1898 invasion of Cuba. The disease first appeared among American troops at Siboney on July 9, and by August 2 there had been 4,298 cases of fever in Santiago. In retrospect, most of these were probably not yellow fever, but military surgeons in Cuba lacked an accurate diagnostic test for the disease and were quick to call them that. The increasing incidence of fever and the fear of a generalized outbreak led Major General William Shafter's general officers and Colonel Theodore Roosevelt to write the Round-Robin Letter demanding an immediate withdrawal of American troops from the island.

It was generally assumed that yellow fever was caused by filth, a conviction that led the army to burn Siboney to the ground after the first outbreak. When the Spanish surrendered Santiago, one of the first actions by Brigadier General Leonard Wood as military governor was to institute a draconian public sanitation program. To his great disappointment, 200 new cases appeared in the city in the summer of 1899 with a 22.8 percent mortality rate. Wood was forced to quarantine the city to control the epidemic.

Beginning as early as the June 25 Battle of Las Guásimas, all American wounded were screened for signs of yellow fever before they were allowed to return to the United States. Anyone suspected of having the disease was held in Cuba. By May 22, every returning ship was inspected by the Marine Hospital Service, and anyone with fever was quarantined. Following the Round-Robin Letter, however, public opinion forced the War Department to remove the men from Cuba, and on August 7, ships began moving them to Camp Wikoff, on the eastern end of Long Island, where they could be held in quarantine until free of the risk of yellow fever.

Proof that the *Aedes aegyptii* was the yellow fever vector and that the disease could be controlled by removing mosquito-breeding areas did not come for another three years but did ultimately result in virtual eradication of the disease in Cuba. Yellow fever was not endemic in either Puerto Rico or the Philippines and was not a problem for the American military in either place.

Jack McCallum

Further Reading

Cirillo, Vincent J. *Bullets and Bacilli: The Spanish-American War and Military Medicine.* New Brunswick, NJ: Rutgers University Press, 2004.

Gillett, Mary C. *The Army Medical Department, 1865–1917.* Washington, D.C.: Center of Military History, United States Army, 1995.

Yellow Fever Board

The Yellow Fever Board consisted of four physicians appointed by Surgeon General George Sternberg on May 23, 1900, to study infectious disease in Cuba. The board, composed of Major Walter Reed and contract surgeons Jesse W. Lazear, Aristides Agramonte, and James Carroll and also known as the Reed Commission, was encouraged by Major Jefferson Keen, a military surgeon who had recently recovered from yellow fever, to concentrate on that disease.

Carroll, who had previously worked with Reed at the Army Medical School, was placed in charge of bacteriology. Lazear, who had trained in entomology with the Italian malaria expert Giovanni Battista Gussi, was eventually given charge of the group's mosquito experiments. Agramonte supervised autopsies and was the group's pathologist.

After a series of false starts, the Yellow Fever Board, as it came to be known, directed its attention to the *Stegomya fasciata* (later renamed *Aedes aegyptii*) mosquito that had been suggested as the disease's vector by Cuban physician Carlos Finlay in 1881. The board designed a remarkable series of controlled experiments that definitively proved not only that the disease was transmitted by the mosquito but also that it was caused by an infectious organism smaller than a bacterium and was therefore the first human infection shown to be viral in origin.

German scientist Robert Koch's postulates requiring passage of an identifiable agent through an experimental animal to prove responsibility for an infectious disease could not be satisfied because no laboratory animal was known to be susceptible to yellow fever. The board was therefore required to design its experiments using human subjects. Since yellow fever at the time had an approximately 30 percent mortality and since there was no treatment for the disease once it was contracted, any human experiment posed significant ethical difficulties. For that reason, the board elected to perform the first experiments on themselves. However, Agramonte was exempted because he had grown up in Cuba and was assumed to have contracted the disease as a child and to be immune. Reed opted out, arguing that at age 47 he was too old to participate safely. Carroll contracted the disease after allowing himself to be bitten by a mosquito that had fed on a yellow fever victim, and although he survived, his health was permanently impaired, and he died seven years later. Lazear also allowed himself to be bitten and did not survive. The board subsequently recruited a series of newly arrived Spanish immigrants and American soldiers as subjects. The ethical questions remained, and the board obtained a written permission—the first formal informed consent—from each potential experimental subject.

Carroll, Agramonte, and Reed—encouraged and funded by military governor Brigadier General Leonard Wood—designed experiments in which they first proved that exposure to clothing, bedding, vomitus, and feces from yellow fever victims did not cause the disease. Next, they divided a small house in half by a screen and placed infected mosquitoes on one side and none on the other with all other conditions being identical. Experimental subjects on the mosquito side contracted yellow fever, while those on the other side of the screen did not. Carroll went on to inject plasma from infected subjects that had been filtered through porcelain known to have small enough pores to capture all bacteria. The filtrate still caused the disease, proving that the responsible agent was smaller than a bacterium.

The results were inconvertible, and Wood promptly used them to justify a draconian anti-mosquito campaign supervised by Major William C. Gorgas. Within three months, yellow fever, which had plagued Havana for almost 400 years, had disappeared from the city. The Yellow Fever Board's defeat of yellow fever was unquestionably the Army Medical Department's greatest triumph during the Spanish-American War and may well have been the greatest achievement of the war altogether. The methods used in the experiments generated much controversy, however, especially after the death of nurse Clara Maass, who allowed herself to be reinfected after recovering from yellow fever in an effort to determine if prior exposure to the disease produced immunity.

Jack McCallum

Further Reading

Altman, Lawrence. *Who Goes First: The Story of Self-Experimentation in Medicine.* New York: Random House, 1987.

Cirillo, Vincent J. *Bullets and Bacilli: The Spanish-American War and Military Medicine.* New Brunswick, NJ.

DOCUMENTS

Valery Havard, Description of the Medical Corps in the Santiago Campaign

When U. S. forces landed in Cuba in 1898, medical science did not yet comprehend the nature of tropical diseases. During the Santiago campaign, about half of General Shafter's army fell ill with malaria, typhoid, and yellow fever. After the capture of Santiago the army's health continued to deteriorate. Seven senior officers, including Theodore Roosevelt, drafted a letter — known as the 'round-robin letter' — recommending the immediate evacuation of U.S. troops from Cuba. Its publication by the press embarrassed political and military leaders and influenced the decision to recall many of the disease-ravaged American forces from Cuba to Montauk Point, Long Island. Here the Army had established an isolated detention camp where those who suffered from tropical diseases received better care. The Cuban experience motivated the Medical Corps to begin a project to determine the cause of yellow fever. It marked the beginning of a long-term trend toward a forward-looking, modern military medical service. The following account was written by an army medical corps officer who served as Chief Surgeon for the American forces in Cuba. It relates the incidence and treatment of sickness in Cuba and the army's response to the Reed Commission's findings on the role of mosquitos in disease transmission.

The number of fever cases continued to increase in the entire command. A careful examination at this time led to the conclusion that from ten to twenty percent (perhaps less) of the sick were yellow fever in the infantry divisions, and less than five percent in the cavalry division. These cases were sent to the yellow fever hospital or otherwise segregated and did not spread, but the malarial and bilious types of fever steadily increased to an alarming extent, amounting to sixty, seventy, or more, percent of the command. This situation placed a very anxious responsibility upon the Medical Department, and presented a problem which has never been satisfactorily solved, namely: Why should the command (5th Corps) remain in good health during the hardships of the campaign (heat, fatigue, scant and indifferent food, lack of shelter), and as soon as the enemy surrendered and our troops began to enjoy rest, comfort and plenty of food, malarial and other undefined forms of fever rapidly spread to such a frightful degree? Opinions differ. Mine is that yellow fever and malarial fever were never widespread, and that most of the sickness thus following a short but exhausting campaign, was the result of improper diet, overeating and intemperance in a tropical climate.

The indications for treatment were, without doubt, after excluding yellow fever, to send back the 5th Corps to the United States and replace it by fresh troops, as was subsequently demonstrated. But the fear of importing yellow fever was so great that the decision to do so was very slowly and grudgingly arrived at by the War Department, and only after a "round-robin," in which all medical officers joined, was formulated and forwarded to Washington.

The Spanish army had also a high percentage of sickness after the surrender, but much smaller than that of our own army. It included a number of malarial and typhoid cases, but consisted chiefly of cases resulting from unhygienic conditions, such as fatigue, overheating, bad and deficient food. The Spanish sick also improved more rapidly than our own and were all deemed (justly or not) well enough to return home with the troops. Doubtless many would have had their lives saved by more prolonged rest and treatment before embarking.

[. . ..]

In September, 1898, the 5th Corps was ordered back to the United States, volunteer troops taking its place. The Department of Santiago and Puerto Principe was organized, with Brigadier General Lawton as Commanding General, but almost immediately replaced by Brigadier General Leonard Wood. I remained as Chief Surgeon of the Department.

One of my principal endeavors, thereafter, was the instruction of the medical officers of the volunteer regiments in the special sanitary duties which tropical conditions imposed upon them. Military posts, each with hospital or dispensary, were established or reestablished in all the principal towns and visited as often as possible, generally with the Commanding General.

[. . ..]

In 1899 a new yellow fever hospital was constructed on an ideal site, and island in the bay of Santiago, placed in charge of Dr. Fabricius, expert bacteriologist, and later of Dr. Orlando Ducker.

Sad and gloomy was the summer of 1899 in Santiago, through the breaking out of a virulent epidemic of yellow fever from which a number of Americans were victims. Surgeon Clendennin, U.S.A., who was in command of the general hospital and devoted to his arduous work died from it in a few days. Dr. Fabricius, as before stated on duty at the Yellow Fever Island, was another victim at about the same time. Assistant Surgeon Newgarden, U.S.A., had a severe attack but recovered. This epidemic was so successfully fought that it had entirely disappeared in November. Since then, it is believed that not a single case has originated in that city. It should be noted that this result was obtained before the agency of the mosquito as transmitter of yellow fever had been suspected.

In April of 1900, upon the recommendation of General Wood, I was transferred to Havana as Chief Surgeon of the Department of Cuba, my duties including not only the administration of the medical department of the troops of occupation, but also the supervision of all infectious diseases on the island. Yellow fever prevailed to an unusual extent in Havana during the year 1900, especially among Americans. Much of my time was accordingly devoted, in concert with Major Gorgas (then health officer of Havana) to the study and application of measures of prevention, isolation and disinfection.

During the same year there were three other outbreaks of yellow fever, namely, at Pinar del Rio, Santa Clara and Quemados, towns which I personally visited as often as was advisable to insure the carrying out of all necessary regulations.

In October of that year, I myself suffered from an attack of yellow fever.

As soon as the Reed Commission had conclusively proved the transmission of yellow fever by mosquitoes, Major J.R. Kean, then Acting Chief Surgeon of the Department of Cuba, recommended the issue of G.O. No. 6, December 21, 1900, in which he stated that: "It is now well established that malaria, yellow fever and filarial infection are transmitted by the bites of mosquitoes,"—the first official publication of this fact. On my return from leave to Havana, in April, 1901, having likewise become convinced of the scientific accuracy of the experiments of the Reed Commission, and with the approval of the Surgeon General, it became necessary to lay greater emphasis upon the new measures of prophylaxis and treatment imposed by the Commission's conclusions. Instructions were accordingly sent (Circular No. 5, April 27, 1901) to all military posts and civil hospitals on the Island, directing explicitly the institution and correct operation of these measures. Thus it was first and fully applied on a large scale, by Major Kean and myself, the wonderful and epoch-making discovery of Reed and his colleagues.

Source: United States. Adjutant-General's Office. *Correspondence Relating to The War with Spain...* Washington, D.C.: Center of Military History, 1993, pp. 249–250.

George Kennan on Medical Care of the Army in Cuba

The American public devoured the many published eyewitness accounts of the Cuban Insurrection and the ensuing Spanish-American War. News correspondents were on hand when U.S. forces landed in Cuba and throughout the war and its aftermath. Among them was the noted explorer, lecturer, and author George Kennan (a distant relative of the famous twentieth century diplomat with the same name). Kennan had gone to work at the age of twelve for a telegraph company, and subsequently traveled to Siberia to lay out telegraph lines. During his travels he met and wrote about political dissidents exiled by the tsarist regime, thus giving voice to his true talents. Kennan came to Cuba in a dual capacity—as a journalist and a Red Cross volunteer. Here he describes in graphic detail the sufferings of wounded U.S. soldiers, including their long waits for medical attention, or even a sip of water. In one instance, five army surgeons worked round the clock to perform more than three hundred operations in just under 24 hours. Before and after treatment, wounded soldiers had to lie outdoors with no protection from pouring rain and baking sun. The outspoken Kennan also published his assertion that General Shafter was entirely to blame for the high incidence of yellow fever in his command, noting that, in contrast, the marines suffered almost no tropical disease.

At sunset the five surgeons had operated upon and dressed the wounds of one hundred and fifty-four men. As night advanced and the wounded came in more rapidly, no count or record of the operations was made or attempted. Late in the evening of Friday, division and regimental surgeons began to come back to the hospital from the front, and the operating force was increased to ten. More tables were set out in front of the tents, and the surgeons worked at them all night, partly by moonlight and partly by the dim light of flaring candles held in the hands of stewards and attendants. Fortunately, the weather was clear and still, and the moon nearly full. There were no lanterns, apparently, in the camp, at least, I saw none in use outside of the operating- tent, and if the night had been dark, windy, or rainy, four fifths of the wounded would have had no help

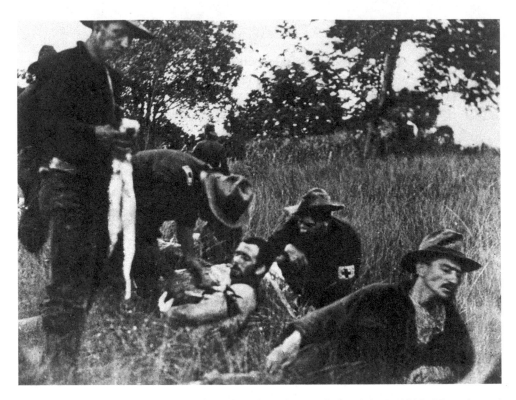

Casualty evacuation following the Battle of El Caney, Cuba, July 1, 1898. Note the red cross patch on kneeling soldier. (National Library of Medicine)

or surgical treatment whatever until the next day. All the operations outside of a single tent were performed by the dim light of one unsheltered and flaring candle, or at most two. More than once even the candles were extinguished for fear that they would draw the fire of Spanish sharp-shooters who were posted in trees south of the camp, and who exchanged shots with our pickets at intervals throughout the night. These cold-blooded and merciless guerrillas fired all day Friday at our ambulances and at our wounded as they were brought back from the battle-line, and killed two of our Red Cross men. There was good reason to fear, therefore, that they would fire into the hospital. It required some nerve on the part of our surgeons to stand beside operating-tables all night with their backs to a dark tropical jungle out of which came at intervals the sharp reports of guerrillas rifles. But there was not a sign of hesitation or fear. Finding that they could not work satisfactorily by moonlight, brilliant although it was, they relighted their candles and took the risk. Before daybreak on Saturday morning they had per formed more than three hundred operations, and then, as the wounded had ceased to come in, and all cases requiring immediate attention had been disposed of, they retired to their tents for a little rest. The five men who composed the original hospital force had worked incessantly for twenty-one hours.

Of course the wounded who had been operated upon, or the greater part of them, had to lie out all night on the water-soaked ground; and in order to appreciate the suffering they endured the reader must try to imagine the conditions and the environment. It rained in torrents there almost every afternoon for a period of from ten minutes to half an hour, and the ground, therefore, was usually water-soaked and soft. All the time that it did not rain the sun shone with a fierceness of heat that I have seldom seen equaled, and yet at night it grew cool and damp so rapidly as to necessitate the putting on of thicker clothing or a light overcoat. Many of the wounded soldiers, who were brought to the hospital from a distance of three miles in a jolting ambulance or army wagon, had lost their upper clothing at the bandaging-stations just back of the battle-line, where the field-surgeons had stripped them in order to examine or treat their wounds. They arrived there, consequently, half naked and without either rubber or woolen blankets; and as the very limited hospital supply of shirts and blankets had been exhausted, there was nothing to clothe or cover them with. The tents set apart for wounded soldiers were already full to overflowing, and all that a litter-squad could do with a man when they lifted him from the operating-table on Friday night was to carry him away and lay him down, half naked as he was, on the water-soaked ground under the stars. Weak and shaken from agony under the surgeon's knife and probe, there he had to lie in the high, wet grass, with no one to look after him, no one to give him food and water if he needed them, no blanket over him, and no pillow under his head. What he suffered in the long hours of the damp, chilly night I know because I saw him, and scores more like him; but the reader, who can get an idea of it only through the medium of words, can hardly imagine it.

When the sun rose Saturday morning, the sufferings of the wounded who had lain out all night in the grass were intensified rather than relieved, because with sunshine came intense heat, thirst, and surgical fever. An attempt was made to protect some of them by making awnings and thatched roofs of bushes and poles; but about seven o'clock ambulances and wagons loaded with wounded began again to arrive from the battle-line, and the whole hospital force turned its attention to them, leaving the suffering men in the grass to the care of the camp cooks and a few slightly wounded soldiers, who, although in pain themselves, could still hobble about carrying hard bread and water to their completely disabled and gasping comrades.

The scenes of Saturday were like those of the previous day, but with added details of misery and horror. Many of the wounded, brought in from the extreme right flank of the army at Caney, had had nothing to eat or drink in more than twenty-four hours, and were in a state of extreme exhaustion. Some, who had been shot through the mouth or neck, were unable to swallow, and we had to push a rubber tube down through the bloody froth that filled their throats, and pour water into their stomachs through that; some lay on the ground with swollen bellies, suffering acutely from stricture of the urinary passage and distention of the bladder caused by a gunshot wound; some were paralyzed from the neck down or the waist down as a result of injury to the spine; some were delirious from thirst, fever, and exposure to the sun; and some were in a state of unconsciousness, coma, or collapse, and made no reply or sign of life when I offered them water or bread.

They were all placed on the ground in a long, closely packed row as they came in; a few pieces of shelter-tenting were stretched over them to protect them a little from the sun, and there they lay for two, three, and sometimes four hours before the surgeons could even examine their injuries. A more splendid exhibition of patient, uncomplaining fortitude and heroic self-control than that presented by these wounded men the world has never seen. Many of them, as appeared from their chalky faces, gasping breath, and bloody vomiting, were in the last extremity of mortal agony; but I did not hear a groan, a murmur, or a complaint once an hour. Occasionally a trooper under the knife of the surgeon would swear, or a beardless Cuban boy would shriek and cry, "Oh, my mother, my mother!" as the surgeons reduced a compound fracture of the femur and put his leg in splints; but from the long row of wounded on the ground there came no sound or sign of weakness. They were suffering, some of them were dying, but they were strong. Many a man whose mouth was so dry and parched with thirst that he could hardly articulate would insist on my giving water first, not to him, when it was his turn, but to some comrade who was more badly hurt or had suffered longer. Intense pain and the fear of impending death are supposed to bring out the selfish, animal characteristics of man; but they do not in the higher type of man. Not a single American soldier, in all my experience in that hospital, ever asked to be examined or treated out of his regular turn on account of the severity, painful nature, or critical state of his wound. On the contrary, they repeatedly gave way to one another, saying: "Take this one first he's shot through the body. I've only got a smashed foot, and I can wait." Even the courtesies of life were not forgotten or neglected in that valley of the shadow of death. If a man could speak at all, he always said, "Thank you," or "I thank you very much," when I gave him hard bread or water. One beardless youth who had been shot through the throat, and who told me in a husky whisper that he had had no water in thirty-six hours, tried to take a swallow when I lifted his head. He strangled, coughed up a little bloody froth, and then whispered: "It's no use; I can't. Never mind!" Our Dr. Egan afterward gave him water through a stomach-tube. If there was any weakness or selfishness, or behavior not up to the highest level of heroic manhood, among the wounded American soldiers in that hospital during those three terrible days, I failed to see it. As one of the army surgeons said to me, with the tears very near his eyes: "When I look at those fellows and see what they stand, I am proud of being an American, and I glory in the stock. The world has nothing finer."

[. . ..]

Late in August it was decided that the marines should return to the United States, notwithstanding their satisfactory state of health, and on the 26th of that month they reached Portsmouth, New Hampshire, with only two men sick. They had been gone a little more than eleven weeks, ten of which they had spent in Cuba, and in that time had not lost a single man from disease, and had never had a higher sick-rate than two and one half per cent.

In view of this record, as compared with that of any regiment in General Shafter's command, we are forced to inquire: What is the reason for the difference? Why should a battalion of marines be able to live ten weeks in Cuba, without the loss of a single man from disease, and with a sick-rate of only two and one half per cent, while so hardy and tough a body of men as the Rough Riders, under substantially the same climatic conditions, had become so reduced in four weeks that seventy-five per cent, of them were unfit for duty, and fifty per cent, of them fell out of the ranks from exhaustion in a march of five miles?

The only answer I can find to these questions is that the marines had suitable equipment and intelligent care, while the soldiers of General Shafter's command had neither.

When the marines landed in Guantanamo Bay, every tent and building that the Spaniards had occupied was immediately destroyed by fire, to remove any possible danger of infection with yellow fever. When General Shafter landed at Siboney, he not only disregarded the recommendation of his chief surgeon to burn the buildings there, but allowed them to be occupied as offices and hospitals, without even so much as attempting to clean or disinfect them. Yellow fever made its appearance in less than two weeks. The marines at Guantanamo were supplied promptly with light canvas uniforms suitable for a tropical climate, while the soldiers of General Shafter's army sweltered through the campaign in the heavy clothing that they had worn in Idaho or Montana, and then, just before they started North, were furnished with thin suits to keep them cool at Montauk Point in the fall. The marines drank only water that had been boiled or sterilized, while the men of General Shafter's command drank out of brooks into which the heavy afternoon showers were constantly washing fecal and other decaying organic matter from the banks. The marines were well protected from rain and dew, while the regulars of the Fifth Army-Corps were drenched to the skin almost every day, and slept at night on the water-soaked ground. The marines received the full navy ration, while the soldiers had only hardtack and fat bacon, and not always enough of that. Finally, the marines had surgeons enough to take proper care of the sick, and medicines enough to give them, while General Shafter, after leaving his reserve medical supplies and ambulance corps at Tampa, telegraphs the adjutant- general on August 3 that " there has never been sufficient medical attendance or medicines for the daily wants of the command." In short, the marines observed the laws of health, and lived in Cuba according to the dictates of modern sanitary science, while the soldiers, through no fault of their own, were forced to violate almost every known law of health, and to live as if there were no such thing as sanitary science in existence.

Source: Society of the Army of Santiago de Cuba. *The Santiago Campaign: Reminiscences...* Richmond, VA: Williams Printing Company, 1927, pp. 217–219.

Curtis V. Hard on American Yellow Fever Victims in Cuba, 1898

Curtis V. Hard of Wooster, Ohio was born in 1845. At the age of nineteen he enlisted in an Ohio regiment that fought in the Civil War. Hard was a prosperous banker, 53 years old, married with three children, when the United States declared war on Spain. President McKinley was from Ohio and had himself fought in the Civil War. McKinley's background helped influence the state of Ohio to mobilize rapidly some 8,000 volunteers. Within 24 hours of the declaration of war, the 8th Ohio Volunteers, with 1,021 officers and men, reported for duty. Later, two of McKinley's nephews joined the regiment. The regiment joined Major-General William Shafter's Fifth Corps for the Santiago campaign in June 1898. On July 11, medical officers detected the first cases of an illness they believed was yellow fever. The sick list quickly grew to alarming proportions. Neither the military nor the civil authorities understood the cause of the fevers that spread through the American forces. Officers and men alike knew that September marked the usual onset of the dreaded yellow fever season. Everyone, including the medical officers, confused the symptoms Colonel Hard described with the symptoms of yellow fever. In fact, the cause was malaria spread by mosquito bites. By August, sickness was so widespread that Shafter's command was withdrawn from Cuba. The 8th Ohio Volunteers never saw combat, but a total of 25 soldiers died from sickness.

Chaplain Campbell arrived in camp on the morning of August 3 and thereafter took charge, of course, of all matters of this kind. Although personally known to only a few of the officers and men he received a hearty greeting. After a hurried introduction and a brief explanation of the situation, he pulled on his rubber boots and rubber coat and started out in the rain and mud to cheer the sick and get acquainted with the well. Inside of two or three hours he had said something to every man, and from that time until the end of his service he was busy caring for the sick, comforting the dying, and burying the dead.

Before we left the island to return to the States fourteen more deaths occurred in the Eighth, eight of them at Sevilla Hill and six at Siboney. Privates William K. Adams and Moses McDowell of Company H died at Sevilla Hill August 3 and Sergeant Charles Thoman of Company A, Bucyrus, at the same place August 4.

On the fifth Private George Coleman, of Company M, died at Sevilla, and Private Frank Gibler of Company I died and was buried at Siboney. There were three deaths again on the seventh of August, all of them at Siboney: Privates George L. Happer, of Millersburg, of Company H, Ora N. Royer of Company K, Alliance, and Corporal Dudley Wilson of Company G, Wadsworth. Captain John A. Leininger of Company F had been unfit for duty much of the time after landing but never went to the hospital. At length on the seventh of August it was thought best to send him into Santiago to the officers' hospital where it was thought he could have better care. We were shocked on the evening of the eighth when his colored servant came into camp with the news that the captain was dead. The officers of his company, with a detail of men, at once went into the city and carefully interred the remains in the Santiago cemetery.

Private Ebbie Bland of Company A died on the eleventh of August at Siboney. Private Irwin Lautzenheiser of Company D, Wooster, died at Sevilla Hill August 13. His brother, also a member of Company D, was with him during his sickness and at his death, which occurred only a few days before our departure for the north. Corporal John S. Lee of company G, a cousin of Captain Lee, died August 15 at Siboney, and on the sixteenth Corporal Charles E. Tarner of Company L died in the camp on San Juan Hill, only a few hours before the orders for our embarkation were delivered. He was buried in the trenches—one of the last things the men of his company did before starting into the city. The next day before we went on board the Mohawk we learned that Ward A. Wilford of Akron, a member of Company B, had died on the sixteenth at Siboney. This made a total of twenty-two men whose bodies we left on the island of Cuba as we sailed away, the Eighth Ohio's contribution to its freedom from Spanish domination.

The death rate was not alarming. But the sickness was appalling. The percentage of sick reported each day by the regiments varied all the way from twenty to forty. Of those not reported sick a very large proportion were weak, emaciated, and unfit for duty. It is safe to say that if the emergency had arisen not five thousand men in that whole army could have marched five miles and carried their accouterments and a single day's rations. Just what ailed us it is difficult for us laymen to determine when the doctors disagreed so widely. Our surgeons did not believe it was yellow fever, and in this opinion they were supported by many, perhaps a majority of the surgeons on the island. But whatever name it may be designated it was an exceedingly debilitating and depressing ailment. Its victims lost appetite, ambition, and sometimes nerve. Many were afflicted with dementia of various degrees, and there were not a few sad cases of extreme insanity. And then there was before us continually the fear that after the whole army had become exhausted and enervated by this fever, whatever it was, when September came the genuine, unadulterated, sure-enough yellow fever would assail us, and then no man would have the physical strength to withstand the siege.

Source: Clara Barton. *The Red Cross in Peace and War.* Meriden, CT: The Journal Publishing Co., 1912, pp. 569–575.

Report of the Yellow Fever Commission (1906)

When U. S. forces landed in Cuba in 1898, medical science had not yet penetrated the nature of tropical diseases. During and after the Santiago campaign, numerous U.S. soldiers fell ill and died of yellow fever and other diseases. Major Walter Reed was appointed in 1900 to lead a commission to study the spread of yellow fever in Cuba. Reed came to believe that a certain species of mosquito was the means by which yellow fever was transmitted. He requested and received from Major General Leonard Wood, military governor of Cuba, permission and funding to conduct human experiments. Reed's two colleagues, Dr. James Carroll and Dr. Jesse Lazear, along with a number of soldiers and civilians, volunteered to be exposed to yellow fever. They either submitted to mosquito bites, received injections of infected blood, or slept in bedding used by infected persons. Twenty-three of the volunteers fell ill with yellow fever, infected by either the mosquito bites or the injected blood. Dr. Lazear received a mosquito bite and died of the ensuing yellow fever, the only fatality in the course of the experiment. The commission's discovery of the means of transmission brought with it the ability to prevent the spread of the deadly disease. It was a historic contribution to public health.

Experiments Conducted For The Purpose Of Coping With YELLOW FEVER. [Senate Document No. 10, Fifty-ninth Congress, second session.]

To the Senate and House of Representatives:

The inclosed papers are transmitted to the Congress in the earnest hope that it will take suitable action in the matter. Maj. Reed's part in the experiments which resulted in teaching us how to cope with yellow fever was such as to render mankind his debtor, and this nation should in some proper fashion bear witness to this fact.

Theodore Roosevelt.

The White House, *December, 5, 1906.*

[Inclosure 1.]
[Memorandum for the President, through The Military Secretary of the Army.]

War Department,
Office Of The Surgeon General,
Washington, August 30,1906.

The persons taking an important part in the investigations in Cuba, which resulted in the demonstration of the fact that yellow fever is transmitted by a species of mosquito, were three members of the board appointed to investigate epidemic diseases in Cuba— Walter Reed, James Carroll, and Jesse W. Lazear—and the individuals who submitted themselves for experimentation by receiving the bites of infected mosquitoes, by receiving injections of mood from yellow-fever patients, and by sleeping in bedding which had been used by yellow-fever patients.

When the Yellow Fever Commission, composed of Walter Reed, James Carroll, Jesse W. Lazear, and A. Agramonte, assembled in Habana they had no thought of investigating the connection of the mosquito with the spread of yellow fever. This idea came to Dr. Reed after the board had demonstrated that the claim of Sanarelli, concurred in by Wasdin and Geddins, that the *Bacillus icteroides* was the cause of yellow fever was without foundation. Dr. Reed then determined to investigate the theory of Dr. Carlos Finlay, that the mosquito was instrumental in conveying yellow fever, which theory Finlay had failed to demonstrate, and which was not then accepted by scientific men. This determination was reached for the reasons which are well stated in Dr. Kelly's biography, and was original with Reed, not being suggested to him by anyone. The final determination to investigate the mosquito theory was arrived at during an informal meeting of the board (Dr. Agramonte being absent) at Columbia Barracks on the evening before Dr. Reed's departure for the United States, early in August, 1901. It was agreed by these members of the board that in making the experiments on human beings, by which alone the demonstration could be made, that they should submit themselves as subjects for experimentation. To Dr. Lazear, who was familiar with mosquito work, was assigned the duty of breeding and infecting the mosquitoes; while Dr. Carroll was to continue the bacteriological work on which the board had been engaged.

On August 2, 1900, before the mosquitoes were ready for the experiment, Dr. Reed was called back to Washington to prepare for publication the abstract of the report of the board appointed in 1898 to investigate the spread of typhoid fever in the volunteer camps in the United States, of which board he was president. This vast work, of which the full report was published by special authority of Congress about a year after Dr. Reed's death, by the only surviving member of the board, Prof. Victor C. Vaughan, of the University of Michigan, was one of the most valuable contributions to science which has been made by the Surgeon General's Office. The work of preparation of the abstract report had been brought to a standstill by the sudden death of the third member of the board, Dr. Edward O. Shakespeare, of Philadelphia, and Dr. Reed's presence at this time was essential for its completion.

During Dr. Reed's absence the inoculations by means of the mosquito were begun. On August 11, Dr. Lazear made the first experiment, but nine distinct inoculations on persons, including himself and Acting Asst. Surg. A. S. Pinto, were unsuccessful. We know now that these failures were clue to two facts—first, that patients after the third day of the disease can not convey the infection to the mosquito, and second, that after having bitten a yellow-fever case the mosquito can not transmit the disease until after an interval of at least 12 days. On August 27 one mosquito was applied to Dr. Carroll, one which happened to fulfill both of these conditions. The result was a very severe attack of yellow fever, in which for a time his life hung in the balance. This was thus the first experimental case. The fever developed on the 31st of August, on which day Dr. Lazear applied the same mosquito which bit Dr. Carroll with three others to another person. This man came down with a mild but well-marked case.

On September 13 Dr. Lazear, while on a visit to Las Animas Hospital (for the purpose of collecting blood from yellow-fever patients for study) was bitten by a mosquito of undetermined species, which he deliberately allowed to remain on the back of his hand until it had satisfied its hunger. Five days thereafter he came down, without other exposure, with yellow fever, which progressed steadily to a fatal termination. These three cases established in Reed's mind the proof of the mosquito theory and made it, in the opinion of his friends, an unnecessary and foolish risk for him, at his age, to submit himself to inoculation. These cases, with his deductions therefrom, were reported by the board in a paper called "The etiology of yellow fever—A preliminary note," read before the American Public Health Association at Buffalo, N.Y., October 22–26, 1900. He then immediately returned to Cuba to undertake a second and more elaborate series of experiments which were made possible by the promise made to him by Gen. Wood on October 12, when told by Reed of the experiments already made, to assist him with whatever money was necessary. This, the second series of experiments, began November 20 at an experimental camp near Quemados, called Camp Lazear, and embraced 14 cases, of which the last was taken sick February 10, 1901. Of these, 10 were mosquito infections and 4 were infected by injection of the blood of yellow-fever patients. All of these cases recovered.

A third series of 6 cases was produced by Dr. James Carroll the next fall to settle certain undetermined facts as regards the etiology of the disease. The first of these cases came down with the fever September 19, 1901, and the last on October 23, 1901. Of these cases 2 were caused by mosquitoes and 4 by blood injections. None of them resulted fatally. The highly dangerous character of these experiments and the good fortune of the board in its second and third series of cases is shown by the fact that Dr. Guiteras, of Habana, in a series of 7 cases inoculated in Habana lost 3, bringing his experiments abruptly to an end.

No enumeration of unsuccessful cases—namely, those which failed to cause the disease—has been made, although it is obvious that the persons undergoing such experiments exhibited as much courage as those in which the disease was transmitted. This is especially true of the cases occurring after the severe case of Dr. Carroll and the fatal case of Dr. Lazear. Certain ones of these unsuccessful cases deserve special mention, being those made with infected bedding at Camp Lazear. In a specially constructed house at that camp, which was intentionally ill ventilated and kept continually at a summer temperature, was placed a large quantity of bedding taken from the beds of patients sick with yellow fever in Habana and soiled with their discharges. In this house Acting Asst. Surg. R. P. Cook and two privates of the Hospital Corps slept continuously from November 30 to December 19. Each morning they packed the various soiled articles of bedding in boxes and unpacked them at night, when they were used to sleep on.

From December 21, 1900, to January 10, 1901, the building was again occupied by two nonimmune Americans under the same circumstances, except that an additional stock of very much fouled bedding and clothing had been added to the collection, and these men slept every night in the very garments worn by yellow-fever patients throughout their entire attacks, besides making use of their much soiled pillow slips, sheets, and blankets. A third couple of Hospital Corps men succeeded these for an, equal length of time. None of these seven individuals contracted yellow fever, but the courage and fortitude shown by them certainly equal that of those who submitted to the bites of the mosquitoes, it being borne in mind that belief in the transmission of yellow fever by infected bedding and clothing was at that time practically universal, whereas the mosquito theory had still very few converts.

After this brief history of this great discovery a statement of the part borne by each of the more important participators in it is necessary to a determination of the reward which would be appropriate to each.

Maj. Walter Reed, surgeon, United States Army, president of the commission to investigate and study the epidemic diseases in Cuba, died in Washington from appendicitis, November 23, 1902, at the age of 51. At the time of his death the Secretary of War had said in his report, which was then in press but not yet given out:

> The brilliant character of this scientific achievement, its inestimable value to mankind, the saving of thousands of lives, and the deliverance of the Atlantic seacoast from constant apprehension, demand special recognition from the Government of the United States.
>
> Dr. Reed is the ranking major in the Medical Department, and within a few months will, by operation of law, become lieutenant colonel. I ask that the President be authorized to appoint him Assistant Surgeon General with the rank of colonel.

Gen. Leonard Wood said of him in an address delivered at a memorial meeting of scientific men in Washington, D. C., shortly after his death:

> I know of no other man on this side of the world who has done so much for humanity as Dr. Reed. His discovery results in the saving of more lives annually than were lost in the Cuban war, and saves the commercial interests of the world a greater financial loss each year than the cost of the Cuban war. He came to Cuba at a time when one-

third of the officers of my staff died of yellow fever, and we were discouraged at the failure of our efforts to control the disease.

In the months when the disease was ordinarily worst the disease was checked and driven from Habana. That was the first time in nearly 200 years that the city had been rid of it. The value of his discovery can not be appreciated by persons who are not familiar with the conditions of tropical countries. Hereafter it will never be possible for yellow fever to gain such headway that quarantine will exist from the mouth of the Potomac to the mouth of the Rio Grande. Future generations will appreciate fully the value of Dr. Reed's services. His was the originating, directing, and controlling mind in this work, and the others were assistants only.

In a letter from Prof. Welch to the Secretary of War he said:

Dr. Reed's researches in yellow fever are by far the most important contributions to science which have ever come from any Army surgeon. In my judgment they are the most valuable contributions to medicine and public hygiene which have ever been made in this country with the exception of the discovery of anaesthesia. They have led and will lead to the saving of thousands of lives. I am in a position to know that the credit for the original ideas embodied in this work belongs wholly to Maj. Reed.

Prof. Welch was Dr. Reed's teacher in bacteriology and was his intimate and confidential friend, with whom he consulted about the details of the work in Cuba.

A bill prepared in this office for a pension for his widow, equal in amount to his monthly pay, was passed, but the amount was so cut down that while it keeps the wolf from the door it does not provide an adequate and comfortable income. It is not probable, however, that Congress would increase this pension, and an effort has been made to supplement it by the raising of a fund of $25,000 by the Walter Reed Memorial Association, incorporated for this purpose in the District of Columbia. The interest on this fund will be given Mrs. Reed during her lifetime, and the principal, after her death, will be devoted to some form of memorial. This fund lacks at present about $6,000 of completion. The existence of this association, should its hopes be attained, does not, however, absolve the nation from the obligation of a fitting recognition for this great work, and it is the opinion of the undersigned, which, it is believed, is shared by the vast majority of physicians in the United States, that Congress should erect a statue to Walter Reed in Washington. The assistance of the President in inducing Congress to do so is requested.

The second member of the commission was Dr. James Carroll, at that time acting assistant surgeon, United States Army.

Dr. Carroll is now 52 years old. He entered the military service June 9, 1874, and served as private, corporal, sergeant, and hospital steward from that date to May 21, 1898, when he was appointed acting assistant surgeon. He was appointed first lieutenant and assistant surgeon in the Medical Corps October 27, 1902, which rank he still holds.

Dr. Carroll was Dr. Reed's truest assistant and coadjutor from the inception of the work which resulted in the discovery of the method of propagation of yellow fever. As stated above, the third series of experiments were performed by Dr. Carroll alone, Dr. Reed having been refused permission to return to Cuba to complete his work.

Dr. Carroll was the first experimental case of yellow fever, and he suffered a very severe attack, to which he attributes a heart trouble from which he now suffers. At the time of undergoing this experiment he was 46 years old, an age at which the risk from this disease is very great, as its mortality rapidly increases with age of patient. He had at that time a wife and five children who had no other means of support except his pay as an acting assistant surgeon.

It is recommended that Congress be asked to pass a special act promoting Dr. Carroll, on account of his services in connection with this discovery and the courage shown by him in subjecting himself to experiment, to the rank of lieutenant colonel, the number of medical officers in that grade being increased by one for that purpose; also his name and effigy should appear on the monument to Walter Reed.

Dr. Jesse W. Lazear was the third member of the commission.

Dr. Lazear was a native of Baltimore and a graduate of Johns Hopkins University, afterwards getting his professional degree at Columbia University and Bellevue. At the time he incurred his death in the course of these experiments, as above mentioned, he was 34 years old. He left a wife and two young children, the younger a little son born a few months before his death, whom he never saw. Mrs. Lazear received from Congress a pension of $17 a month with $2 additional for each of two minor children until they reach the age of 16. Also a battery in Baltimore Harbor was, by direction of the Secretary of War, named in his honor. It is believed that this recognition on the part of the nation for his services is utterly inadequate. His widow's pension should be increased to $100 a month, and steps should be taken to perpetuate his name in connection with the Walter Reed monument above suggested.

Dr. A. Agramonte was the fourth member of the Yellow Fever Commission. He was a Cuban by birth, an immune to yellow fever, and having been assigned other work, took no part in the first series of experiments with regard to the conveyance of the disease by the mosquito, of which, in fact, he was not at the time cognizant. Being an immune, he ran no risk in connection with this work, and it is believed that his contributions to it have been sufficiently recognized in the association of his name with the other members of the commission who brought about this great discovery.

Twenty-three of the men who submitted themselves for experiment by the board contracted yellow fever, beginning with Dr. James Carroll, who was taken sick August 31, 1900, and ending with John R. Bullard, who was taken sick October 23, 1901.

Conspicuous among them was John J. Moran, a civilian clerk employed at the headquarters of Gen. Fitzhugh Lee, at Quemados, who was one of the earliest volunteers for the second set of experiments, and whose action was dictated by the purest motives of altruism and self-devotion. Mr. Moran disclaimed, before submitting to the experiments, any desire for reward, and has never accepted any since, although he was offered the $200 which the liberality of the military governor enabled the commission to give to each experimental patient, the members of the board excepted. Such was his modesty that he has made no effort, so far as known to this office, to make known his connection with these experiments and reap the credit which is so justly due him. Mr. Moran was a native of Ohio. His present address is not known to this office. The first inoculations in the case of Mr. Moran were for some reason unsuccessful, on November 26 and 29. He did not suffer an attack until after the third inoculation, on December 21.

The same remarks apply to the first experimental case of the second set, Pvt. John R. Kissinger, Hospital Corps, who volunteered at the same time with Moran and equally disclaimed any desire for reward.

Pvt. Kissinger did not leave Cuba immediately after the experiments, as did Mr. Moran, and therefore the military authorities were able to reward him in some measure along with other enlisted men who volunteered for these experiments. He was promoted acting hospital steward, presented with a gold watch by the chief surgeon of the department in the presence of all the medical officers and Hospital Corps men on duty at Columbia Barracks, and also received a present of $115 in cash. He took his discharge November 14, 1901, and has since (on December 17, 1903) made application for pension. This was refused for lack of evidence that his ill-health was incident to the service.

Of the other experimental cases, seven were Spanish immigrants who submitted to experiments purely for the money which they were promised. With regard to those who were American soldiers, however, 10 in number, in addition to those already mentioned, it can not be doubted that, although they received pecuniary rewards, a desire to assist in what they appreciated was a great and glorious work, together with a spirit of adventure, was the most powerful motive. The same is true of the last experimental case, Mr. John R. Bullard, a graduate of Harvard, where he was a distinguished athlete and captain of the university crew. The names of these men, with the dates of their attack, are appended with this report.

It remains to mention Dr. Robert P. Cook, acting assistant surgeon, and the six privates of the Hospital Corps, who were for 20 nights shut up in the infected bedding house at Camp Lazear. These experiments, which were absolutely necessary to demonstrate that yellow fever could not be carried otherwise than by the mosquito, had for these men, so far as they knew, an equal element of danger with the other experiments and had in addition such repulsive and disagreeable features as to test to the full their hardihood and patience. Much of the bedding upon which they slept and which they were required daily to handle, was so soiled with the discharges of the sick as to be very repulsive to the nose and eye, and the last experimenters actually slept in the pajamas and sheets which had been worn by severe cases of yellow fever. The names of these men are appended to the list given below of experimental cases of yellow fever.

It will be observed that three of these men—Folk, Jernegan, and Hanberry—afterwards submitted to the mosquito inoculation or blood injection in order to demonstrate their nonimmunity at the time of the first experiment.

It is believed that the names of all the Americans on this list should be placed on a tablet in connection with the monument to Walter Reed.

From the foregoing it will be seen that the total disbursements of this great nation in the way of rewards for those who made possible this discovery and their families, amounts to $146 a month. As to its value to the American people attention is invited to the quotations from Gen. Wood and Prof. Welch given above, and others given in the inclosed circulars published by the Walter Reed Memorial Association.

How discreditable appears this niggardly provision when compared with the action of the English Government which more than a century ago, when the purchasing power of money was far greater than at present, gave to Jenner, the discoverer of vaccination, grants amounting to £30,000 sterling. He also received from a subscription in India £7,383 sterling, while the Reed Memorial has so far succeeded in raising only a little over half that sum.

It is believed that if the President would exert his great personal influence in furtherance of the aims of that association its task would be soon completed.

R. M. O'REILLY,
Surgeon General, United States Army

Source: Senate Documents, 61st Congress, 3rd Session, December 5, 1910–March 4, 1911. Vol 61. Yellow Fever (Doc 822). Washington, D.C.: Government Printing Office, 1911, pp. 17–23.

■ CHAPTER 6
World War I

INTRODUCTION

World War I was the first major conflict in which scientific principles of surgery, anesthesia, asepsis, and infection control were widely adopted. In contrast to previous wars, doctors had the knowledge and ability to control infections and prevent communicable diseases.

In 1914, Americans had provided hospital and transportation services on the Western Front with several voluntarily manned and funded motor ambulance services and a series of university-based teams of physicians and nurses operating primarily under the auspices of the American Hospital in Paris. The first Americans officially to enter the war were medical personnel assigned to the British Army the month after the United States entered the war, in May 1917. Before any U.S. soldiers had been sent to Europe, 1,400 physicians, 1,000 nurses and 2,600 enlisted men had been deployed in addition to six base hospitals. This gave the American military the priceless ability to learn from its allies who had already been fighting for three years.

They observed significant advances in military medicine with consequent better outcomes. The earliest improvements were in transportation and triage. Litter bearers retrieved men from the field and took them to aid stations just behind the front lines. After bandaging and stabilization, the men were transported—increasingly by motor ambulance—to casualty clearing stations (CCSs) just beyond the reach of artillery fire where wounds were débrided (dead tissue removed) and redressed, fractures braced, and minor injuries definitively treated. From the CCS, men were taken to field hospitals where surgical teams could perform emergency operations. Field hospitals were usually adjacent to a rail line allowing further transport to base hospitals where more complex surgery, convalescence, and rehabilitation could take place. For the most severely wounded there were specialized hospitals in the zone of the interior where long-term rehabilitation and complex reconstructive procedures could be accomplished.

Initiating treatment at CCSs made it possible to manage wounds within minutes to hours rather than the one to two days that had been usual early in the war. Early treatment decreased blood loss and the risk of infection, and survival rates improved. The heavily fertilized fields of northern France were rife with *Clostridium perfringens* and the related *Clostridium tetani*, responsible for gas gangrene and tetanus, respectively. Early wound débridement decreased the incidence of gas gangrene, and an effective antiserum (11 million doses of which had been administered by war's end) virtually eliminated tetanus.

Chemical sterilization of wounds also contributed to the decrease in secondary infection. Direct application of chlorine was replaced by continuous irrigation with a combination of hypochlorites and boric acid developed by French physician Alexis Carrel and British chemist H. D. Dakins. In the absence of antibiotics, which were not developed until the interwar years, the Carrel-Dakins method provided a remarkably effective way to limit wound infections. The death rate in hospital from wounds was 4.5 per 1,000 as compared to 10.48 per 1,000 in the American Civil War of 1861–1865.

Trench warfare with machine guns, shrapnel, high explosives, land mines, grenades, and mortars caused a unique assortment of injuries. Wounds to the head came from exposure over trench rims, and extremity injuries came from mines protecting the space between opposing lines. The prevalence of extremity injuries necessitated improvements in orthopedic reconstruction and prostheses and in diagnosis and repair of nerve injuries. The high number of head injuries led to better intracranial surgery (particularly under the auspices of American Harvey Cushing), and the complex facial injuries engendered innovative techniques in plastic and reconstructive surgery. Improvements in anesthesia and the general application of aseptic surgical techniques benefited all areas of surgery. Although the case mortality rates of head, chest, and extremity wounds improved during World War I, the lack of antibiotics meant that improved survival from penetrating abdominal wounds would have to wait until the next war.

Unlike prior wars, the rate of death from injury was more than twice that from disease in World War I, even when the high mortality of the 1918 influenza epidemic is included. Although not as lethal as in prior conflicts, disease was still a serious problem in World War I. Recruits, many of whom came from sparsely populated rural areas, were thrown together in close quarters with urbanites whose immune systems were accustomed to high population density and carried protection against many contagious diseases. The nonimmune recruits were subject to and suffered in great numbers from measles, mumps, scarlet fever, and meningitis. Diseases such as smallpox, typhoid, tetanus, diphtheria, and some forms of dysentery that had previously devastated armies were effectively controlled with vaccines. Some diseases carried by arthropods, such as louse-borne typhus and trench fever, were at least partially controlled by chemical pest control.

American soldiers in World War I received better medical care than those in any previous war. For the first time in a major war, combat casualties exceeded non-combat deaths. Among the major improvements in military medicine during World War I were generalized use of hypodermic syringes, retractors, forceps, rubber gloves, thermometers, sterile gauze, motor ambulances, mobile laboratories, diagnostic X-rays, vaccinations, trained nurses, and iodine solutions. A much better understanding of neuropsychiatric casualties arose. Care for veterans evolved from the custodial care that had characterized previous periods into a commitment to rehabilitation. This would lead to the 1930 consolidation of veterans' agencies into a single entity, the Veterans Administration, which provided care for both service- and non-service related disabilities.

James R. Arnold

ENTRIES

American Field Service and Other World War I Volunteer Ambulance Services

A group of volunteers, the best known of which was the American Field Service, played a significant role in evacuation of the wounded on the Western Front and comprised the first organized American presence during World War I.

At the outset of the war, the French ambulance service was primarily composed of horse-drawn wagons; with only 40 motorized medical transports, the Allies were desperately short of both cars and drivers. Within weeks of the war's onset, H. Herman Harjes, an American partner in the Paris banking firm Morgan-Harjes, collected five Packards and a group of volunteer drivers and began moving French wounded from rear-area receiving points to various hospitals, primarily in

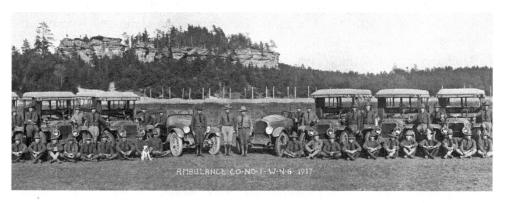

The development of motorized vehicles provided a new way to move casualties during World War I. This American Ambulance Company proudly displays their equipment in a 1917 photo. (Library of Congress)

and around Paris. Thereafter, Harjes concentrated his efforts in building an ambulance service that eventually came under the aegis of the American Red Cross.

At about the same time, Richard Norton, set up a similar volunteer corps for the British expeditionary force. Norton and his brother managed to garner significant donations of money and equipment and to recruit a broad range of primarily upper-class volunteers for what became the Anglo-American Volunteer Motor-Ambulance Corps. Norton's corps was temporarily subsumed under the British Red Cross. By 1916, Norton found himself at odds with the British Red Cross and merged with Harjes into the unit that bore both their names and was assigned to the American Red Cross. When the unit dissolved in 1917, it comprised 13 sections with more than 100 cars and in excess of 200 drivers and mechanics.

The best known of the American volunteer units was the American Field Ambulance Service (later shortened to American Field Service, or AFS), organized and directed by Abram Piatt Andrew, a Princeton doctoral graduate, former Harvard professor, and recent assistant secretary of the treasury. In 1914 Andrew, a dedicated Francophile, decided to go to Paris to offer whatever help he could to the war effort. The venerable American Hospital in the upper-class Paris suburb of Neuilly had established an ancillary military hospital. Like other volunteer hospitals, the Neuilly facility's directors realized they could not get patients without the transport to bring them in and so had formed a motor ambulance corps. (The French term *ambulance* actually referred to the entire organization rather than just to the vehicles that brought the wounded to the hospital.) Andrew took over that service and, with the help of his friend Henry Sleeper began soliciting money and volunteers.

The initial AFS volunteers came overwhelmingly from among Sleeper's and Andrew's circle of friends and were predominantly undergraduates from Harvard and Yale Universities. Later volunteers included undergraduates and recent alumni of other New England colleges as well as from Stanford University; the Universities of California, Chicago, Michigan, Wisconsin, and Illinois; and Washington University in St. Louis.

Unlike Norton and Harjes, who used whatever donated vehicles they could get, Andrew decided early on that efficiency dictated use of a uniform car, and he settled on converted Model T Fords. The first American Hospital Fords were donated by Harold White, manager of Ford Motor Company's Paris assembly plant. Canvas-covered wooden frames were bolted to the back of the chassis for carrying the *blessés* [French for wounded] while the driver's compartment was left open to the air. Henry Ford, a dedicated pacifist, refused to contribute to the war effort in any way and, throughout almost all of the AFS's short life. Andrew and Sleeper were forced to buy their Fords and their replacement parts at retail prices. The $360 cost was small enough and donations were large enough that they were able to accumulate several hundred vehicles. The chassis were bought in Detroit and shipped to France in wooden crates for local assembly, and the wood from the crates was salvaged to build the ambulance bodies.

The Fords proved a fortuitous choice for more than just reasons of economy. They were easy to assemble and simple enough mechanically that even the inexperienced American volunteers became adequate mechanics. Most of the parts were interchangeable, and the frame was built of remarkably durable vanadium steel. The engine was a single block with the pistons and valves mounted on top where they could be easily removed and cleaned or replaced. Although they could only carry two to six wounded (depending on whether they sat or required stretchers), the Fords were more maneuverable and took up less road space than the larger Packards, Cadillacs, Peugeots, and Bentleys used by other units. The semielliptical rear springs gave the ambulances a comparatively smooth ride and made them a favorite of the French soldiers.

Like Norton's and Harjes's units, the AFS cars initially operated as behind-the-lines transports, but all the Americans wanted to be more closely involved in the actual war. In April 1915, Andrew convinced the French general staff to allow his cars to go to the *postes de secours*—collecting stations just behind the lines—so they could move the wounded from the actual front to evacuation hospitals. What began as an experiment proved so effective that Andrew's cars and the Norton-Harjes units became the sole transport in parts of the front from Amiens to the Vosges.

Andrew eventually separated himself from the American Hospital in a dispute over allocation of donated funds, and the AFS continued as an independent effort until the United States entered the war in April 1917. The U.S. Army decided from the time of American entry into the war that the volunteer ambulance units would be under control of the Army Medical Corps, and they assigned Colonel Jefferson Randolph Keen to effect that change. Norton and virtually all his drivers refused to be "militarized," but Andrew accepted a commission as major in the U.S. Army and, with a majority of his drivers, submitted to military control. The AFS role was expanded to include transport of military materiel as well as the wounded, and the Ford Model A replaced the little "flivvers" on the Western Front.

Norton, disillusioned and intensely disliked by General John J. Pershing, left France. While passing through London on his way home, he succumbed to meningitis at the age of 46 on August 2, 1918. Herman Harjes joined the U.S. Army and became Pershing's liaison to the French.

Jack McCallum

Further Reading

Hansen, Arlen J. *Gentlemen Volunteers: The Story of the American Ambulance Drivers in the Great War, August 1914–September 1918*. New York: Arcade Publishing, 1996.

History of the American Field Service in France "Friends of France" 1914–1917. Told by Its Members. Boston: Houghton Mifflin Co., 1920.

Morse, Edwin. *The Vanguard of American Volunteers: In the Fighting Lines and in Humanitarian Service, August 1914–April 1917.* New York: Charles Scribner's Sons, 1919.

Crile, George Washington (1864–1943)

An American surgeon famous for his studies on shock and surgical anesthesia and founder of the Cleveland Clinic, George Washington Crile was born on a small farm near Chili, Ohio, on November 11, 1864. He entered the Ohio Normal School at age 17, where he paid his expenses by teaching elementary school students. After graduation, he took a job as principal of the Plainfield, Ohio, School, where he was befriended by Dr. A. E. Walker, who allowed him to come along on patient visits and to perform simple procedures. Crile enrolled in the proprietary Wooster Medical School in Cleveland in the spring of 1886 and graduated with honors a year later. After graduation, Crile became a house officer at the University Hospital of Cleveland, where he was taught by Frank Weed. After graduation, he joined Weed and Frank Bunts, another Wooster graduate, in private practice.

Crile became interested in shock and spent three months at Columbia University's College of Physicians and Surgeons studying physiology, histology, and pathology. In 1892 and 1895, he traveled to Europe, where he studied with Theodor Bilroth and Sir Victor Horsley. While in Horsley's laboratory, he met Charles Scott Sherington, Britain's preeminent physiologist, who was also studying shock. After returning to Cleveland, Crile won the Cart-wright Prize for his essay "An Experimental Research into Shock," which became the first of his 24 books.

Crile joined the faculty of the Western Reserve Medical School in 1900. Three years later, he described an inflatable rubber suit for treatment of shock on which the pressurized flight suits of World War II were later based. That same year he joined Johns Hopkins University Medical School surgeon Harvey Cushing in a presentation to the Boston Medical Society urging routine monitoring of blood pressure during surgery. A committee of the society considered the recommendation and decided such monitoring was unnecessary.

In 1910, Wooster and Western Reserve merged, and Crile joined the faculty of the new institution as clinical professor of surgery. He continued with a busy private practice, performing as many as 20 operations a day, and developed a special interest in procedures on the thyroid. He described the first radical neck dissection and, in August 1906 at Cleveland's St. Alexis Hospital, performed the United States' first successful human-to-human blood transfusion.

Crile had a lifelong interest in improving the safety of surgical procedures. In order to prevent lethal endocrine storms in anxious patients about to have thyrotoxic goiters removed, he often performed "steal" procedures in which he would come into a hospital room without warning and remove the patient's tumor while he or she was still in bed to save them the psychological stress of being taken to an operating room. Crile supplemented gas anesthesia with morphine, scopolamine, and locally infiltrated cocaine—a combination still used with only minor modification.

Crile helped form the American College of Surgeons in 1912 and was named Honorary Fellow of the Royal College of Surgeons of England in 1913. When the United States entered World War I, he formed the Lakeside unit that became Base Hospital 4 and came to France with the first detachment of the American Expeditionary Force on March 25, 1917.

In 1921, Crile joined Bunts, William Lower, and John Phillips to form the Cleveland Clinic. In December 1942, Crile suffered a stroke related to an episode of endocarditis and died the following month.

Jack McCallum

Further Reading

Crile, Grace, ed. *George Crile: An Autobiography*. Philadelphia: J. B. Lippincott, 1947.

Herman, Robert. 1994. "George Washington Crile (1864–1943)." *U2* (May): 28–83.

Cushing, Harvey Williams (1869–1939)

Doctor Henry Williams Cushing is widely recognized as the father of neurological surgery and also been credited with being the first endocrinologist. Cushing was born on April 8, 1869, in Cleveland, Ohio, to a family descended from a long line of New England physicians. After graduating from Yale, Cushing went to Harvard Medical School, from which he graduated in 1895. In the late 19th century, it was customary for medical students to administer ether during surgery, and Cushing had the misfortune of losing a patient from an overdose of the anesthetic gas. This incident led him to begin charting pulse and respirations. It marked the first use of the graphic anesthetic record that remains standard practice. Cushing's interest in intra-operative monitoring also led to his introduction of the Riva-Rocca blood pressure measuring apparatus to the operating room in 1901.

In 1897, Cushing went to the new Johns Hopkins Medical School to work with William Halsted and to become the first American surgeon to devote himself entirely to brain surgery. At the time the mortality rate for intracranial surgery was so great that Halsted warned Cushing he would be unable to earn a living if that was all he did. In 1900, Cushing traveled to Europe, where he worked with Charles Sherrington, Sir Victor Horsley, and Theodor Kocher. While in Kocher's laboratory, Cushing studied the elevation in blood pressure and decrease in pulse rate that accompany increased pressure on the brain.

On returning to Hopkins, Cushing helped form the Hunterian Laboratory, which became a world-renowned center of surgical and physiological research. Cushing's interest in pituitary tumors led to his development of techniques to reach the gland through the nose and to the development of endocrinology as a specialty. In 1912, Cushing moved to the Peter Bent Brigham Hospital in Boston as Harvard's Moseley Professor of Surgery.

Cushing was a committed Francophile and, in 1915, took the Harvard Ambulance Hospital to France to work with the American Hospital of Paris in treating wounded French soldiers. When the United States entered World War I on the Allied side in April 1917, Cushing became director of Base Hospital 5 and senior consultant in neurosurgery to the American Expeditionary Forces. His monograph on neurosurgery (which had been initially published as a section of W. W. Keen's *Surgery*) was reprinted by the surgeon general of the U. S. Army and became the standard neurosurgery reference for American military surgeons. Cushing's meticulous technique and concentration on hemostasis were credited with halving the mortality rate of intracranial surgery during the war. Cushing also introduced innovative methods of using X-ray to localize metallic foreign bodies and magnets to remove them from the brain.

Cushing was a notoriously slow surgeon who was fanatical about hemostasis. In 1911, he invented a silver clip that replaced the painstaking technique of individually tying off even very small severed blood vessels. In 1926, in cooperation with engineer Frank Bovie, he popularized the use of electrical currents to coagulate bleeding vessels, thus reintroducing heat cauterization to surgery.

Cushing took a position as professor of medical history at Yale after his retirement from Harvard—an involuntary termination occasioned by Cushing's own rule that no surgeon could operate past age 62. He left one of the world's finest collections of antique medical books to the Sterling Library following his death on October 7, 1939.

Jack McCallum

Further Reading

Fulton, John. *Harvey Cushing: A Biography.* Springfield, IL: Charles C. Thomas, 1946.

Sweet, William. "Harvey Cushing: Author, Investigator, Neurologist, Neurosurgeon." *Journal of Neurosurgery* 50 (January 1979): 5–12.

Thomson, Elizabeth. *Harvey Cushing: Surgeon, Author, Artist.* New York: Schuman's, 1950.

Walker, A. Earl. *A History of Neurological Surgery.* Baltimore: Williams & Wilkins Co., 1951.

Influenza Pandemic (1918–1920)

A major, worldwide influenza outbreak occurred at the end of World War I, causing more deaths than from all other causes during the entire war. Estimates of total mortality from the pandemic range from a conservative 20 million to nearly

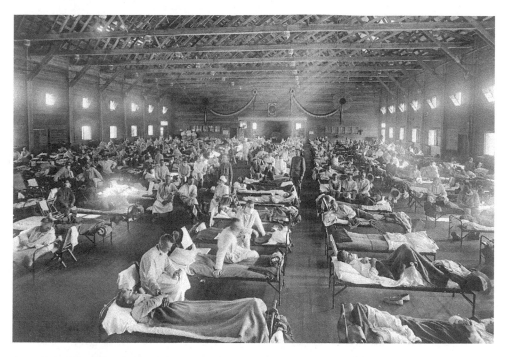

A world-wide influenza epidemic began in 1918. Fatalities may have reached 20 million. Here an emergency hospital at Camp Funston, Kansas, during the epidemic. (Otis Historical Archives Nat'l Museum of Health & Medicine)

100 million worldwide, compared to 9.2 million combat fatalities and 15 million total deaths from other causes. The average lifespan in the United States in 1917 and 1919 was 51 years. In 1918, as a result of the pandemic, the average dropped to 39 years. There were 729,381 cases of flu in the U.S. armed forces, with 7.2 percent mortality. Forty percent of the U.S. Navy and 36 percent of the U.S. Army were infected in 1918.

The 1918 pandemic was caused by a variant of the influenza A virus. The virus has the ability to stick first to the outer surface of the cells lining the lungs and then to penetrate those cells, co-opt the intracellular machinery, and cause the cell to manufacture new virus particles that can be egested and coughed up, then infect a new host.

Influenza epidemics occur regularly and usually cover a restricted geographic area. Although exposure to a particular variant of the virus confers life-long immunity, the pathogen has the ability to subtly alter its protein structure so that it can appear to be an organism the immune system does not recognize. Occasionally, it will develop a whole new gene, allowing it to look like a unique organism to which the body has no immunity whatsoever. These drastic changes, known as antigenic shifts, lead to pandemics, or worldwide disease outbreaks.

The first recorded cases of the influenza pandemic were in the Spanish town of San Sebastian in February 1918, accounting for the disease's most common eponyms—the Spanish Flu or the Spanish Lady. The first U.S. military case occurred on March 4 at Camp Funston (an adjunct of Fort Riley, Kansas) and cases were reported in British and French troops on the Western Front in early April. A curious aspect of the disease was its ability to traverse long distances faster than could be accounted for by existing ground or sea transportation.

By mid-summer, the disease mysteriously disappeared, having primarily affected Europe and North America, sparing Asia and the Southern Hemisphere. Although it had caused relatively debilitating illness, the first wave of the pandemic typically caused an illness that abated after about three days and was rarely fatal.

The disease returned with a vengeance in the early fall of 1918. This time, it seemed to arise in Asia, sweeping through India (where fatalities, although poorly recorded, may have reached 20 million), Southeast Asia, China, Japan, the Pacific Islands, and South America. By September the disease had broken out in Boston and, shortly thereafter, in the eastern Massachusetts military facility at Fort Devens.

The second wave was an entirely different disease. Unlike the usual influenza that shows a predilection for the very young and the very old, this pandemic had three peaks of age preference: birth to 5 years, 70–74 years, and, atypically, 20–40 years. Young adults—specifically those of military age—were a primary target.

The new disease was of remarkably rapid onset. Stories abound of people being unexpectedly found dead sitting in chairs, dying on the subway going home from work, or being well on arising and dying before sundown. The illness began with sudden onset of flushing, chills, and fever followed by a cough with thick, bloody sputum. Within hours the patients would be cyanotic and, unable to move air, would suffocate. Those who survived the early stages would often develop a superimposed bacterial pneumonia a few days later and die from the complication.

There was understandable public panic in reaction to the disease. Cities passed laws mandating stiff fines for citizens venturing out in public without masks. Theaters and churches (but rarely saloons) were closed, and the provost marshal general of the U.S. Army canceled the planned 142,000-man draft for September. Rumors circulated that the disease had been released by a combination of poison gas and rotting bodies from the battlefield, that the Germans had contaminated the U.S. East Coast from submarines, and that Germany's Bayer chemical company had contaminated aspirin with a new germ.

There was no treatment, but, just as it had earlier in the year, the disease spontaneously disappeared. It re-emerged in an attenuated form in 1920 before again disappearing, this time for good. The disease has not been seen again, although fear of its recurrence led directly to the Swine Flu panics and vaccination efforts of 1976 and 2009–1010.

Jack McCallum

Further Reading

Barry, John M. *The Great Influenza: The Epic Story of the Deadliest Plague in History.* New York: Penguin, 2005.

Collier, Richard. *America's Forgotten Pandemic.* London: Allison and Busby, 1996.

Crosby, Alfred W. *The Plague of the Spanish Lady.* Cambridge: Cambridge University Press, 1989.

Kolata, Gina. *Flu: The Story of the Great Influenza Pandemic of 1918 and the Search for the Virus That Caused It.* New York: Farrar, Strauss and Giroux, 1999.

Levine, Arnold. *Viruses.* New York: Scientific American Library, 1992.

Keen, William Williams (1837–1932)

William Williams Keen was one of the most famous late 19th-century American surgeons and arguably the founder of American neurosurgery. Born in 1837, Keen graduated from Brown University in 1859, and enrolled in Jefferson Medical College in 1860. He took time off to serve as a surgeon in the Union Army in 1861 before returning to his studies and graduating from Jefferson in 1862.

After graduation, Keen rejoined the Army and was assigned to Turner's Lane Hospital in Philadelphia, where he assisted neurologist Silas Weir Mitchell and participated in studies of gunshot wounds, especially those involving the nervous system.

He returned to Jefferson to teach surgical anatomy in 1866 and remained there until 1875, when he formed the Philadelphia School of Anatomy, where he taught for the next 14 years. In 1889 he was appointed professor of surgery at Jefferson and remained there until his retirement in 1907. During that time he also taught artistic anatomy at the Pennsylvania Academy of Fine Arts and was professor of surgery at the Women's Medical College of Pennsylvania.

Keen's *Surgery: Its Principles and Practice* was the standard textbook of that specialty for decades. In 1893, Keen assisted at the operation to remove a cancer from President Grover Cleveland's lower jaw. The procedure was performed on the president's yacht anchored in Long Island Sound and was kept secret for fear of disturbing already unsettled American financial markets. In 1917, Keen rejoined the Army as a consultant in surgery and was, with William Halsted, a major advocate of sterile technique in military surgery and wound care.

After retirement, he became an outspoken advocate for the theory of evolution and animal experimentation and died in Philadelphia at the age of 95.

Jack McCallum

Further Reading

N.a. 1932. "William Williams Keen." *Canadian Medical Association Journal* 27 (August): 181–182.

Shell Shock

Shell shock was the name applied in World War I to an assortment of symptoms including anxiety, an exaggerated startle response, tremors, nightmares, hallucinations, delusions, withdrawal, and catatonia. During World War I, psychiatric casualties were common among British, French, and German soldiers from the outset of trench warfare on the Western Front.

Throughout the war, 20–30 percent of battlefield casualties were psychiatric. The combination of a relatively static front, agonizingly long battles, atrocious living conditions, and high incidence of injury and death contributed to the prevalence of mental breakdown.

Early in the war the British diagnosed psychiatric casualties as shell shock with a "W" (wounded) appended to the diagnosis, possibly under the mistaken idea that the symptoms resulted from small brain hemorrhages caused by explosive concussions. The "W" entitled men to a wound stripe and disability with a pension. The alternative diagnosis, neurasthenia, was a sickness with an "S" designation, no honors, and no pension. The British established neurasthenia centers in the home islands, and prior to 1917, medical officers were liberal with the diagnosis of shell shock and transfer home for rest and hypnotherapy.

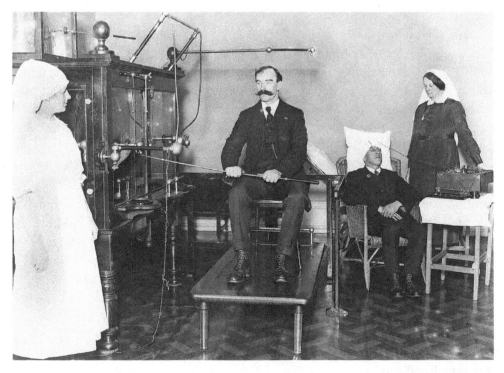

In World War I, the British diagnosed psychiatric casualties as "shellshock." In this 1917 image, nurses at a British hospital use experimental electrotherapy to treat soldiers suffering from shellshock. (Hulton-Deutsch Collection/Corbis)

By 1917 the drain on frontline manpower for psychiatric reasons became serious, and medical officers were encouraged to use the "S" designation. The Royal Army Medical Corps established designated casualty clearing stations near the front where psychiatric casualties were treated for up to a month with sedatives, rest, and reassurance. Using this scheme, 55 percent of men returned to their units, 29 percent were reassigned to labor brigades (mostly working on French farms), and only 16 percent were evacuated to base hospitals. Just before the Third Battle of Ypres (Passchendaele, July 31–November 10, 1918), the British General Staff issued General Routine Order Number 2384 forbidding the diagnosis of shell shock and ordering that all psychiatric casualties be sent to a single designated hospital with a diagnosis of "NYDN" (Not Yet Diagnosed, Nervous) with the dual intent of returning as many men as possible to the front and of discouraging malingering.

The Germans were more punitive and inclined to view shell shock as a character defect, which they managed with a variety of painful treatments including electroshock therapy. The United States adopted the British scheme, and even though the number of psychiatric casualties distressed American Expeditionary Forces (AEF) commander General John Pershing, 85 percent of his men with shell shock returned to their units and only 1 percent were evacuated to the United States.

Postwar treatment of the psychiatrically injured was a difficult and expensive problem. In 1921, 65,000 British veterans were on a pension for psychiatric disability, and there were still 30,000 on pension in 1938. In the United States as late as 1940, 27 of 90 veterans' hospitals were designated as psychiatric facilities, and treatment of shell shock victims had cost in excess of $1 billion.

Jack McCallum

Further Reading

Eksteins, Modris. *Rites of Spring: The Great War and the Birth of the Modern Age*. Boston: Houghton Mifflin, 1989.

Fenton, Norman. *Shell Shock and Its Aftermath*. St. Louis: The C. V. Mosby Company, 1926.

Macdonald, Lyn. *The Roses of No Man's Land*. New York: Atheneum, 1989.

Transfusion

Transfusion is the administration of blood or blood products obtained from one person into another. The earliest historical reference to transfusion was in 1492, when three young clerics volunteered to have blood removed and given to Pope Innocent VIII, who was comatose from a recent stroke. It is likely that the pope actually drank the blood rather than receiving it intravenously, and neither he nor his donors survived the experiment.

William Harvey's demonstration in 1628 that blood circulated from the heart to the arteries and then back through the veins was the crucial piece of information that made transfusion in the modern sense possible. In 1665, English surgeon John Wilkins and, shortly thereafter, Richard Lower of Oxford successfully transfused blood collected from one dog into the vein of another. The success of that experiment led Lower to attempt administration of dog blood into a human, and, in 1667, French surgeon Jean Baptiste Dénis described transfusion of sheep blood into humans. The practice was tried by a number of other Parisian practitioners, but the complication rate was so high that the city's Society of Physicians outlawed the practice 11 years later, effectively stopping experiments in animal to human transfusion.

In 1795, Philadelphia physician Philip Syng Physick successfully transfused blood from one person to another, but he did not publish the results of his experiment, and the practice did not become general. The next documented transfusion was in 1818, when English obstetrician James Blundell saved an exsanguinating patient by giving her blood collected from her husband. Difficulties with clotting and deterioration of collected blood as well as lack of knowledge of blood typing continued to make transfusion impractical throughout the 19th century. Milk (obtained from cows, goats, and humans) was tried as a substitute for blood but had a high rate of unacceptable complications, and that practice was replaced with the first saline transfusion in 1884.

The modern era of transfusion began in 1901 when Karl Landsteiner discovered the three major blood groups—A, B, and O—for which he was awarded the 1930 Nobel Prize for Physiology or Medicine. In 1907, Reuben Ottenberg successfully typed and cross-matched blood between donor and recipient and recognized that people with type O blood were universal donors, able to give blood to those with all other types. In 1908, Alexis Carrel successfully transfused blood directly from the artery of a donor to the recipient's vein, thus avoiding the problem of clotting.

The clotting problem was partially solved in 1915 when Dr. Richard Lewisohn of New York's Mount Sinai Hospital discovered that addition of sodium citrate to whole blood kept it from clotting. The following year, Francis Rous and J. R. Turner developed a citrate-glucose combination that allowed blood to be stored for several days. American Army officer Oswald Robertson, recognizing the importance of that discovery for the British war effort, organized "blood depots" to supply military hospitals.

Interest in transfusion continued after the war, and, in 1926, the British Red Cross started the world's first formal transfusion service. The first blood bank opened in Leningrad in 1932, and the first hospital blood bank was organized by Bernard Fontus at Chicago's Cook County Hospital five years later.

In 1939, Landsteiner, Alex Weiner, Philip Levine, and R. E. Stetson discovered the Rh blood groups (named for the Rhesus monkey) and removed what had been the major cause of transfusion reactions after Landsteiner's original discovery. Edwin Cohn's demonstration that blood plasma could be broken into albumin, gamma globulin, and fibrinogen using cold ethanol fractionation gave military surgeons a new way to resuscitate the severely injured.

University of Pennsylvania surgeon Isidor Ravdin successfully resuscitated severely wounded soldiers and sailors after the Pearl Harbor attack in 1941, using albumin rather than whole blood. In response to the need for whole blood during World War II, J. F. Loutit and Patrick Mollison developed acid citrate dextrose solution, which anticoagulated blood without significantly adding to its volume and which significantly extended its shelf life. The replacement of glass bottles with plastic bags for storage in 1950 and the discovery of CDPDA-1 anticoagulant, which allows refrigerated blood to be safely stored for 35 days, bring the technology to date.

Jack McCallum

Further Reading

Schmidt, P. J. 1968. "Transfusion in America in the Eighteenth and Nineteenth Centuries." *New England Journal of Medicine* 279: 1319–1320.

Starr, Douglas. *An Epic History of Medicine and Commerce.* New York: Alfred A. Knopf, 1998.

Trench Fever (Volhynian Fever)

Trench fever, also known as Volhynian fever, is a disease caused by *Rochalimaia quintana* (named for its discoverer, H. da Rocha Lima, and the disease's typical five-day course). Rochalimaia is a rickettsial organism related to that which causes typhus and Rocky Mountain spotted fever. Humans are the only reservoir for the disease, which is transmitted when the louse bites a carrier and defecates on the skin of another host. When the new host scratches and breaks skin contaminated by the feces, the microorganism enters the bloodstream.

Trench fever is typically manifested as a rash, fever, and bone and joint pain. The bone pain lasts for several weeks after the illness has subsided and is often incapacitating. True typhus, although common and lethal on the Eastern Front during World War I, was virtually nonexistent in France during the war. Trench fever, on the other hand, accounted for one-fifth of the illness in the German and Austrian armies and as much as one-third of that in the British army between 1915 and 1918.

By 1916, experiments on human volunteers had confirmed the role of the body louse in transmission of trench fever, and delousing became a priority. Men were rotated to rear areas as often as possible, where they were bathed, shaved, and chemically deloused. Clothing was also rotated, with uniforms traded for those left by the preceding group, which had been steam cleaned for reuse.

After World War I, trench fever largely disappeared until the 1990s, when it re-emerged among homeless alcoholics in France and the United States; in impoverished populations in Russia, Mexico, and Poland; and in patients with AIDS.

Jack McCallum

Further Reading

Biddle, Wayne. *A Field Guide to Germs*. New York: Anchor Books, 1995.

Schaechter, Moselio, Gerald Medhoff, and Barry I. Wisenstein. *Mechanisms of Microbial Disease*. Baltimore: Williams & Wilkins Co., 1993.

Trench Foot

Trench foot is an incapacitating deterioration in the skin of the foot that was particularly common in the trenches of the Western Front during World War I. Trench foot became a serious problem on the Western Front as soon as the battle lines became fixed and the weather turned cold. Men in the trenches stood for hours in cramped spaces, often up to their ankles in nearly freezing mud. Their tightly wrapped puttees around the lower leg further hampered blood circulation, and the men went for weeks without removing wet, filthy socks and shoes. When they did leave the trenches and took off their socks, soldiers often found white, swollen, insensate feet and, in the worst cases, rotting toes were left behind in their shoes.

By the winter of 1916, up to one-fifth of some units were incapacitated by trench foot. Senior officers initially viewed the problem as self-inflicted, and it became the responsibility of every junior officer to ensure that his men carried dry socks at all times and removed their shoes and socks and rubbed their feet with whale oil daily. When the English recognized that Belgian soldiers—who did not wear tight leg wraps—rarely got trench foot, they abandoned puttees. Still, the problem was severe enough that many men, when they were rotated to the rear, found it impossible to walk and had to be carried out on their comrades' backs. Nurses in rear-area hospitals massaged the dead feet with warm oil, and military surgeons removed necrotic toes as necessary while waiting for the extremities to turn from white to pink. By 1917, military surgeons recognized that trench foot carried an exceptional risk of associated tetanus, and sufferers were routinely vaccinated.

Jack McCallum

Further Reading

Fauntleroy, A. M. *Report on the Medico-Military Aspects of the European War*. Washington, D.C.: Government Printing Office, 1915.

Keen, W. W. *The Treatment of War Wounds*. Philadelphia: W. B. Saunders Co., 1918.

MacDonald, Lyn. *1914–1918: Voices and Images of the Great War*. London: Michael Joseph, Ltd., 1988.

X-Ray

X-ray is short wavelength, high-energy radiation that can be used to visualize internal body structures.

German physicist Wilhelm Conrad Röntgen first noted on December 28, 1895, that a wave form different from electrons could be generated from a cathode ray tube. Shortly thereafter, he noticed that those rays penetrated skin more easily than bone and would leave a shadow of the bone on a photographic plate. He described the finding to a friend, who communicated it to a relative who edited *Die Presse* in Vienna, and the newspaper ran a front-page story about the discovery on January 5, 1896. Within days, the story was repeated in newspapers around the world.

Both the public and medical professionals realized almost immediately the medical potential of X-rays in defining fractures and locating foreign bodies. On February 3, the first clinical X-ray image in the United States was produced at Dartmouth College on a child with a fractured forearm. Two days later, scientists at the U.S. Military Academy at West Point experimented with the penetration of X-rays through steel, bronze, and copper. Within the following month, Giuseppe Alvaro used X-rays to find bullets in two soldiers. Both bullets were successfully located and removed. During the Greco-Turkish War of 1897, the German Red Cross put an X-ray machine at the Turkish Yildiz Hospital in Constantinople, and the British put a machine near Athens to use on Greek wounded. Both were restricted to rear-area facilities because of the delicacy of the X-ray tubes and difficulty getting reliable power sources.

Although the British Surgeon Major Walter C. Beevor managed to haul an X-ray machine and a hand-operated dynamo to the front during the 1897–1898 Tirah campaign in India, military surgeons continued to take the point of view that X-rays were best used in a delayed fashion. There was widespread feeling that making it easy to locate bullets inside the body might encourage young surgeons to operate more often than was actually necessary. Still, X-ray imaging made it much less necessary to probe deep in body cavities for lost projectiles, and X-rays were regularly employed during the British Nile expedition in September 1898. During the Spanish-American War, U.S. Army and Navy surgeons used a total of 17 X-ray machines manufactured by the Edison Company and General Electric, among others, which were kept on the hospital ships sailing off the coast of Cuba. Physicians on these vessels were also the first to describe burns from X-ray overdose.

By World War I, X-ray had become a standard tool in the military surgical armamentarium, and Marie Curie personally operated a unit near the French lines. Interestingly, forward surgical teams in Iraq and Afghanistan have forgone X-ray in advance surgical units under the assumption that fractures can be treated based on physical examination and surgery extensive enough to require X-ray diagnosis is best done elsewhere.

Jack McCallum

Further Reading

Bruwer, André, ed. *Classic Descriptions in Diagnostic Roentgenology*. Springfield, IL: Charles C. Thomas, 1964.

Cirillo, Vincent. *Bullets and Bacilli: The Spanish-American War and Military Medicine*. New Brunswick, NJ: Rutgers University Press, 1999.

Eisenberg, Ronald. *Radiology: An Illustrated History*. St. Louis: Mosby Year Book, 1992.

DOCUMENTS

Answering the Call: The U.S. Army Nurse Corps, 1917–1919

Although female nurses had long served with the military, not until 1901 were they formally accepted into the U.S. Army Medical Department. The Army Nurse Corps was not formally organized until 1918. During World War I, about 10, 660 nurses went to Europe with the American Expeditionary Force. The following excerpts include a schematic diagram showing how wounded were evacuated from the front lines back to the advance base hospitals. Most nurses served away from the front in rear-area hospitals. The printed excerpts, written by two female nurses, relate their experience at these hospitals. The statement about dealing "with the inevitable infection" describes the reality of military medical care before the advent of antibiotics. Medical personnel fought infection in gaping wounds with tetanus antitoxin, debridement, and irrigation. Nurses irrigated open wounds with various antiseptics, usually Dakin's solution. For broken limbs, nurses used bed frames (Bradford or Balkan) with extensions for traction of broken limbs, and hung bottles of Dakin's solution for irrigation. All of these procedures marked tremendous improvements over past eras of military medical care.

"Our census increases day by day. We receive and evacuate every other day, more arrive than are sent away, my floor is fairly quiet after mid-night. Most of the patients sleep through Dakin irrigations, yet when they are awake they fuss considerably about treatments. Last Thursday we received a large convoy at an early morning hour and we stayed on duty until after our evening meal. That evening 16 of our patients went to surgery, no operating done after 11 PM. These are busy nights and busier days ... our patients are coming directly from The Front and they say it is terrible, lying there waiting for help to come. All come in awful condition, no previous care has been given to their wounds. It takes a lot of soaking to clean their wounds, dried blood, filth and dirt and lice. The bath house is not able to cope with the situation and neither can our limited staff and walking patients.

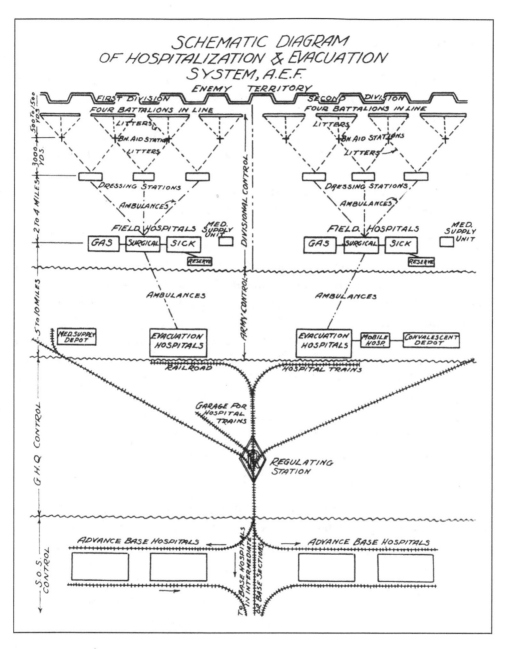

FIGURE 6.1. A schematic of doctrinally ideal evacuation from the battlefield. In practice, the American Expeditionary Forces (AEF) deviated from this model when the situation warranted. (Ireland, Major General M.W. The Medical Department of the United States Army in the World War, Vol. VIII, U.S. Government Printing Office: Washington, D.C., 1927, p. 262.)

Four of our nurses left for the Front, conditions are worse there. We do have a roof, a floor and everyone is fed after a fashion. No one works less than 12 hours in 24 and most of us do more. I see no one these days but my patients. I am happier than any time since in France, I feel I am really needed." (Essig, Maude Frances. *My Trip Abroad With Uncle Sam: 1917–1919. American Expeditionary Forces in France, Reserve Army Nurse Corps, American Red Cross Nurse #4411 ("How We Won World War I"). Undated. Photocopied collection in Army Nurse Corps Archives, Office of Medical History, The Office of the Surgeon General, Falls Church, VA. July 29, 1918.)

"Battle casualties with open wounds required yet another plan of care in the pre-antibiotic era of World War I. Their treatment included extensive wound debridement and irrigation through perforated red rubber tubes with Carrel-Dakin solution (sodium hypochlorite) to deal with the inevitable infection. Staff administered tetanus antitoxin to all such patients routinely. Nurses cared for those with orthopaedic injuries in Bradford frames and extension devices for traction." (Sarnecky, Mary T. *A History of the U.S. Army Nurse Corps.* University of Pennsylvania Press: Philadelphia, PA, 1999, p. 96.)

"Venereal diseases have been subject to control by policies, medical, educational, and disciplinary, so different from those applied in any Army heretofore. . .It is not too much to say that the official attitude of the Government as expressed in orders from the War Department and from the commander in chief supported by a logical medical service for the prevention and treatment of venereal diseases, have resulted in a smaller loss of man power to the Army, a lower incidence rate of the diseases, and a small number of permanently disabled and invalided men from these diseases than has been recorded in any other army up to the present time . . .

These diseases, when treated according to the information available through medical science, can be controlled, and to a greater degree than ever before have been controlled, by applying the principles of preventive medicine, namely, diminution of contact with human sources of infection, prophylactic treatment promptly after exposure, and segregation with intensive treatment for those in the communicable stages of the diseases." *Report of the Surgeon General U.S. Army to the Secretary of War, 1919, Vol.* II. (Government Printing Office: Washington, D.C., 1919, p. 1312.)

Army nurse Helen Fairchild, from Pennsylvania, volunteered to go overseas with 63 other nurses from Pennsylvania Hospital just one month after the United States declared war in April 1917. She was 32 years old when she served with Base Hospital No. 10, stationed at Le Treport, France.

Fairchild had had a history of abdominal pain before she left for France, and during November 1917 she suffered from a recurrence. By Christmas she was vomiting after every meal, and in January X-rays and exploratory surgery revealed a massive gastric ulcer, caused or worsened by exposure to mustard gas used by the enemy. She underwent a gastro-enterostomy on January 13, 1918, and initially did well but became jaundiced on the third day postoperative and deteriorated rapidly. She died in a coma on January 18, 1918.

Fairchild's cause of death was initially attributed to acute atrophy of the liver, but a post-mortem examination showed the final cause of death to be hepatic complications of the chloroform used for her general anaesthetic.

Fairchild received a full military funeral attended by an entire garrison of English, Canadian, French, and American officers, nurses, and troops. She was buried first in Mont Huron Cemetery, Le Treport, and later reburied in the American Cemetery at Bony (Somme), France. (Rote, Nelle Fairchild. *Nurse Helen Fairchild,* WW1 1917–1918, Fisher Fairchild Publishing Co.: Lewisburg, PA, 2004.)

Source: Lisa M. Budreau and Richard M. Prior. *Answering the Call: The U.S. Army Nurse Corps, 1917–1919.* Washington, D.C.: Office of the Surgeon General, U.S. Army, Borden Institute, Walter Reed Army Medical Center, 2008, pp. 68, 102, 183, 192.

■ CHAPTER 7
World War II

INTRODUCTION

When Japan attacked Pearl Harbor on December 7, 1941, America was thrust in World War II. Thereafter, about 16.1 million Americans served in the armed forces. The Army Medical Department expanded rapidly from 13,000 officers and men in 1939 to 664,000 by war's end. In the United States military, including the Merchant Marine, about 292,000 died in battle during the war. About 670,000 soldiers, sailors, airmen, and marines were wounded. Whereas in World War I, between 8 and 11 of each 100 wounded who reached forward hospitals alive subsequently died, in World War II this figure declined to 4.5 per 100 wounded. The major reasons for this reduction in death rates included improvements in transportation and triage, the use of antibiotics, and the use of blood plasma and whole blood for transfusions.

Better transportation and triage were made possible by improvement in systems first tried in World War I. By 1939 military surgeons recognized the importance of early management of battlefield trauma. Medics trained and equipped to control blood loss and administer analgesics at the initial site of injury were regularly attached to individual combat units. About one in twelve U.S. Army soldiers were trained as combat medics. They employed injectable morphine on the battlefield to reduce both pain and shock during evacuation.

Transport from the field was organized in stages, with each step assigned a specific range of duties.

The first stop after field stabilization was the regimental collecting station, where hemostatic bandages and splints could be applied. The collecting stations also had plasma or blood available to manage shock and could secure adequate ventilation, including tracheotomy if needed. From the collecting station, men could be moved to semimobile field hospitals equipped to perform emergency surgery. The field hospitals were the first stage fully staffed with physicians. From the field hospital, men could be moved to fixed-station or general hospitals where more complex procedures (neurosurgery, chest surgery, orthopedic reconstructions, and the like) could be performed and where men expected to return to duty could convalesce. General and rehabilitation hospitals in the zone of the interior provided major reconstruction (predominantly orthopedic and plastic surgical procedures) and long-term rehabilitation if necessary. Depending on the severity of injury, a wounded man could exit the system and return to duty at any point in the chain. The war featured a low morality rate in large part because of the rapidity with which seriously wounded men moved through the evacuation system to receive appropriate specialized care.

Development of the freely moveable hospital blossomed in World War II. These "auxiliary surgical teams" remained somewhat difficult to transport and limited in the services they could provide but were an important interim step toward the mobile army surgical hospitals of Korea and Vietnam. Aeromedical evacuation, although tried in a crude way in World War I, came into its own in World War II. It largely involved use of fixed-wing aircraft to move men from field or general hospitals to facilities in the zone of the interior. Medical air transport became especially sophisticated in the long distances of the Pacific war, where the Army Nurse Corps developed the expertise in managing patients during prolonged transit that presaged current civilian and military flight nurses.

The island war in the Pacific presented unique problems in medical evacuation; the distances were inordinately long, and there was almost never an accessible general hospital to augment basic field hospital care. The U.S. Navy employed hospital ships to unprecedented advantage in World War II. At the beginning of the war, the Navy had only two hospital ships, and only one of these was in the Pacific. During the war, the United States commissioned an additional eight hospital ships and developed an entire class of troop transports equipped to provide limited hospital services. The Navy also deployed a series of adapted landing craft manned with four surgeons and 27 corpsmen and capable of serving as field hospitals for up to 350 wounded. Hospital ships were held well back from areas of direct combat and served essentially the same role as land-based general hospitals.

Although some new surgical techniques, particularly in vascular surgery, were developed during World War II, the primary advances were in early management and treatment of physiologic effects of trauma. Medics made almost immediate hemostasis and pain management a standard. Better understanding of the mechanisms and treatment of shock came early in the war. Shock is clinically characterized by a fall in blood pressure, a rise in the pulse, coolness and discoloration of poorly perfused extremities, and mental changes ranging from anxiety through confusion to coma. The syndrome's common denominator is failure of the heart and circulatory system to supply adequate blood to the body's organs. In the early years of the war clinicians realized that poor perfusion was the common factor in a variety of types of shock. Blood loss, loss of body fluid such as that caused by weeping burn wounds, sepsis with its toxic bacteriologic by-products, and extreme cold can all cause the circulatory system to fail. The physiologic effects of that failure can (at least temporarily) be ameliorated by increasing the amount of fluid in the system.

Soviet scientists in the 1930s had shown that plasma—blood with red cells removed—could be effectively used to treat shock. Plasma had two signal advantages: unlike whole blood, it was not type specific, and it could be readily stored for long periods. Plasma could be started by medics at the front, and it was widely administered from the early days of the war. Recognizing the need for blood and plasma, the British started a national blood banking program early in the war, a collection and storage system the Americans later enlarged and improved. As the war progressed, plasma's limitations as a replacement for lost blood became evident, and use of whole blood to treat shock became more prevalent. Although civilian donors played a major role in supplying the blood banks, most donations came from combatants themselves, with medics providing a disproportionate share. In addition to whole blood, military surgeons had cardiac stimulants and vasoconstrictors, such as adrenaline and ephedrine to augment perfusion.

Military medicine also saw significant advances in management of infectious diseases during World War II. These improvements primarily involved treatment and control of tropical diseases, control of diseases resulting from poor sanitation aggravated by dietary deficiency, and chemical treatment of infections.

The Pacific war forced Japanese and Allied soldiers to fight in areas where tropical infections, especially malaria, were endemic. In the latter part of 1942 and early 1943, American soldiers in the Solomon Islands were hospitalized for malaria at a rate of 970 per 1,000 per year, with 100,000 men ultimately contracting the disease. The unacceptable loss of fighting men led General Douglas MacArthur to form the Combined Advisory Committee on Tropical Medicine, Hygiene, and Sanitation. The committee instituted preventive measures that brought an 85 percent decrease in the hospitalization rate within six months.

Quinine was the agent of choice in treating malaria at the beginning of the war, but the Japanese captured the drug's major sources of supply. The antimalarial Atabrine was developed as a synthetic substitute, and, although soldiers had to be forced to take it because of its bitter taste and tendency to turn the skin yellow, 2.5 billion doses had been dispensed by war's end. Vigorous efforts were used to control the Anopheles mosquito that carried the disease, including oil coating of breeding ponds and spraying with the newly developed chemical insecticide DDT. As a result of these preventive measures, less than one percent of hospitalized American personnel had malaria by the end of 1943. Besides malaria, soldiers in the Pacific Theater suffered from dengue fever (an untreatable, incapacitating, but usually self-limited viral disease), various forms of infectious diarrhea, and fungal skin diseases (collectively termed "jungle rot").

DDT was also used to kill body lice that carried typhus. Typhus, a louse-borne rickettsial disease, was the most threatening infectious disease in the European

Theater. When the Allies launched the North African offensive, the area was in the midst of a typhus epidemic that ultimately infected more than 500,000 civilians. The U.S. Army received a vaccine mass-produced by a process developed in the U.S. Department of Agriculture, and only 11 men out of a force of nearly half a million contracted typhus. Allied troops arrived in Europe vaccinated against typhus, typhoid, paratyphoid, and smallpox, but malaria remained a significant problem, especially in Italy, because Allied soldiers resisted taking Atabrine.

One of the most important advances in treatment of wartime trauma was the use of antibiotics. Following the attack on Pearl Harbor, the National Research Council reported that the use of sulfanilamide and sulfathiazole reduced morality and controlled infection. In contrast to World War I, when about 80 percent of men with perforating abdominal wounds died, most of the Pearl Harbor casualties who survived shock to undergo surgery and sulfonamide therapy recovered. Shortly thereafter, sulfa drugs became routine treatment for pneumonia, gonorrhea, meningitis, dysentery, and streptococcal infections. Only after the war did scientists realize that sulfa drugs were an effective antimicrobial agent that limited bacterial growth whereas penicillin killed bacteria.

Improvements in aviation and submarine technology outstripped the ability of humans to adapt to newly accessible environments. The extremes of temperature, pressure, and atmosphere became acute concerns as great depths and nearly stratospheric altitudes were reached. Warplanes had service ceilings well beyond the survival capabilities of humans without artificial pressurization. Supplemental oxygen was required above 10,000 feet, and daytime bombing missions at altitudes in excess of 25,000 feet were the rule in the European Theater. At these altitudes, temperatures ranged as low as −50°F, posing significant risk of frostbite or even hypothermic shock. A dive-bomber could descend at 30,000 feet per minute (compared with a commercial airliner's 400 feet per minute), a rate that introduced serious risk of barotrauma to the middle ear, sinuses, or intestines. Pooling of blood in the extremities due to extreme gravitational forces from rapid acceleration caused loss of vision and unconsciousness. Allied pilots taped their legs and abdomens to protect against blackouts, and the Germans manufactured the first pressurized bodysuit with the same goal. Rapid ascent, either from the deep ocean to the surface or from the surface to high altitudes, produced intravascular nitrogen bubbles leading to the syndrome of joint pain and stroke, collectively referred to as the bends.

World War II proved a transformational event for American society. Those changes affected the military medical establishment in numerous ways. Penicillin served as a catalyst for the rapid development of the worldwide pharmaceutical industry. The success of medical air transport stimulated the further development of a modern system utilizing helicopters for emergency evacuations. The field of psychiatry made major advances. The military's medical departments expanded into a complex health care organization featuring specialists in new areas including diet, physical therapy, and pharmacology. All of these improvements paved the way for subsequent advances in treating the physical and psychological casualties of war.

In broad terms, World War II featured advances in triage and transport, management of shock, and treatment of infectious diseases, as well as the emergence of aviation and submarine medicine. Nazi Germany had used human captives to perform medical experiments including extending exposure to cold and high altitude under the subjects died. This gross misuse of human experimentation led to new international standards for medical research.

James R. Arnold

ENTRIES

Combat Fatigue

The term "combat fatigue" was coined during World War II; in other wars, the symptoms that comprise it have been variously referred to as battle fatigue, war neurosis, exhaustion, shell shock, and posttraumatic stress disorder. Combat fatigue is a group of ill-defined symptoms including excessive fatigue, an exaggerated startle response, tremors, violence, nightmares, delusions, hallucinations, withdrawal, and catatonia.

Ancient historians described combat-induced mental illness, but diagnosing battle-related behavioral abnormalities as a disease was rare prior to the 20th century. In World War I, the problem was termed "shell shock" under the mistaken theory that explosive concussions caused small brain hemorrhages, leading to cerebral dysfunction. By World War II it was widely understood that the symptoms were psychiatric in nature, were similar to traumatic neuroses seen in the civilian population, and were not associated with identifiable anatomic brain damage.

In spite of an early British emphasis on battlefield psychiatry during World War II and an American attempt to exclude men with psychiatric illness from military service, mental illness remained a major cause of combat disability, with about 30 percent of Allied combat zone casualties being psychiatric in nature. Although physicians in World War I had shown that treatment close to the front lines made it possible to return a number of psychiatrically disabled soldiers to combat, the lesson had been forgotten. Early in World War II, patients with what was now called combat fatigue were routinely evacuated to rehabilitation hospitals, and most were discharged from the military. As manpower became scarce, more of these men were placed in pioneer or labor details in the rear area, but few returned to combat.

Captain Frederick R. Hanson, an American neurologist and neurosurgeon who had joined the Canadian Army early in the war and participated in the landing at

Dieppe, transferred to the U.S. Army and developed what became a successful and widely employed treatment for combat fatigue, also euphemistically referred to as "exhaustion." The essential parts of the regimen included sedation, brief periods of rest, and treatment in a facility close to the front where the patients and staff continued to wear combat uniforms. Hanson realized that treating these patients as if they were mentally ill and physically separating them from their units made it unlikely that they would return to duty. Using his treatment protocols, the British and American armies were able to return 70–80 percent of combat fatigue victims to their units, and only 15–20 percent of patients requiring evacuation to the zone of the interior were psychiatric.

Shortly after the Italian invasion, the U.S. Army established the post of division psychiatrist, and Hanson produced a manual for internists so nonpsychiatrists could use his methods. As the war went on, Allied military psychiatrists became convinced that no soldier was immune from combat fatigue. They hypothesized that any man subject to continuous combat for a long enough time would become nonfunctional and estimated that 200 days of constant action was about the maximum a soldier could be expected to tolerate. The British adopted a system of unit rotation to give their men regular periods of rest and were able to stretch the length of tolerance to nearly 400 days, but the Americans, except in the Army Air Corps, adopted a more haphazard approach of rotating individuals with the longest periods of service rather than rotating units as a whole. Individual rotation worked poorly and was finally replaced with the British system late in the war.

Military physicians, mindful of the heavy clinical and financial burden of long-term psychiatric illness after World War I, correctly predicted that the true cost of combat fatigue would not become evident until well after the soldiers returned to civilian life.

Jack McCallum

Further Reading

Cowdrey, Albert E. *Fighting for Life: American Military Medicine in World War II.* New York: Free Press, 1994.

Slight, David. "Psychiatry and the War." In William H. Taliaferro, *Medicine and the War.* Chicago: University of Chicago Press, 1944.

DDT (Dichlorodiphenyltrichloroethane)

Dichlorodiphenyltrichloroethane (DDT) is an insecticide introduced in 1940 that was key to the control of insect-borne diseases in the later years of World War II. Louse-borne typhus had killed 2.5 million soldiers and civilians on the Eastern Front during World War I and had broken out in Eastern Europe and North Africa when the United States entered the war in 1941. Insect-borne disease was not just a problem on the European fronts: American military surgeons estimated

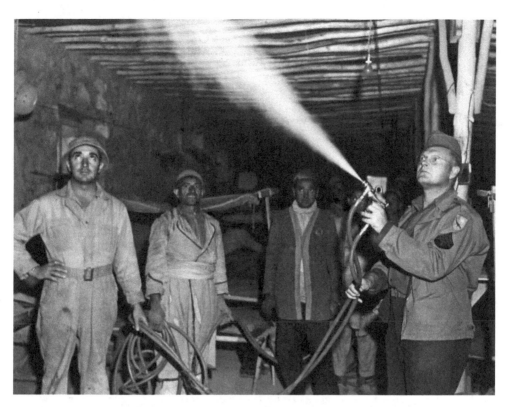

Introduced in 1940, DDT (Dichlorodiphenyltrichloroethane) greatly helped control insect-borne diseases during World War II. Here DDT is sprayed in a field hospital barracks. (National Library of Medicine)

that up to half of all troops deployed in the Pacific Theater of Operations might be infected by malarial mosquitoes. With those risks in mind, the War Department enlisted civilian and governmental research agencies including the Rockefeller Institute and the Department of Agriculture's Orlando, Florida-based Bureau of Entomology and Plant Quarantine to develop an insecticide that could be effective at low concentrations, that would be easily spread, that would persist in the environment, and that did not harm humans.

The Rockefeller louse lab and the Bureau evaluated more than 8,000 chemicals using experiments that included infesting conscientious objectors with lice harvested from New York City homeless people. In 1942, pyrethrins derived from the heads of chrysanthemum flowers appeared to be the most effective way to kill lice, and the chemical was distributed to military units beginning in August of that year. However, most chrysanthemum supplies came from Japan or from Dalmatia, which was under German control, so an alternative source for the chemical was necessary.

In August 1942, Geigy Colour Company of Basel, Switzerland, offered use of its insecticide Gesarol. The agent was based on DDT, had been patented in 1940, and had already been proven effective against potato beetles. Because Switzerland maintained neutrality in the war, the chemical was made available to both the Allies and to Germany, but German scientists showed little interest. American investigators, on the other hand, quickly demonstrated that DDT powder admirably satisfied all their requirements. It did, however, have distressing side effects at high concentrations in some animals, particularly when used as a solution rather than as a powder. Army physicians ultimately decided that the risk of insect-borne disease outweighed the risk of side effects and started general distribution of the insecticide in May 1943.

During the remainder of that year, American laboratories produced 193,000 pounds of the chemical, and, by June 1945, production had reached 3 million pounds a month. DDT was hailed as the war's greatest contribution to human welfare and as equivalent in importance to penicillin and sulfa. Geigy's Paul Müller received the Nobel Prize for Physiology or Medicine in 1948 for his work with DDT.

When the insecticide was widely used after the war, a variety of undesirable effects, particularly on wildlife and the environment, became evident, and use of DDT in the United States was almost entirely banned in 1972.

Jack McCallum

Further Reading

Perkins, John. *Insects, Experts and the Insecticide Crisis: The Quest for New Pest Management Strategies*. New York: Plenum Publishing Corp., 1982.

Russell, Edmund. *War and Nature: Fighting Humans and Insects with Chemicals from World War I to Silent Spring*. Cambridge: Cambridge University Press, 2001.

Stapleton, Darwin H. 2005. "A Lost Chapter in the Early History of DDT: The Development of Anti-Typhus Technologies by the Rockefeller Foundation's louse laboratory, 1942–1944." *Technology and Culture* 46 (3): 513–540.

Field Hospitals

Field hospitals are mobile treatment facilities that began as rudimentary shelters near the front lines and have evolved into containerized modules with beds, laboratories, X-ray facilities, and operating suites.

In the 18th century, field hospitals served as dressing stations and places to stabilize wounds. Large operations and amputations remained the province of fixed, rear-area hospitals. The principal change in field hospitals through the middle of the 19th century was their increased use for performance of larger surgical procedures. French surgeons Baron Dominique-Jean Larrey and Pierre François Percy recognized that wounds, especially those inflicted by artillery or bullets, healed best if treated early. They introduced organized retrieval of the wounded by designated litter bearers and designed ingenious self-contained wagons with the equipment necessary to perform major surgical procedures that could follow armies and be deployed close to the front lines. Although the development of anesthesia, antisepsis, and X-ray in the latter half of the 19th century brought new opportunities for field surgery, mobile hospitals were less important in the static trench warfare of World War I than in the more mobile conflicts that had preceded it.

Field hospitals again became important in World War II. By the 1940s it was possible to load laboratories, blood banks, X-ray machines, and fully equipped operating rooms onto trucks, so field hospitals could follow the troops and were typically set up a few miles behind the front. The wounded were taken directly from forward-area dressing stations and all but the largest surgical procedures could be done in them. Convalescents could even be held for several days of post-operative observation. By the Korean Conflict, the field hospitals had grown into mobile army surgical hospitals (M.A.S.H. units) of up to 60 beds and were nearing the size and status of evacuation hospitals.

In the Vietnam War, helicopter transport and improved management of shock and multiple trauma resulted in a death rate for soldiers who arrived at a field hospital of only 2.6 percent. Current U.S. Army practice is to staff field hospitals with forward surgical teams typically composed of three general surgeons, one orthopedist, two nurse anesthetists, three nurses, and various medics and other support personnel. These teams travel with the troops and can set up a fully functioning hospital with four ventilator-equipped beds and two operating suites in 60 minutes. The entire facility, including three deployable rapid-assembly shelter units that can be joined to form a 900-square-foot facility, is carried in six Humvees. Surgical and laboratory facilities are sufficient to perform surgery on up to 30 wounded soldiers. Modern field hospitals have also become a major element in planning for nonmilitary disasters, and civil authorities around the world have stockpiled these units.

Jack McCallum

Further Reading

Gawande, Atul. 2004. "Casualties of War—Military Care for the Wounded from Iraq and Afghanistan." *New England Journal of Medicine* 351 (December): 2471–2475.

Heizmann, Charles. 1917–1918. "Military Sanitation in the Sixteenth, Seventeenth and Eighteenth Centuries." *Annals of Medical History* 1: 281–300.

Stewart, John, and Frank Warner. 1945. "Observations on the Severely Wounded in Forward Field Hospitals: With Special Reference to Wound Shock." *Annals of Surgery* 122 (August): 129–146.

Gonorrhea

Gonorrhea is an infection of the mucous membranes of the male or female urogenital tracts caused by *Neisseria gonorrhoeae*. The gonococcus and its close relative the meningococcus are responsible for virtually all human disease from gram-negative cocci. The disease is characterized by burning and pain on urination and may be accompanied by a genital ulcer. In rare cases, gonorrhea may progress to septicemia with involvement of joints and widespread, pustular skin rash. Although penicillin was, at one time, the main treatment, most gonorrheal organisms are now resistant and must be treated with third-generation cephalosporins.

Until the late 17th century, medical writers failed to distinguish between syphilis and gonorrhea, a situation made more confusing when English military surgeon John Hunter deliberately injected himself with material from the pustule of a patient with gonorrhea. The man had syphilis as well and, when Hunter acquired both diseases, he incorrectly concluded that the two were one illness.

With control of syphilis, gonorrhea became the predominant venereal infection among soldiers. During World War II, venereal disease accounted for as many admissions as all other infections combined, with the majority being from gonorrhea. Among American troops, 1,250,846 soldiers were treated for sexually transmitted diseases. Because penicillin was still effective in the 1940s, it was used widely among both troops and German prostitutes. When antibiotic supplies were limited, a tactical decision was made to use available penicillin for gonorrhea rather than for wounds on the theory that treating soldiers suffering from the former was more likely to result in an effective combatant than treating the latter. After the war, prostitutes received penicillin preferentially rather than making it available for more serious illnesses in other civilians.

Venereal disease during the Korean Conflict came, in large part, as a result of infection acquired from Japanese prostitutes, 75 percent of whom had gonorrhea. Incidence of venereal disease in Vietnam varied from 196 to 281 per 1,000 troops between 1965 and 1970 and was mostly gonorrhea, making it by far the most common infectious disease during that war.

Jack McCallum

Further Reading

Cowdrey, Albert. *United States Army in the Korean War.* Washington, D.C.: Center of Military History, 1987.

Lada, John. *Medical Statistics in World War II.* Washington, D.C.: Office of the Surgeon General, 1975.

Neel, Spurgeon. *Medical Support of the U.S. Army in Vietnam: 1965–1970.* Washington, D.C.: Department of the Army, 1973.

Head Injury and Cranial Surgery

Head injury remains one of the major causes of death from war wounds. Head injuries can be divided into those caused by acceleration-deceleration (such as falls or vehicular injuries, from chariots to motorized personnel transports), low-velocity impact injuries (rocks, clubs, maces, and swords), and high-velocity impact injuries (bullets, shrapnel, and blast injuries). The first two have been present since before recorded history, while the last is unique to more modern times.

Greek and Roman understanding of cerebral anatomy and physiology was limited and often incorrect, and many of their mistakes persisted well after the Renaissance. In the 17th century, René Descartes pronounced the pineal gland the seat of the soul but continued to believe the animal spirit resided in the ventricles. Those misconceptions notwithstanding, the brain's importance was uncontested and, prior to the late 19th century, surgeons rarely violated it voluntarily.

The range of head injuries changed dramatically in the 15th century with the adaptation of gunpowder to warfare. High-velocity wounds penetrated the brain with a violence previously unimagined. Besides recognizing the direct tissue trauma from projectiles, early military surgeons were convinced that gunpowder itself was toxic.

In the 18th century, Percival Pott and Lorenz Heister independently suggested exploratory trephine in cases of paralysis. With the emerging understanding of cerebral localization, the idea that specific parts of the brain had specific functions, they recognized that relieving pressure from the side of the brain opposite the paralyzed parts might be of benefit, and they recommended drilling exploratory holes looking for blood clots that might cause that pressure. Still, they were only looking for blood between the dura and the skull and, although Pott suggested opening a tense, blue dura to look for deeper blood collections, he held out little hope that the patient with such a problem would survive. No one had the temerity to hunt for clots in the brain substance.

Realistic opportunities for survival from penetrating head injuries came as the result of a flurry of technical advances that began in the mid-19th century and included (roughly in order of development) anesthesia, antiseptic and then aseptic surgery, better diagnostic techniques including localization by physical examination and X-ray, antibiotics, and rapid transport and resuscitation.

Mortality from penetrating head wounds in the Crimean and American Civil wars was 73.9 percent and 71.6 percent, respectively. After 1865, Lord Joseph Lister's antiseptic and Ernst von Bergmann's aseptic surgical techniques and X-ray localization became available. Mortality from penetrating head wounds in World War I dropped to 35 percent. After development of sulfa and penicillin antibiotics, that mortality rate dropped to 14 percent in World War II. Emergency life support with artificial ventilation, better treatment of shock, and helicopter transport from the battlefield to well-equipped surgical facilities became standard during and after the Korean Conflict. Mortality from penetrating head injuries in Korea was 9.6 percent and that in Vietnam was 9.7 percent.

Jack McCallum

Further Reading

Coats, J. B., and A. M. Meirowsky. *Neurological Surgery of Trauma.* Washington, D.C.: Office of the Surgeon General, Department of the Army, 1965.

Cushing, Harvey. 1918. "Notes on Penetrating Injuries of the Brain." *British Medical Journal* 1: 221–226.

Gurdjian, E. S. *Head Injury from Antiquity to the Present with Special Reference to Penetrating Head Wounds.* Springfield, IL: Charles C. Thomas, 1973.

Hamman, W. H. 1971. "Analysis of 2187 Consecutive Penetrating Wounds of the Brain from Vietnam." *Journal of Neurosurgery* 34: 127–131.

Malaria

Malaria is a protozoal disease caused by one of five subspecies of plasmodium. Although 80 percent of the world's cases of malaria occur in tropical Africa, the disease has also been seen throughout Asia, Europe, and the Americas and has been endemic in both Europe and North America. The organism is transmitted by the female of one of several species of Anopheles mosquito that bite humans and ingest malarial gametocytes, one of the stages of the organism's complex developmental cycle. The protozoan multiplies in the mosquito's abdominal cavity before migrating to the insect's salivary glands, from which it is injected into a new victim. Once in the human bloodstream, the organism migrates to the liver, where it multiplies before returning to the bloodstream to enter red cells and feed on hemoglobin. When the victim is bitten by another mosquito, the malaria organism is ingested and the cycle begins again.

The genus *Plasmodium* has four species of which *falciparum* is the most lethal. An inoculation with the *falciparum* parasite can lead to cerebral malaria and death within a few days of infection. The three other species, sometimes popularly referred to as "baby" malaria, can lead to decades of recurring fever but are rarely fatal.

Malaria has been a recurrent problem for military forces and that problem fully emerged in World War II.

Java produced 95 percent of the world's quinine. When that island fell under Japanese control, the Allied forces were left without a reliable source of the drug. In the early stages of the Pacific campaign malaria disabled five times as many troops as did the Japanese, although subsequent development of the synthetic anti-malarial drug Atabrine alleviated the problem. Because malaria was endemic in the southern United States where many troops were being trained, local wetlands were drained and hundreds of thousands of acres were treated with insecticides.

Malaria again emerged as a major problem during the Vietnam War. It has been estimated that 70 percent of hospital admissions in the Vietnam War were for arthropod-borne diseases including malaria. Beginning with the U.S. invasion of Panama in the early 1990s, American military forces deployed to endemic malaria areas have been issued uniforms, tents, and bedding impregnated with permethrin, a synthetic form of the natural insect repellent produced by chrysanthemums. Still, of the 725 members of the U.S. Army Ranger task force deployed to eastern Afghanistan between June and September 2002, 38 were infected with *Plasmodium vivax.*

There is no vaccine to prevent malaria, and, although there is chemoprophylaxis to prevent the disease and chemotherapy to treat it, resistance to those drugs is increasingly common. Malaria remains the world's most common cause of death from infectious disease.

Jack McCallum

Further Reading

Cartwright, Frederick, and Michael Biddis. *Disease and History.* New York: Dorset Press, 1972.

Karlen, Arno. *Man and Microbes: Disease and Plagues in History and Modern Times.* New York: Simon & Schuster, 1996.

McNeil, William H. *Plagues and Peoples.* Garden City, NY: Anchor Press, 1976.

Nuclear Warfare and Radiation Injury

The first nuclear weapon to be used in warfare was dropped on Hiroshima, Japan, on August 6, 1945. The uranium-235 bomb was detonated at an altitude of 570 meters above ground level, had the destructive force of 12.5 kilotons of TNT, destroyed every structure within a five-square-mile area, and killed approximately 64,000 people during the subsequent 30 days. Three days after the first explosion, a second bomb was dropped on Nagasaki. This was a 29-kiloton plutonium-239 bomb that killed 40,000 people within 30 days. By comparison, the total number of fatalities was less than those in the Allied firebombing of either Dresden or Tokyo in 1945, and the United States dropped bombs with three times the explosive force of the two Japanese bombs combined on Vietnam in 1972 alone. Nevertheless, the atomic weapons came in single packages, were relatively cheap to produce and deliver, and provided no opportunity for flight or protection.

Immediate damage to the human body from atomic weapons is of three kinds: blast injury, burns, and radiation damage. The temperature in the 15-meter radius of the Hiroshima fireball was 300,000°C, so the primary injuries close to detonation were from blast effect and burns. Bare skin was burned as far as 3.5 kilometers from the blast site. About 70 percent of those who died had blast injury, 65 percent had burns, and 30 percent had radiation injury—many, of course, having more than one kind of injury.

The type of injury varies with the size of the weapon. A 1-kiloton device (typical for a tactical battlefield weapon) would produce lethal blast effect to an average radius of 0.55 kilometers from detonation, lethal burns to 0.35 kilometers, and

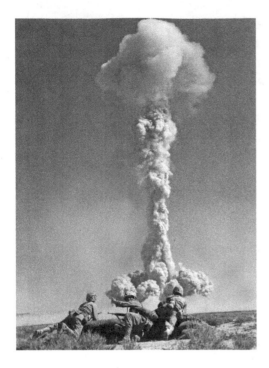

Nuclear weapons introduced a new challenge to military medicine. To familiarize soldiers with nuclear blasts, the military deliberately deployed units to observe nuclear blasts such as this one in Nevada in 1952. (Marine Corps Historical Center)

lethal radiation to 0.7 kilometers, making the last the most deadly. On the other hand, a 1-megaton device would have lethal thermal effect to a radius of 2.6 kilometers, while the blast would be lethal to 5.5 kilometers and radiation death would occur as far away as 9 kilometers.

While radiation would be irrelevant as a cause of death immediately after detonation, its residual effects would be devastating. A fissile explosion produces multiple unstable isotopes that emit primarily beta particles and gamma rays as they decay to stability. The radioactive half-lives of these isotopes vary from as little as a few seconds to as much as 10 million years. Ultimately, most of those within an area of 450 square miles around a 1-megaton detonation would become ill. In an air burst, about half of the radioactive particles produced will fall to earth within 24 hours, but smaller amounts will continue to be carried in the wind and will fall on virtually every part of the planet over the subsequent six months. Radiation dose can be acquired externally from either the air or ground or internally by ingestion or inhalation and can damage a number of organs including the skin, eyes, bone marrow, thyroid, lungs, liver, and sexual organs.

Acute radiation sickness affects primarily the gastrointestinal and neuromuscular systems. It begins with anorexia, nausea, vomiting, diarrhea, abdominal cramps, and dehydration. At high doses, radiation causes apathy, fatigue, fever, sweating, hypotension, shock, and death from cardiovascular collapse. About 90 percent of people with an exposure greater than 390 rads will get radiation sickness, and virtually all those with a dose of 500 rads will die. Delayed effects include asphyxia from pulmonary edema and widespread bleeding and inability to fight infection related to bone marrow failure and loss of platelets and white blood cells.

Much of our knowledge of the long-term effects of radiation comes from following survivors of the Japanese bombs and from sporadic inadvertent human exposures. Information on local effects of radiation fallout was gleaned from an episode in which a 15-megaton device was detonated over Bikini Atoll in the Pacific Ocean. Wind carried a radiation plume over inhabited parts of Micronesia, including the island of Rongelap, 105 miles away, where the inhabitants absorbed doses in excess of 175 rem in the 48 hours after the explosion. They suffered skin and corneal burns, had abnormal blood counts for 15 years, and had a high incidence of hypothyroidism and neoplastic thyroid nodules.

The Atomic Bomb Casualty Commission began collecting information on Japanese atomic bomb survivors in 1947 and continued to do so until it was replaced by the binational Japanese-American Radiation Effects Research Foundation in 1975. These groups studied life span and disease in survivors and in people who were in utero at the time of the explosions and compared them with matched controls. Nearly 80 percent of survivors came for annual checkups and almost 45 percent of those who subsequently died came to autopsy. The most striking late effect was leukemia, which peaked in incidence in 1952 and 1953. Those less than 10 years old at the time of exposure were most likely to develop one of the acute leukemias, while those over 50 in 1945 were susceptible to one of the chronic forms. Incidence of both increased with exposures as low as 20 to 30 rads. Multiple myeloma and cancers of the thyroid, breast, lung, and stomach developed for up to 20 years. Those exposed in utero were subject to microcephaly, mental retardation, and growth failure.

Jack McCallum

Further Reading

Adams, Ruth, and Susan Cullen, eds. *The Final Epidemic: Physicians and Scientists on Nuclear War*. Chicago: University of Chicago Press, 1981.

Penicillin

Penicillin was the first biologically derived antibiotic, and its application marked the beginning of a new era in battlefield surgery. Molds had been recommended for wound treatment for more than 1,500 years, but never in a systematic or generally effective way. In an 1897 dissertation, French medical student Ernest Duchesne, had shown that extract from the mold *Penicillium glaucum* protected laboratory animals subsequently inoculated with the bacterium that produces typhoid fever.

In 1928, bacteriologist Alexander Fleming returned to his laboratory at St. Mary's Hospital in London's Paddington suburb to find that cultures of staphylococcus that he had left scattered about had become spoiled by airborne molds.

On the verge of dipping them in Lysol, he noticed that some had a ring of killed bacteria around the clumps of cultured mold. Fleming incorrectly identified the mold as *Penicillium rubrum* (it was really *Penicillium notatum*) and reported his findings in the *British Journal of Experimental Pathology*, in which he named the active agent penicillin. Penicillin, however, proved to be extraordinarily difficult to extract and almost impossible to stabilize, and his mold cultures completely stopped producing the substance after about eight days. Unable to produce usable quantities of penicillin—and, in fact, unable to reproduce his original accidental experiment—Fleming moved on to other areas of research.

In 1938, Oxford University's Howard W. Florey assembled a research team that included immigrant bacteriologist Ernst Chain and Norman C. H. Heatley to look for effective antibacterial agents. Florey had been taught by Cecil Paine, who had been one of Fleming's students and had been an editor of the journal that published Fleming's original paper, so it is likely he already had some knowledge of penicillin when he adopted it as one of his areas of interest. By 1940 Florey's team extracted enough penicillin to test it on four laboratory mice with four more animals serving as controls. All the controls died while half of the treated mice survived. This result persuaded the team of penicillin's efficacy. The first human—a healthy volunteer—was injected with 100 milligrams of penicillin on January 27, 1941, but she suffered a severe febrile reaction from a contaminant in the preparation. The first actual clinical use of penicillin was February 1, 1941, when it was administered to London policeman Albert Alexander, who had cut himself shaving and gotten staphylococcal sepsis with osteomyelitis, pneumonia, and a necrotizing infection of his eye. Alexander initially improved, but Florey did not have enough penicillin to continue treatment in spite of recovering and reusing crystallized drug from the patient's urine. When the drug was stopped, Alexander relapsed and died. With the thought that children, being smaller, would need less drug, Florey next treated five children with sepsis that would have previously proven fatal. Four survived, and the fifth died of a brain hemorrhage without autopsy evidence of remaining infection.

By this time, the Battle of Britain was occupying the country's attention and all of its industrial capacity, leaving no resources for production of penicillin, so the Rockefeller Foundation paid for Florey and Heatley to come to the United States in July 1941, where Department of Agriculture officials put them in touch with the Northern Regional Research Laboratory at Peoria, Illinois. That laboratory was a national center of research on fermentation. At Peoria, three signal developments occurred. First, it was shown that addition of corn steep liquor (a by-product of corn syrup production) to Penicillium cultures could increase penicillin output by a factor of 10. Then, a strain of Penicillium retrieved from a moldy cantaloupe found in a Peoria market was shown to increase penicillin production by a factor of 200. Mutations of that organism induced by X-ray and ultraviolet radiation increased that rate to a factor of more than 1,000. Finally, cultures that had previously only grown on the surface of milk bottle–sized flasks were induced to grow throughout aerated 25,000-gallon tanks. That application made commercial production possible, and Alfred N. Richardson of the Office of Scientific Research and Development's Medical Research Committee enlisted Merck and Company, Charles Pfizer Company, and E. R. Squibb and Sons to the effort. It is likely that Richardson and the U.S. government were already considering the possible military uses of penicillin should the U.S. enter World War II.

In early 1943, only enough penicillin was produced to treat 100 people, even with urine recovery and reuse of the drug. By summer of that year, more drug was available, but it still cost more than $20 a dose. By 1944, American pharmaceutical companies were producing 300 billion units a month, and, by D-Day, enough penicillin was available to treat every British and American casualty from the invasion. In May 1945, when the drug was released to the civilian population, the price had dropped to $0.55 a dose.

By the end of the war, a previously unimaginable 95 percent of battlefield injuries that came to treatment were surviving, the death rate from pneumonia had dropped from 18 percent to less than 1 percent, and syphilis could be reliably treated. As Fleming had predicted, however, resistant strains of staphylococci began emerging almost as soon as penicillin became available. The bacteria acquired the ability to produce an enzyme—penicillinase—that broke the drug down and passed that trait from generation to generation. The first penicillin-resistant staphylococcus was identified in 1942, and, by 1952, 60 percent of staphylococci were resistant to even massive doses of the drug. In addition, widespread use of the drug led to allergic reactions; the first fatal case of penicillin-induced anaphylaxis was reported in 1949. Resistance and allergies triggered a search for variants of penicillin and entirely new drugs that is ongoing.

Jack McCallum

Further Reading

Boetcher, Helmuth M. *Wonder Drugs: A History of Antibiotics*. Philadelphia: J. B. Lippincott, 1963.

Maurois, André. *The Life of Sir Alexander Fleming, Discoverer of Penicillin*. New York: E. P. Dutton and Co., 1959.

Sheehan, John C. *The Enchanted Ring: The Untold Story of Penicillin*. Cambridge, MA: MIT Press, 1984.

Sulfonamides

Sulfonamides were the first class of chemical agents with wide applicability as specific antibiotics.

The story of synthetic antibiotics begins with German chemist Paul Ehrlich, who reasoned that, if histological dyes would selectively attach themselves to parts of bacteria, there might be other chemicals that would behave in a similar fashion and be toxic to the organisms instead of simply changing their color. His experiments with organic arsenicals led to discovery in 1909 of arsphenamine (or Compound 606, as it was the 606th compound his laboratory had tested), which had some activity against syphilis. Ehrlich's success encouraged I. G. Farbenindustrie to investigate possible antibacterial activity of the aniline dyes they manufactured. Farben chemist Gerhard Domagk found Prontosil in 1934 after empirically testing thousands of compounds. In 1935, French chemist Ernest Fournou of the Pasteur Institute showed that Prontosil was hydrolyzed to sulfanilamide, the actual antibacterial chemical, after administration.

After Fournou's discovery, sulfanilamide's importance was almost immediately recognized by researchers and clinicians, and a rush ensued to develop variants that eventually included sulfapyridine, sulfathiazole, and sulfaguanidine. Sulfa drugs were used by both sides in the Spanish Civil War, and they were a regular part of every modern army's supplies when World War II started in 1939. Sulfa powder was widely distributed and used to dust fresh wounds early in the war. American production of sulfa drugs started at 350,000 pounds in 1937 and rose to more than 10 million pounds by 1942. The indiscriminate use of the antibiotic led to early development of bacterial resistance and, by the end of the war, parenteral penicillin had largely replaced it. Nonetheless, sulfa drugs were used to treat President Franklin Roosevelt's skin infection and Prime Minister Winston Churchill's pneumonia during the war, and they played a major role in lowering the death rate from penetrating wounds, especially those involving the head. Sulfa drugs were also widely used against gonorrhea, and their effectiveness against dysentery gave Americans a significant advantage over their Japanese opponents in the Pacific who had only limited access to the drug.

By the end of World War II, bacterial resistance had rendered sulfa drugs largely ineffective in treating penetrating wounds, although they continued to have a role in treatment of burns, venereal disease, and urinary tract infections.

Jack McCallum

Further Reading

Miller, C. P., and M. Bornhoff. 1950. "The Development of Bacterial Resistance to Chemotherapeutic Agents." *Annual Review of Microbiology* 4 (October): 201–222.

Mohler, Henry K. 1941. "The Therapeutic Use of Sulfanilamide and Related Compounds." *The Military Surgeon* 88 (January): 473–486.

DOCUMENTS

Urology in World War II

In 1944, Brigadier General Hugh J. Morgan was the United States Army's Chief Consultant in Medicine. At a meeting of the Executive Committee of the American Urological Association, Morgan criticized the way urologists had historically dealt with gonorrhea. Gonorrhea had seriously afflicted thousands of American soldiers in World War I. The first excerpt provides part of the Surgeon General's report, submitted in 1919, that examined venereal diseases among American soldiers in Europe during World War I. At that time, the only reliable treatment was prevention. About 30 years later, medical personal could use a newly developed "miracle drug", penicillin, to treat venereal diseases. Morgan's criticism of urologists produced the following exchange of letters between Morgan and an urologist, Dr. David M. Davis. The letters allude to how medical personal treated venereal diseases before the discovery of penicillin as well as providing insight into the state of medical knowledge as antibiotics emerged as the treatment of choice. It is particularly noteworthy to find in Davis's second letter discussion of resistance to sulfonamide and his accurate prediction that resistance to penicillin would occur in the near future.

August 21, 1963

My dear John:

Here is the whole dossier on l'affaire Morgan. Now, almost twenty years later, the most amusing thing seems to me to be the 1944 papers delivered at the A.U.A. convention by Army Urologists on the treatment of gonorrhoea by penicillin.

The recent book by Laurence Stallings on the A.E.F. in World War I gives extensive notice to the conquest of venereal disease at that time by effective prevention according to the gospel of Young and Pershing. I still think the palms for the improved treatment in World War II will have to go to the chemists and urologists rather than to old Hugh Morgan, God rest his soul.

Keep the letters as long as you wish, but when you are through with them send them back unless you want them to remain in the Archives.

Kindest regards.
Sincerely,
DAVID M. DAVIS, M.D

June 24, 1944

My dear Hugh:
At a meeting of the Executive Committee of the American Urological Association in St. Louis this year it was alleged that you had stated in an address before an

Orthopedic Society that the treatment of gonorrhoea had been taken away from the Urologists in the Army as they were nothing but "rectal chiropractors". I stated that I could not believe that you would make any such statement; nevertheless, I think this allegation requires a categorical denial. It was further reported that in most of the Army hospitals the cooperation between the medical and urological departments was good, but that in some of them patients with complications, those with acute infections superimposed upon chronic infections or the results thereof, and sulfonamide-resistant and penicillin-resistant cases suffered from being under the care of medical officers unfamiliar with the natural history of the disease gonorrhoea, and further that the criteria of cure were in some cases inadequate. At present the treatment of acute gonorrhea consists of the injection of penicillin or the administration of sulfonamides, either of which may be performed by any physician. I am sure that most urologists are happy to be freed of this routine work, yet we must perforce continue to insist most emphatically that there be no failure or inadequacy in the treatment of soldier patients due to indifference or ignorance. It would seem desirable therefore to require at all times the closest cooperation between those charged with the treatment of gonorrhoea and the Urologists.

Sincerely,
David M. Davis, M.D.

29 June 1944

Dear David,
This is what I said in a facetious vein at the College of Physicians' Meeting:

> "What of the omnipresent problem of the venereal diseases in the Army? You will be relieved to learn that in this war the venereal diseases have finally made good their escape from the awkward and, as we now view it, medieval clutches of the urological surgeon who, armed with sound, syringe, silver salts, irrigating can. and a long, strong index finger, indulged his naive faith in irrigations and dilatations of the posterior urethra and chiropractic manipulations of the prostate and seminal vesicles. Nowadays gonorrhea is being allowed to remain a simple pyogenic infection of the anterior urethra, and secretions from which are provided, by the good God, with natural drainage and with frequent physiological irrigation. I am happy to report that at last in the Army the venereal diseases are officially assigned to the beneficent care of the internist. As a result, the complications of gonorrhea have become practically nonexistent."

I might have added that it is my sincere belief that few diseases have been so over-treated and, in the light of recent experience, mishandled in the past as gonorrhea. There isn't the slightest doubt in my mind but that practically all of the local 'complications' of gonorrhea (post-urethritis, seminal vesiculitis, prostatitis, stricture, etc.) and most of the metastatic complications (arthritis, endocarditis) stem from ill-advised irrigations and manipulations of the past era. These complications of gonorrhea were present in about one-fourth of Army cases before the advent of the sulfonamides. They have practically disappeared since. Of course, one can say that this proves nothing except that the sulfonamides cure gonorrhea. Nevertheless, circumstantial evidence (and, I suspect, your own good judgment) indicates that it isn't this alone which is responsible for the disappearance of complications. They have occurred in sulfonamide-treated gonorrhea when sounds and massage have been employed to supplement chemotherapy and to satisfy criteria for cure. Moreover, some of you urologists emphasized this long before 1935. It appears obvious to me that the pre-sulfonamide, local methods of treatment were responsible for the vast majority of the complications of gonorrhea.

I agree heartily that the urologist can and does contribute most helpfully in the management of local complications of gonorrhea. In Army practice this involves less than 1 percent of cases on many posts. I cannot agree that urologists in general are familiar with the "natural history of the disease". In the past they have been too busy treating it—and, in my opinion, encouraging its extension up the urinary tract. It is my opinion that rest and fluids would have been much better treatment in the pre-sulfonamide era than the usual urological practices. Of course, hindsight is often better than foresight, but I do think that we should be frank and admit our mistakes. When we are frank, we must admit that the use of surgical techniques afforded the patient few, if any, advantages in the past and many disadvantages. As I see it, the urologist will have little opportunity in the future to apply surgical techniques to the treatment of gonorrhea.

I wish we could sit down and talk this out. I have had little or no opportunity to discuss this matter with enlightened urologists. In the Army I have talked with a good many who simply would not give up the traditional attitude. Charlie Howe and I did have a chance to talk together once and I think we see eye to eye—and I suspect you and I would be in general agreement. I honestly think the urologists would be wise to close the chapter on gonorrhea. It's out of the urological field now, and I think you should let it stay out without protest – for the record isn't too good.

My 'dukes are up' and I'm braced for the attack!

With my good wishes and the hope that our paths will cross again soon, I am,

Sincerely,
HUGH J. MORGAN

July 3, 1944

My dear Hugh,
Many thanks for your prompt and enlightening reply to my recent letter. I am grateful for your attitude, and that your dukes are up. I feel that we can now slug it out, with no hard feeling, but pulling no punches.

I shall not contradict your statement that your remarks at the College of Physicians meeting were in a facetious vein, but I fail to find any evidence of facetiousness in the quotation. It sounds very serious and indeed official to me. I cannot forget that you occupy a position of eminence and great authority, and that you have made a violent and scornful attack on a whole branch of the medical profession, without any qualifications or exceptions. I believe that such a procedure was unworthy of the Chief Consultant in Medicine for the United States Army. I further believe that such an attack is, even without considering the details of the therapeutic problems involved, unjustifiable in that it is based on criticism of methods which at the time they were advocated were the best that were known. It would be just as easy to criticize internists for the futile treatment of pneumonia before the discovery of serum, sulfonamides, and penicillin, and of typhoid by the starvation treatment, or of diabetes before the discovery of insulin. I would not do so, because I know they were doing the best they could. Have you any evidence to prove that urologists as a whole are more unprogressive, stupider and more dishonest than internists as a whole? I do not believe that Osler, Thayer, Llewellys Baker, Warfield Longcope or Arthur Bloomfield would have handled the matter in this way.

You confess that you have had little or no opportunity to discuss this matter with enlightened urologists. That, my dear Hugh, is not my fault, nor the fault of any other enlightened urologist, but solely of yourself. Yet without such consultation you have gone ahead and made this very vital decision for the whole army, and have added a gratuitous attack on the sincerity and intelligence of the entire urological profession. I shall be quite frank to say that I think you should, after properly informing yourself, offer a wholehearted apology, just as public as the attack.

I do not know whether there is a Chief Consultant in Urology in the Army, and if there is, I do not know his name. I do know that the man who claims to control the Urological personnel is young, inexperienced, and only slightly acquainted with the Urological profession. I also know that all the urologists with sufficient age and experience, and with suitable character to fill this office acceptably are still at their civilian, and usually professorial, jobs. I do not know why Urology has been treated so contemptuously. I suspect that it is because those who have made the decisions are uninformed, and prejudiced because of things that are now ancient history.

While I cannot hope to cover all of the technical points involved in the treatment of gonorrhoea, I would like to mention a few. The treatment by bed-rest and fluids has been advocated by a good many men, but carried out more extensively in the United States Army than elsewhere, for the obvious reason that it is easier to subject soldiers than civilians to this regimen. The results showed no appreciable diminution in complications. Statistics available in your own office will confirm this. For many years the constant effort of all good Urologists has been to avoid overtreatment. The popular book of Pelouze is an example of this. The plain fact is that complications occur less frequently now because modern drug therapy quickly destroys the etiological agent. Complications are just as frequent as ever in drug-resistant cases. Thanks to the survival of sulfonamide-resistant strains, the failure rate after sulfonamide treatment has already risen to about twenty percent. The advent of penicillin was a God-send to the internists. Without it, they would be saddled with a steadily increasing number of sulfonamide-resistant cases. The failure rate after both sulfonamide and penicillin is now between one and two percent. It is an excellent prediction that this rate will rise as drug resistant strains are disseminated. Chronic urethritis is often due to old strictures, congenital, traumatic, or inflammatory, or to congenital stenosis of the meatus. Internists are scarcely in a position to discover these lesions. Chronic prostatitis is usually due to congenital contracture of the vesical orifice. The treatment of this disease by protracted prostatic massage is completely outmoded.

I am as anxious to be frank as you are. It is frank to say that all methods of treatment of gonorrhoea before the advent of sulfonamides were practically without any effect whatever. Gonorrhoea in the hands of the competent urologist, who sedulously avoided overtreatment, ran its natural unaffected course, just as it did in the Army hospitals under bed-rest and fluids. Urologists regretted this, but could not help it. They attempted to free patients from the results of their complications, and assist them to a complete and permanent cure. Why the discovery of new drugs, which has changed all this, should be made the occasion for condemning and humiliating all Urologists is beyond me.

I too wish we could sit down and talk this out. I should be happy to have you spend a day at my Clinic (we now have from two to ten cases of acute gonorrhoea per month in the dispensary), and to devote all the time you wish to discussion. I am proud of my specialty, and I think you will be too when you learn the facts.

Sincerely,
David M. Davis, M.D.

Source: John F. Patton. Medical Department, United States Army, Surgery in World War II: Urology. Office of the Surgeon General and Center of Military History, United States Army, Washington, D.C., 1987, pp. 70–74.

Nursing in World War II

Lillian Dunlop entered the Army Nurse Corps in November 1942. She served in the Pacific theater during World War II. The Pacific theater presented unique challenges for medical care. Many battles involved amphibious landings against fortified islands defended by fanatical Japanese soldiers. American casualties often were high. Wounded soldiers had to be evacuated to hospital ships since there were no nearby land-based hospitals. Thereafter, critical cases were transported by air so they could receive specialized care. Dunlop rose steadily through a series of increasingly important leadership positions culminating in her appointment as the 14th Chief of the Army Nurse Corps. The following excerpt relates her memories of nursing care given to the marines and soldiers who fought against the Japanese.

Treatments and Medications

I'd like to describe more of the treatments and medications that we used. In those days we gave a lot of sulpha, which was administered every four hours. The penicillin was a powdered concoction and had to be mixed up at the time we gave it. In other words, we couldn't mix it up in the morning for all the dosages we were going to give during the day. We had to mix it up just before we were going to give it. The powder and mixing solution had to be kept over in the laboratory. So the corpsman would go over to the laboratory and get the penicillin and we'd sit there and mix it up. We'd then draw up our syringes for the dosage we were going to give and fix up our tray with our penicillin. The corpsman would take a water pitcher and those envelope paper cups and the sulpha pills. The two of us would go around to the cots and we'd tap on the mosquito net. We used to laugh, because they'd stick a hand out for the sulpha and stick out their rear end where we'd poke it to give the penicillin. Then we'd go on to the next patient. So you can imagine what it was like each time the penicillins were given, some as often as every three or four hours. We were constantly mixing penicillins and getting our sulpha ready to give to the patients. They began to get some penicillin in the beeswax that was longer lasting. We'd only have to give that twice a day. But we didn't have much of that. The sulphas and penicillin were about all we had. Of course, there was atabrine for malaria and aspirin.

In addition to that we were busy doing dressings. I can remember our experience at Tacloban. We'd come on duty—this again was one long ward and one nurse covering two wards, maybe even covering 200 patients or so. We came on duty, and the dressing cart would be perhaps halfway down the ward. That's as far as they had gotten that day with changing dressings. So we'd start from that point, changing dressings and doing treatments that still needed to be done.

I saw my first gangrene in the Admiralties. Some of the Marines who had been on Cape Gloucester were sent down to us. They had received immediate medical care—morphine, bandages, and all—on the beaches, and then they were put on landing craft and sent down to us. Some of them had gangrene. They had received the antitoxin but it was outdated. Also, I saw my first scrub typhus. There is so much kunai grass up in Cape Gloucester that the sharp edges of the kunai grass cut the soldiers. The little mites had gotten into them. We saw scrub typhus and the malarias and, of course, hepatitis.

Patient Evacuation

We also had a lot of amputees, orthopedic patients, and neurosurgical patients. We did not have a means for quick evacuation of the patients. There was no scheduled evacuation. Sometimes we heard that there was a ship coming in. It took supplies on up ahead of us and it was coming back and was able to take out some patients to Australia. Well, naturally we tried to get the most critical patients we had, like the paraplegics, out. But some of the patients stayed for months before we could get them on a hospital ship to get them out to Australia. All of the transportation that they had was needed to get troops and supplies up and to bring casualties back as soon as they could. It was quite a challenge for nursing.

Source: Cynthia A. Gurney. *33 Years of Army Nursing: An Interview with Brigadier General Lillian Dunlap.* United States Army Nurse Corps, Washington D.C., 2001, pp. 28–29.

■ CHAPTER 8
Korean War

INTRODUCTION

The Korean War began on June 25, 1950, when North Korean forces crossed the 38th Parallel to invade South Korea. It ended in stalemate on July 27, 1953, with the 38th Parallel again serving as the line dividing the two Koreas. Because of its treaty commitment to South Korea and its zeal to contain the spread of Communism, the United States entered the war as soon as the North Koreans invaded. Although it began only half a decade after the end of World War II, the Korean conflict engendered signal advances in American military medicine, including the refinement of the Mobile Army Surgical Hospital (MASH), helicopter transport of the sick and wounded, and improvements in the treatment of vascular injuries, head injuries, and shock. Many of these techniques ultimately were translated to civilian medicine and have since become standards of care.

As had been the case in all of America's previous wars, military medicine was ill-prepared for the conflict. After World War II, military doctors were rapidly demobilized. Between June 1945 and June 1950, the Army Medical Corps lost 86 percent of its officers and 91 percent of its enlisted personnel. In an attempt to replenish the supply, residencies were opened at a number of army hospitals with the intent that, in return for being paid during postgraduate training, the new specialist physicians would serve for a time in the military. Unfortunately the program was new. The program's participants were still in training when the war began. In addition, civilian physicians were in relatively short supply, and those in domestic practice were busy and prosperous. Consequently, they were not keen to serve in Korea. A specific draft for physicians was not instituted until August 1950, and it produced no direct help in Korea until January 1951. By 1952, 90 percent of physicians serving in Korea were draftees.

The first military medical contingent in Korea was the Advance Command and Liaison Group of 15 officers and 2 enlisted men dispatched by the Far East Command (FEC) on June 27, 1950. Its mission was to care for American refugees fleeing the fighting and to begin replenishing supplies lost in the fall of Seoul.

Thereafter, the medical aspect of the war can be divided into three parts: offensive operations, defensive operations against invading forces and during withdrawal, and static defensive operations. These distinctions are important because the rate and type of injury differed among the three.

For the first time in the history of military medicine, data on battle and non-battle (further subdivided into disease and injury) casualties were collected on punch cards and returned to Washington for computer analysis by the Medical Department and the Surgeon General. The Adjutant General collected an entirely separate set of data, and the two sets do not uniformly agree. Surgeon General records report 18,769 killed in action, 77,788 wounded in action and admitted to treatment facilities, and 14,575 with wounds not requiring admission. The Adjutant General's records report 19,658 killed in action and 79,526 wounded in action. Only the Surgeon General collected data on disease and non-battle injury. A total of 443,163 patients were admitted to treatment facilities during the war; this included 365,375 non-battle admissions (82.4 percent). Of these, 290,210 were for disease, and 75,165 were for non-battle injury. Over the course of the war, 30 of each 1,000 active-duty personnel were killed in action, 121 of each 1,000 were admitted for battle injury, and 570 of each 1,000 were admitted for disease or non-battle injury. In general all of these incidences declined as the war progressed.

The most common battle injuries were penetrating wounds (57 percent) and fractures (23 percent), although the specific mechanism of injury varied with the type of combat. Average casualties per division per day were 119 in withdrawal, 77 in defense against a main force, and 67 in offense against a main force. In addition, the death rate among casualties was 25.2 percent in defense and only 14.6 percent in offense. Death rates also varied according to the weapon with which the casualty was inflicted: 28.4 percent for small arms, 23.8 percent for mines and booby traps, 18.4 percent for artillery, and 10.8 percent for hand grenades.

Army hospitals in Korea performed 89,974 surgical procedures throughout the duration of the conflict. Fifty-nine percent of those admitted with battle wounds required some sort of surgery, and the case-fatality rate was 2.5 percent (compared to 4.5 percent during World War II). Many patients required more than one operation, with the average being 1.2 procedures per wounded patient admitted. Surgery in Korea tended to be quick and of the salvage variety, with definitive treatment left to rear-area hospitals.

One of the most important technical advances during the war was the increased use of whole-blood transfusions to resuscitate patients in shock. A wounded soldier received an average of 3.3 pints of whole blood, although transfusions of 15 to 30 units were not unusual. This practice placed a predictable strain on the donation system, with 21,188 pints collected in the United States and 22,099 pints collected in Japan in 1950 alone. Caucasian and native Japanese blood supplies were segregated, although it is not known whether this was done for medical or racial reasons.

Neurosurgery posed a particularly challenge, because of both the complexity of the injuries and the extreme shortage of trained personnel. By 1952 a special evacuation path through the 8209th (and later the 8063rd) MASH units, commanded by Lieutenant Colonel Arnold Meirowsky, was established to care for wounds of the head and spinal cord. Vascular injuries posed another technical challenge. Use of vein grafts to repair arterial injuries was a significant advance, and by 1951 these repairs resulted in salvaging 85 percent of limbs with major vascular disruptions. Cold injuries were an especially common cause of non-battle traumatic admissions. During 1950 there were 1,791 cases of cold injury, for an incidence of 34 per 1,000. Medics were particularly hampered in the actions around the Changjin and Pujon reservoirs when the cold caused medicine, intravenous fluids, and plasma to freeze and become unusable.

Infectious disease was a persistent problem. Of those treated for non-battle-related causes and not requiring admission, 90 percent had infectious or parasitic disease. Most common were respiratory disease (20 percent), ill-defined febrile illnesses, and diarrheal disease. The latter was especially severe early in the war when hygienic facilities were lacking. Gastrointestinal disease (especially shigellosis) occurred at a rate of 120 per 1,000 per year in August 1950. Other common infectious ailments were encephalitis, polio, hemorrhagic fever, hepatitis, and venereal disease.

Malaria and plague were locally endemic but never became a serious problem for United Nations (UN) troops including the American contingent.

The third most common medical problem was neuropsychiatric (NP) illness. The frequency of disability from psychiatric illness varied greatly with the stage of the war. Early in the war, young psychiatrists were stationed at the rear. Inexperienced and far removed from the battlefields, these doctors tended to be liberal in sending home soldiers with psychiatric complaints. As the war progressed, physicians were moved closer to the front and became less sympathetic, and the rate of psychiatric disability dropped. A second factor was the kind of fighting going on at the time. The rate of NPs dropped from 249 per 1,000 before August, 1950, to 18.4 per 1,000 during the UN offensive that began in mid-August, 1950. It rose again when the winter weather set in.

Deployment of medical facilities proceeded rapidly in the fall of 1950. By November, four MASH units, with bed capacities increased from a planned 60 to 150, had been established in Korea, along with three 400-bed semi-mobile evacuation hospitals, four 400-bed field hospitals, one station hospital, and three hospital ships. Two additional MASH units were deployed in 1951, and one of the evacuation hospitals was moved to Japan in December 1950. After the Chinese entered the war in October 1950, three additional evacuation hospitals were committed,

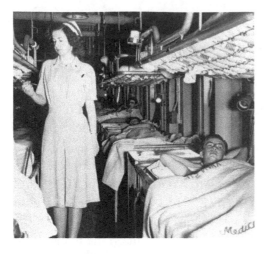

A nurse administers to her hospital ward aboard the USS *Consolation,* one of seven hospital ships that served during the Korean War. (Department of the Navy, Bureau of Medicine and Surgery)

but they functioned as immobile station hospitals. The field hospitals were converted to treat prisoners of war (POWs).

The evacuation sequence from facility to facility was from battalion aid station, to regimental collecting station, to division clearing station, to evacuation hospital at Pusan, to Korean airfields, to the 118th Station Hospital at Fukuoka (Kyushu, Japan), to other army hospitals in Japan (Osaka and Tokyo), to Tripler Army Hospital (Hawaii), to either Travis Air Force Base (California) or Lackland Air Force Base (Texas), to zone-of-the-interior hospitals. Patients requiring emergency stabilization or surgery could be sent from either the regimental collecting stations or the division clearing stations to the MASH units. From there, the stabilized patients were sent on either to the evacuation hospital at Pusan or directly to Fukuoka. Of admissions for battle injury, 10 percent received final disposition at a forward unit (aid, clearing, or collecting station), 57 percent at army hospitals in the FEC, 6 percent at non-army hospitals (navy or air force), and 26 percent at hospitals in the United States. These figures include both discharge and death, although 96 percent of all deaths occurred in one of the FEC hospitals. Eighty percent of division wounded eventually returned to duty.

Transport changed as the war progressed. Because the terrain in Korea was difficult, the initial stages of transport were by hand-carried litter, especially when combat units were moving either in advance or retreat. From the aid and clearing stations, transport was primarily by rail. Early in the war, gasoline-powered rail cars carried patients from the front at Chochiwon to Taejon. They held 17 litters or 50 ambulatory patients and traversed the 30 miles in about 45 minutes. As the front stabilized later in the war, formal rail transport was more frequent. Rail facilities were brought to within 8,000 yards of the front line, and evacuation trains typically comprised eight ward cars, two orderly cars, a kitchen car, a dining car, a pharmacy car, an officer personnel car, and a utility car.

Because of both improved transport (both rail and air) and treatment facilities located relatively close to the front line, a remarkable 58 percent of soldiers wounded in the battle received medical care within two hours of injury, and 85 percent were treated within six hours. The median time from wound to first care was 90 minutes, and 55 percent of casualties were hospitalized the same day they were wounded—a number that rose to nearly 100 percent by 1953.

Early in the war, evacuation from Pusan to Fukuoka was principally by ship, with hospital ships, troop transports, and even ferries pressed into service. This relatively slow and expensive method of transport was quickly replaced by air evacuation. In the first year of the war, Douglas C-47 Skytrains (Dakotas) were utilized, although as the war progressed, Douglas C-54 Skymasters became available. The longer range of the C-54s allowed direct transfer to Japan.

Because there was an initial shortage of all physicians and a persistent lack of some specialists, a tactical decision was made to substitute triage and transport for personnel. The army realized that the best use could be made of scarce personnel by concentrating them in hospitals in rear areas. Patients who were predicted to recover in fewer than 30 days were kept at Pusan; those expected to recover in 30 to 120 days were kept in Japan; and those anticipated to have prolonged recovery were returned to the United States. A complex of evacuation units grew around the 8054th Evacuation Hospital at Pusan. The 8054th was initially in the Pusan Middle School but grew to several buildings with 1,200 beds that handled up to 12,000 admissions a month. It was assisted by the Swedish Red Cross Hospital, the First Prisoner-of-War Hospital, and several hospital ships and specialized units.

The overall record of army medicine in Korea compares favorably to that of World War II. The case-fatality rate for those wounded in battle in the earlier war was 4.5 percent, dropping to 2.5 percent in the latter. In addition, these rates dropped as the war progressed—the rate for 1950 is not known, but for 1951 it was 2.1 percent, and by 1952 it was down to 1.8 percent. Of those wounded but not killed in Korea, 87.9 percent returned to duty, 8.5 percent were separated as disabled, and 1.4 percent were separated for administrative reasons. Overall, medical care in Korea was characterized by rapid transport, effective early resuscitation and surgery, and some advances in surgical technique and decline in mortality rates from battle injury.

Jack McCallum

ENTRIES

Aeromedical Evacuation

Evacuation of the sick and wounded by either fixed-wing or rotary aircraft is known as aeromedical evacuation. Attempts to create a military air ambulance date to 1910, but it was not before 1920 that the first American military aircraft specifically designed as an air ambulance was deployed. By World War II, fixed-wing transport of the sick and wounded was standard military procedure. In 1942 the Fifth Air Force evacuated 13,000 patients from New Guinea to Australia, and 383,676 patients were air evacuated from Europe in the last six months of the war. In 1943 a Sikorsky R-6 helicopter, the first rotorcraft used for air evacuation, was modified to carry a pilot and a medic inside the aircraft and two patients in litters attached to the outside.

When the Military Air Transport Service was chartered after World War II, patient transport was one of its designated missions. In 1949, the secretary of defense declared air transport the method of choice for moving those injured in battle. At the onset of the Korean conflict, the rough terrain and inadequate land transport facilities on the peninsula and the need to transport patients to remote specialized medical facilities proved this decision to have been a good one and hastened its implementation. Late in July 1950 a helicopter detachment of the 3rd Air Rescue Squadron was sent to Korea to retrieve downed pilots. Because the unit was underutilized, its helicopters were instead to transport the sick and wounded. The first trial flight took off from a school yard in Taegu and landed at the 8054th Evacuation Hospital at Pusan on August 3, 1950. After the Chinese offensive of November 1950, General Douglas MacArthur decided helicopters should be a routine part of his medical units' equipment, and he convinced the Surgeon General to establish and equip two helicopter ambulance companies of 24 craft each. The Marines began using helicopter evacuation that month and it was routine in the Army by January 1951.

Sikorsky H-5 helicopters were the most popular for air evacuation from the beginning, but they were fragile, and, because they were no longer in production, parts were scarce. For these reasons, they were initially reserved to move patients from aid stations to MASH units and were used only for those patients deemed unlikely to survive without air transport. As the Korean conflict progressed and the H-5s' unique suitability to their mission became clear, helicopters were used closer to the front lines and for less urgent cases. Ultimately, helicopter transport from the site of trauma to an appropriate treatment facility became a standard of care not only in the military but also in the transport of civilian trauma victims.

U.S. Navy physicians realized that air transport to rear-area hospitals was faster and more efficient than transport by sea. As a consequence, ships that had initially been earmarked to transport and treat patients became floating stationary hospitals with helipads to receive the wounded. Single-engine, fixed-wing aircraft were also used to move patients. The l5-B could carry one litter and one ambulatory patient, and the C-64 could carry three litters and two ambulatory patients. Transport from Pusan to Japan and on to the United States was principally carried out by aircraft of World War II vintage. Late in the Korean conflict, the newer C-119 and C-124 became available. The C-124 could be configured to carry 136 litters, 35 medical personnel, and a portable operating facility. Its lack of soundproofing and insulation and the length of time required to load and unload such a large contingent limited its usefulness in combat situations but did not seriously detract from its ability to transport stable patients the long distance from Japan to the United States.

In the U.S. operations in Iraq and Afghanistan starting in 2001, high-speed jet transports have been used to carry patients whose surgery had been partially completed in field hospitals to base hospitals as far away as Europe to have their operations completed.

Jack McCallum

Further Reading

Cleaver, Frederick. *U.S. Army Battle Casualties in Korea.* Chevy Chase, MD: Operations Research Office, 1956.

Cowdrey, Albert E. *United States Army in the Korean War: The Medic's War.* Washington, D.C.: Center of Military History, United States Army, 1987.

Naval Aerospace Medical Institute. *U.S. Naval Flight Surgeon's Manual.* Washington D.C.: Bureau of Medicine and Surgery, Department of the Navy, 1989.

Smith, Allen D. 1953. "Air Evacuation—Medical Obligation and Military Necessity." *Air University Quarterly* 6: 98–111.

Battle Fatigue

Battle fatigue is military a term used to describe a broad range of psychological and psychiatric symptoms in individuals who had been traumatized by combat and combat-related incidents. Also known as shell shock, battle shock, and battle stress, such adverse reactions to the stress of combat were termed NPs. Battle fatigue should not be confused with acute stress disorder, or post-traumatic stress disorder, which can also be precipitated by combat but are largely chronic, or long-term, illnesses. Unlike the latter, battle fatigue is seen usually as a temporary short-term condition. During the early months of the Korean conflict, when conditions were very bad for United Nations Command troops, NPs were common as exhaustion, despair, and fear of encirclement shattered the morale of many men and some whole units. NPs reached a high point in September 1950, precipitated by the heavy North Korean assault.

A variety of factors contributed to the large number of cases. Many veterans of World War II believed that the Korean fighting was more intense than any they had known, and the landscape of denuded hills gave a sense of no place to hide. The process of fighting up one hill only to be confronted with another beyond was psychologically as well as physically wearing. Many of the newcomers to battle faced the stress of battle suddenly and among strangers. As a result, the ratio of NPs to wounded almost doubled from the World War II norm.

Many mistakes were made in the handling of these types of casualties during the early months of the Korean conflict. Failures by both commanders and medical officers amplified psychiatric losses. The basic lessons learned in World War I and later relearned in World War II—that men suffering from battle fatigue should be held as close as possible to the front line—was, partly from necessity, forgotten.

Men with mild nonpsychotic symptoms were sent by plane or ship to Japan, the worst possible treatment because it took a soldier from the line and taught him the lesson that escape from danger was the reward for this behavior. The result was the loss of many men who, with a few days of rest, a sedative, and a hot meal, could have returned to duty.

With the formation of the Pusan Perimeter, the psychiatric admission rate soared, from 50 cases per 1,000 troops per year in July 1950 to 258 in August. Between July and December 1950, the 8054th Evac Hospital evacuated 85 percent of its NPs and returned only 15 percent to duty. The combination of retreat, poor command decisions, inexperienced doctors, quick evacuation, and lack of bed space contributed to the heavy NP losses in the early days of the war, when personnel losses were critical. An exception to this situation was the 2nd Division, where an effort was made from the first days of the battle to hold NPs at the clearing-station level, where most could be dealt with by granting them several days' rest and then returning them to duty.

Eventually the lessons of World War II were relearned, but the presence of veteran medical officers was the key to revival of the World War II approach. Individual, not institutional, memory resulted in a better record for combat psychiatry that saw more NPs treated and returned to duty.

An interesting new development in handling the stress of combat was a morale-enhancing program of what might be termed preventive psychotherapy. World War II statistics showed that sharp increases in casualty rates of all types occurred when troops experienced combat for more than 180 days without relief. Hence, the Department of the Army authorized temporary duty in Japan for the purpose of rest and recuperation (R&R); personnel serving in Korea were authorized a five-day R&R period.

James H. Willbanks

Further Reading

Cowdrey, Albert E. *United States Army in the Korean War: The Medics' War.* Washington, D.C.: U.S. Army Center of Military History, 1987.

Gabriel, Richard A., ed. *Military Psychiatry: A Comparative Perspective.* New York: Greenwood, 1986.

Casualties

There are no complete, definitive casualty figures for military and civilian losses in the Korean War. A conflict in a country with little governmental or private apparatus for record keeping and involving secretive belligerents, the Korean War defied counting. This condition characterizes many casualty estimates for World War I and World War II and the First and Second Indochina wars as well. Casualty figures are also complicated by postwar attempts by the belligerents to exaggerate their enemies' losses and mask their own, although for the United States a simple error and misleading counting rules have confused historians. Many Americans still believe that 54,246 U.S. servicemen died in the Korean War from all causes. In 2000, the Department of Defense finally went back to original records and concluded that the real figure is 36,914 American war-related deaths from all causes, since adjusted to 36,574.

The 54,246 or 54,000 figure, which routinely appears on monuments and in textbooks, became the received wisdom through its use in the Statistical History of the United States, a compilation that has appeared in various editions since 1945 under the sponsorship of the U.S. Bureau of the Census and the Social Science Research Council. Until 1990 the same figure appeared in the official publications of the Department of Defense.

U.S. casualty statistics are confusing because of two counting errors perpetuated by the Department of the Army and the Census Bureau. During the war, for an American soldier to be counted as killed in action (KIA) or died of wounds (DOW), his body had to be recovered and processed or he had to have been seen by two other soldiers as a corpse. Unidentified remains became "unknown" KIAs. Using such counting rules, the number of battlefield deaths was 19,585 with another 4,544 identified men DOW either in friendly or enemy hands.

Thus, the armed forces had 24,129 identified battlefield deaths, yet eventually settled on the number 33,667 as total battle-related deaths. Where did the additional 9,538 war-related deaths come from? These servicemen were listed missing in action (MIA), and this figure could not be compiled with any accuracy until after the exchange of prisoners of war (POWs) in 1953. POWs identified by name as dying in captivity (all causes) was 2,730, but this figure may not cover all deaths before assignment to POW camps. The Department of Defense (reflecting its dependence on U.S. Army estimates) declared the deceased POWs and remaining MIAs as combat-related deaths, thus raising the figure to 33,667. The Department of Defense still carries the MIA figure as 8,177, but these MIAs are included in the total of war-related deaths.

The difficulty in assessing Korean War deaths is complicated by the category "other deaths," which entered the conventional historical wisdom by 1960 as 20,617. Someone should have been suspicious because this figure would have come close to returning to pre–World War II patterns for the U.S. armed forces, which was that "other deaths" outnumbered battlefield deaths. Yet the service personnel in the Korean War did not endure a major epidemic (like the Spanish flu of 1918–1919) nor did they suffer thousands of deaths, as in Vietnam, from helicopter crashes. When the Department of the Army went back to the surgeon general's records in the 1990s, it determined that its "other deaths" were actually 2,452. The other services' figures had been too small (797) and consistent to be an issue. Thus the "other deaths" figure was really 3,249. How does one explain a differential of more than 17,000 lives? It appears that two things happened: (1) the MIA, including those who died from diseases as POWs, were double-counted, and (2) the U.S. Army's figure for "other deaths" included all noncombat deaths throughout the army, worldwide, during the Korean War era and was reported by the Surgeon General as 10,220. The official casualty figure (all causes) for the U.S. armed forces in the Korean War is now 36,574.

Allan R. Millett

Further Reading

Cole, Paul M. *POW/MIA Issues, Vol. 1, The Korean War.* Santa Monica, CA: RAND Corporation for the National Defense Research Institute, 1994.

Democratic People's Republic of Korea, Ministry of Defense. *The Victorious Fatherland Liberation War Museum.* Pyongyang, North Korea: Foreign Languages Publishing House, 1979.

Nahm, Andrew C. *Korea, Tradition and Transformation: A History of the Korean People.* Elizabeth, NJ: Hollym International, 1988.

Reister, Frank. *Battle Casualties and Medical Statistics: U.S. Army Experience in the Korean War.* Washington, D.C.: Office of the Surgeon General, 1973.

Republic of Korea, Korean Overseas Information Service. "Summary of Damage Caused by North Korea during the Korean War." March 6, 1974, File 620.008, U.S. Eighth Army Historical Files, Eighth Army History Office, Yongsan, Seoul.

Republic of Korea, Ministry of National Defense. *The History of the United Nations Forces in the Korean War.* 6 vols. Seoul: War History Compilation Commission, 1967–1975.

U.S. Department of Defense, American Services Information Service. *Defense 97 Almanac.* Alexandria, VA: U.S. Government Printing Office, 1998.

U.S. Department of Defense, Office of Public Information. "Report of U.S. Killed, Wounded, and Missing in Action." November 5, 1954, Summary no. 160, U.S. Eighth Army Historical Files, Eighth Army History Office, Yongsan, Seoul.

Combat Medics

As had been the case in World War II, for combat soldiers medical treatment started on the battlefield. The first providers were fellow soldiers trained as combat medics. Enlisted men of a regimental medical company were called "medics" in the army and "corpsmen" by U.S. Marine corps units. Marine corpsmen were actually navy hospital corpsmen assigned to Marine units as combat medics. In army units one medic was attached to each rifle platoon, with a total of seven medics in a rifle company. Marine units were similarly manned. Most combat patrols included a medic. These medical personnel had to deal with all manner of wounds and injuries, including those caused by small arms, heavy weapons, mortars, and artillery fire. Depending on the time of year, they also dealt with frostbite and heat prostration, as well as various illnesses and communicable diseases.

Medics, usually unarmed, carried out their duties in the heat of battle. With only small first-aid kits, they often accomplished medical near-miracles. Battlefield casualties, once treated, were evacuated to the battalion aid station by litter bearers. Many of these bearers were men of the Korean Service Corps. Some wounded had to find their own way to the rear if they were judged to be "walking wounded."

Depending on the seriousness of their injuries, the wounded men were then evacuated by jeep, ambulance, or helicopter to the regimental collecting station, the division clearing station, or MASH. Early in the war some fixed-wing liaison aircraft were also used for medical evacuation.

As had been the case in World War II and again would provide so in future wars, American combat soldiers had a high regard for the combat medics. The combat medics routinely and selflessly risked their lives to provide aid to their fallen comrades. The number of medics who received medals for valor attests to their bravery. Medics received 8 of the 131 Medals of Honor awarded in the Korean War. Of these, four (three posthumous) were awarded to army medics and four (all posthumous) went to navy hospital corpsmen serving with marine units.

Norman R. Zehr

Further Reading

Apel, Otto F., Jr. *MASH.* Lexington: University Press of Kentucky, 1998.

Cowdrey, Albert E. *United States Army in the Korean War: The Medic's War.* Washington, D.C.: U.S. Army Center of Military History, 1987.

Jordan, Kenneth N., Sr. *Forgotten Heroes.* Atglen, PA: Schiffer Military/Aviation History, 1995.

Meid, Pat, James M. Yingling, Nicholas Canzona et al. *U.S. Marine Operations in Korea, 1950–1953.* 5 vols. Washington, D.C.: U.S. Marine Corps Historical Branch, 1962–1972.

Hospital Ships

In the spring of 1862, the U.S. Sanitary Commission and Frederick Law Olmsted oversaw conversion of several freighters including the *Daniel Webster* for the transport of sick and wounded from the Chesapeake Bay during the Peninsula Campaign. At the same time, Union forces at Fort Henry converted the river steamer *City of Memphis* and four other commandeered vessels for the same purpose. In April 1862, General Ulysses S. Grant captured four Confederate steamers and converted one, the *Red Rover*, into the first real American hospital ship.

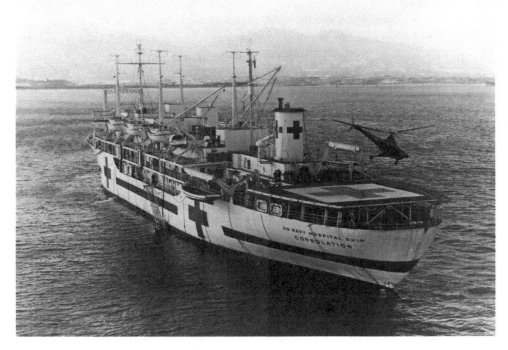

The USS *Consolation*, stationed off the Korean Coast on December 21, 1951, awaits the first air evacuation of casualties directly from the battlefield to the hospital ship. Ships originally intended to transport the wounded became fixed base hospitals with helicopter access. Seven hospital ships served during the Korean War. (Naval Historical Center)

It was equipped with a kitchen and bakery, an elevator, and a fully furnished operating theater.

During World War I, most hospital ships were converted ocean liners, painted white with red crosses, and registered with and presumably protected by the Geneva Convention as adapted to maritime warfare in 1864 and revised in 1907. In World War II, hospital ships supported American operations in the Mediterranean. They truly came into their own in the Pacific campaigns. Here, military operations focused on capturing Japanese-held islands. This resented unique problems in medical evacuation; the distances were inordinately long and there was almost never an accessible general hospital to augment basic field hospital care. At the beginning of the war, the U.S. Navy had only two hospital ships (the USS *Relief* and the USS *Solace*), and only one of these was in the Pacific. Over the next three-and-a-half years, the United States commissioned an additional eight hospital ships and developed an entire class of troop transports equipped to provide limited hospital services. The Navy also deployed a series of adapted landing craft—LST (H)s—manned with four surgeons and 27 corpsmen and capable of serving as field hospitals for up to 350 wounded. Hospital ships, required by the Navy to be held well back from areas of direct combat, served essentially the same role as land-based general hospitals.

A total of seven ships formally served as floating hospitals or patient transports during the Korean conflict. Their role changed dramatically from that originally envisioned as the war progressed. The *New Haven* class were dedicated 500-foot hospital ships first built during World War II. The USS *Consolation* was in commission in 1950 and made a rapid trip from the eastern United States to Korea when hostilities broke out. The rest of the class was in the reserve fleet in San Francisco. Three hospital ships were activated and sent to Korean waters. Almost from the outset, the decision was made to use the ships as stationary floating hospitals. They were initially berthed at Pusan but moved north along both the east and west coasts of Korea after the United Nations forces broke out into the peninsula. In the frantic early days of the war (before organized air evacuation from Korea to Japan was in place) the troop ships USNS *Sgt. George D. Keathley* and USNS *Sgt. Andrew Miller* were pressed into service to move the wounded to rear-area hospitals. Early on, even these resources were overwhelmed and local ferries were used as well.

As helicopter and fixed-wing transport became available, the role of the hospital ships changed dramatically. The C-47 Dakotas and C-54 Skymasters assumed essentially all transport duties, so the ships were moored close to combat areas to serve as fixed base hospitals. At first flat-topped barges were moored next to the ships to allow helicopter access. Later, formal "helo" decks were added so patients could be brought directly on board. At various times, the ships were also moored directly to piers and served as both floating hospitals and outpatient clinics. The upper three decks housed up to 800 inpatients whereas the lower three decks were administrative and clinic spaces. By September 1952, the U.S. Navy hospital ships had admitted 40,662 patients; about 35 percent were battle casualties and the rest were diseases and nonbattle injuries.

Jack McCallum

Further Reading

Cowdrey, Alfred E. *United States Army in the Korean War: The Medic's War.* Washington, D.C.: Center for Military History, 1987.

Coyl, E. B. 1953. "Hospital Ships in Korea." *Military Surgeon* 112: 342–344.

Kimura, S. *The Surgical & Medical History of the Naval War between Japan & Russia.* Tokyo: Toyo Printing Co., Ltd., 1911.

Olmsted, Frederick Law. *Hospital Transports: A Memoir of the Embarkation of the Sick and Wounded from the Peninsula of Virginia in the Summer of 1862.* Boston: Ticknor and Fields, 1863.

Plumridge, John H. *Hospital Ships and Ambulance Trains.* London: Seeley, Service & Co., 1975.

Wilbur, C. Keith. *Civil War Medicine.* Guilford, CT: Globe Pequot Press, 1998.

Mobile Army Surgical Hospitals in the Korean Conflict

Mobile army surgical hospitals or MASH units are fully equipped mobile hospitals complete with tentage, supplies, and personnel with portability that allows them to accompany military units in either advance or retreat. Semimobile medical units that could be placed close to the front and still function as surgical hospitals had been pioneered by the British in World War I as casualty clearing stations. The American Expeditionary Force in World War I had adopted the model, and General Douglas MacArthur deployed mobile surgical units in the Pacific during World War II, although with limited success. Between 1948 and 1949, five MASH units were created, although none were based in the Pacific.

When the Korean conflict broke out, the necessity for such units was evident, and three MASH units were activated—the 8055th on July 1, 1950, the 8063rd on July 17, and the 8076th on July 19. The 8055th left Sasebo for Pusan on July 6 and proceeded by train directly to Taejon. The 8063rd left July 18 for Pohang-dong to support the 1st Cavalry. The 8076th arrived in Pusan July 25 and moved up the Taejon-Taegu corridor to support the Eighth Army. All three would later follow their combat units after the breakout and invasion of North Korea. In 1951 the 8225th MASH unit was deployed, and an additional unit was organized by the Norwegians and sent to Ujongbu the same year. Two additional MASH units, one of which (the 8209th) specialized in caring for neurosurgical cases, were deployed in 1952.

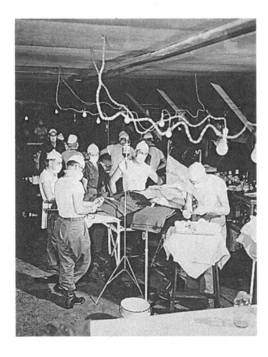

The refinement of the mobile army surgical hospital (MASH) during the Korean War was a major advance in military medicine. Here surgeons at a MASH facility operate twenty miles behind the front in 1952. (National Archives)

The MASH was initially intended to be a 60-bed unit to provide triage and early stabilization prior to transfer to an evacuation hospital farther from the front. Each was to have a headquarters detachment, a preoperative and shock treatment area, an operating section, a postoperative area, a pharmacy, an X-ray section, and a holding ward. It was to be staffed by 14 medical officers, 12 nurses, two Medical Service Corps officers, one warrant officer, and 97 enlisted men. One of the medical officers was assigned as commander, and there were two anesthesiologists, one internist, four general medical officers, and five surgeons. The number of beds, mission, and staffing never exactly fit that plan. Because of the excess of wounded over treaters—especially in the early part of the war—the MASH units actually served as small evacuation hospitals. At one point, just the holding area of the 8076th had 200 beds.

The chain of evacuation had the MASH units receiving patients (usually by rail or helicopter) from aid or collecting stations. After initial treatment, the wounded requiring additional care were transferred to either the evacuation hospitals at Pusan or directly to one of the Far East Command's facilities in Japan.

Early in the war, there was a severe shortage of personnel to staff the MASH units. The residency programs in the Army hospital system were tapped to provide partially trained specialists on temporary duty. These young physicians and dentists were often asked to perform jobs for which they had little or no training; it was not uncommon for dentists to give anesthesia, psychiatric residents to perform surgery, or radiologists to set fractures.

The combination of inadequate training and high patient volume led to less than fastidious surgical technique. Open wounds were often cleaned but not closed, leaving the definitive surgery to hospitals farther down the chain. A typical abdominal operation involved making a large incision for control of any obvious bleeding. Then the gut was examined for visible perforations, which were clamped and repaired. The abdominal cavity was then rinsed to clean out loose food and parasites. The viscera were then replaced and the skin closed with the expectation that further surgery would be necessary to manage unaddressed details.

The doctor shortage was eased by the draft of 1950, but a new set of problems arose. Ninety percent of the military physicians who ultimately served in Korea were drafted, and many had previously served in World War II as enlisted men. They had only recently completed their medical training and begun busy civilian practices, and they had little enthusiasm for their new predicament and little inclination to cooperate with military rules and discipline. Disciplinary and morale challenges worsened as the war progressed and the lines stabilized. The MASH units evolved into fixed hospitals relatively remote from the front lines staffed with female nurses and with access to a variety of recreational facilities and temptations.

Although quirky and often confused, the pattern of care—early stabilization followed by more orderly completion of care in specialized facilities—that began in

Korea's MASH units joined the helicopter transport model (also developed in Korea) to form the template for the shock-trauma services now present in virtually every large city in the United States.

Jack McCallum

Further Reading

Cleaver, Frederick. *U.S. Army Battle Casualties in Korea*. Chevy Chase, MD: Operations Research Office, 1956.

Cowdrey, Albert E. *United States Army in the Korean War: The Medic's War*. Washington, D.C.: Center of Military History, 1987.

Reister, Frank. *Battle Casualties and Medical Statistics: U.S. Army Experience in the Korean War*. Washington, D.C.: Office of the Surgeon General, 1973.

DOCUMENT

MASH: An Army Surgeon in Korea

Otto F. Appel was a 28-years old doctor when he was assigned to the 8076th Mobile Army Surgical Hospital (MASH) in Korea. The MASH concept was designed to provide immediate emergency surgical care for wounded soldiers. The Korean War was the test of the concept. Early in the war, there was a serious lack of trained medical personal. Consequently, residents from the Army hospital system were sent to Korea where they were often called upon to perform jobs for which they had little or no training. The combination of inadequate training and high patient volume led to slipshod surgery. To meet the manpower shortage, the army resorted to the Doctors Draft Act. The draftees, including Apel, had only recently completed their medical training and were just beginning their civilian practices. They resented being drafted and resisted military discipline. Nonetheless, once they went to Korea, they performed amazing feats. Korea was the first conflict where helicopters transported large numbers of wounded soldiers from the frontlines to the MASH units. Surgeons like Apel created a system of emergency care that became the model for modern shock-trauma services.

In Korea the term *air evacuation* included the entire plan to evacuate the wounded from the theater of operations. First, evacuation within Korea meant carrying the wounded from the battle lines to the surgical hospitals. Second, evacuation meant the movement of wounded patients from the surgical hospitals to the field hospitals or evacuation hospitals. Third, evacuation meant flying the wounded in fixed-wing aircraft from Korea to the hospitals in Japan and from Japan back to the United States. All of these were important functions in the medical evacuation schema. In the MASH we saw the first category, the removal of the wounded from the battlefield to the surgical hospital. It was an inspiring sight for all concerned. Even though the vast majority of patients were still transported on the ground, the presence of the helicopter, specialized though it was, changed the face of medical care on the battlefield. The first use of the helicopter for medical evacuation in Korea was during the battle for the Pusan Perimeter. Evacuation in this case meant flying patients from the MASH to a field hospital in Korea and later back to general hospitals in Japan. On August 3, 1950, at the Taegu Teachers College, the location of MASH 8055, a Sikorsky helicopter landed in the yard of the school, a building that was being used as an operating room. Two of the serious patients from the post-op ward were carried to the Sikorsky on litters and strapped to the helicopter behind the pilot's seat. There was a pilot and one passenger, Eight Army surgeon Col. Chauncey Dovell. The wounded were flown from the precarious location of the MASH to the more secure 8054th Evacuation Hospital in the port city of Pusan. Several months later, during the Chinese New Year's offensive, Lieutenants Willie Strawn and Joe Bowler, both flying H-13s, transported four recently wounded soldiers from aid stations at the front to MASH 8063, thus flying the first medical evacuation missions in history. The Third Air Rescue Squadron, an air force unit whose mission was to rescue downed pilots, began to use their helicopters to transport wounded soldiers from the field of battle. Many more medical evacuation flights followed. Later, in Vietnam, such flights came to be known simply as medevac. In Korea we referred to that part of medical evacuation, from the frontline aid stations to the MASH, as copters.

Helicopter evacuation required a much closer selection of evacuees than did evacuation by field ambulance or litter. The battalion surgeon or the medic on the scene decided quickly who was to be evacuated based on several criteria: the extent of the wound itself, the availability of the aircraft, the number of casualties, and other means of evacuation available. Priority went essentially as follows: (1) soldiers in shock or continuing hemorrhage; (2) traumatic amputations; (3) open fractures of long bones, complicated by shock; (4) apparent extreme arterial damage or wounds treated with a tourniquet; (5) extensive muscle damage; (6) abdominal wounds; (7) sucking chest wounds; (8) less severe chest wounds; (9) thoracicoabdominal wounds; (10) face or neck wounds with impaired breathing; (11) head injuries in coma; and (12) suspected gas gangrene. These patients, by any method of evacuation, were directed to the MASH for immediate surgery. Those who were to go by helicopter often received closer attention in preparation for the trip.

As a result of the better preparation that was required for helicopter evacuation, these patients were in better condition when they arrived at the MASH. The gravest threat in many serious wounds in Korea was shock. As it worked out, the additional preparation for helicopter transport improved the chances of avoiding shock as well as trauma during transportation. Before any evacuation the patient had to be completely prepared: all medical care possible should have been given, including stabilization of all wounds, complete security of the patient to the litter, adequate attention to blood pressure, adequate sedation for pain and shock, chest wounds tightly bandaged, and breathing airways cleared and secured against blockage by bleeding or vomit. With this preparation, the helicopter not only moved the patient faster but got him there in better condition.

The helicopter provided economy of personnel by permitting the battalion surgeon to direct the wounded to the appropriate hospital and allowing the army to centralize medical personnel in specialized hospitals. Those in immediate need of surgery went directly to the MASH. Those whose injuries required immediate evacuation but did not require immediate surgery could be sent to other facilities. For example, psychiatric patients or patients dying of complications from illness could be sent directly to a field hospital of the battalion surgeon's choice, thus bypassing the MASH. Helicopters made all the hospitals in the combat zone available to the battalion surgeon.

On the other end, the speed and flexibility of the helicopter permitted the Medical Corps to centralize doctors and nurses in specialized treatment facilities instead of scattering them to different places on the battlefields. At the beginning of the war, each MASH unit did general surgery. When I arrived, the 8076th took all comers. As time went on, each MASH began to specialize. MASH 8076 became known as the place to treat extreme vascular injuries. MASH 8055 was known for its treatment of head injuries. If a head injury came to us at MASH 8076, we would give immediate treatment, stabilize the patient, and transport him to 8055. The other MASH units did likewise with vascular injuries, and by late 1951 we were receiving the lion's share of vascular work. MASH 8063 was known for treating unusual conditions, particularly the mysterious ailment that swept Korea in 1951–52 called, for lack of a better name, hemorrhagic fever. In cases of suspected use of biological or chemical weapons, such as nerve gas, the wounded were taken to MASH 8209, later redesignated MASH 8225, a stable unit that did not move like the other MASH units. Others may have gone to an evacuation hospital. With the reduction in transit time from the battlefield to the MASH, the increase in range, and the flexibility of landing, the wounded could go to a specialized treatment facility where he could receive the best treatment available.

Source: Otto F. Apel Jr. and Pat Apel. *MASH: An Army Surgeon in Korea.* Lexington, KY: University Press of Kentucky, 1998, pp. 68–69, 79–81. Used by permission of the University Press of Kentucky.

■ CHAPTER 9
Vietnam War

INTRODUCTION

Medical advances during the Vietnam War were the culmination of a century of progress in treating trauma and controlling infectious diseases. Additionally, the nature of the conflict engendered a unique spectrum of psychiatric, medical, and traumatic conditions.

Mortality rates among the soldiers in wars since the mid-19th century have generally declined: 15 percent in the Mexican-American War (United States only), 20 percent in the Crimean War (all participants), 14 percent in the American Civil War (Union only), 8 percent in World War I (United States only), 4.5 percent in World War II (United States only), and 2.5 percent in the Korean War (United States only). In Vietnam, the mortality rate among U.S. military personnel from all causes was 2.7 percent. Because a higher proportion of soldiers in the latter conflict were hospitalized, the slight rise in mortality actually represents an improvement in overall survival.

The 20th century was one of dramatic advances in battlefield medicine and surgery. Effective debridement of wounds and the use of intravenous fluids and whole blood to resuscitate wounded soldiers became standards of practice during World War I. During World War II, penicillin and sulfa drugs became available, and techniques were developed for management of some thoracic and vascular injuries. Better vascular surgery and more liberal use of whole blood accounted for most of the improved survival in the Korean War. Helicopter evacuation, more rapid resuscitation, and readily available specialty surgery characterized military medicine in Vietnam.

In 1965 the U.S. Army had a single 100-bed hospital at Nha Trang. At the war's peak in 1968, the U.S. Department of Defense operated 5,283 beds at 19 fixed sites and MUSTs (medical unit self-contained, transportable). Because there was no clearly defined front, medical facilities were geographically dispersed throughout the Republic of Vietnam (RVN, South Vietnam) and tended to remain in the same locations rather than follow troop movements as they had in previous wars.

By June 1969 the Army Medical Corps in Vietnam comprised 16,000 physicians, 15,000 nurses, and 19,000 other officers.

The military medical system was divided into five echelons. The first echelon began with the aid man, usually called a medic, who initiated emergency care and evacuation from the battlefield. He was responsible for arresting hemorrhage, securing an airway, dressing wounds, splinting fractures, relieving pain, and positioning the patient safely for transport. The physician at the battlefield aid station began more definitive resuscitation, including starting an intravenous line (by cut-down, if necessary), doing thoracentesis or tracheostomy, beginning positive pressure ventilation, ligating small bleeding vessels, and starting either salt solutions, plasma expanders (dextran, albumin, or Plasmanate), or uncross-matched whole blood.

The second echelon was the division clearing station, which had a larger staff of physicians, a better supply of whole blood, and oxygen. Antibiotics were begun, and tetanus antitoxin was given at this level.

The third echelon was the mobile surgical or evacuation hospital. Here major hemorrhage could be controlled and patency of difficult airways ensured. Whole blood and bicarbonate to correct acid-base imbalance were used. A major difference in resuscitative practices between the Vietnam War and earlier conflicts was the more liberal use of either uncross-matched or type-specific whole blood.

The fourth echelon was the general hospitals located in Okinawa and Japan. These had facilities for specialty medical and surgical services and psychiatric treatment. Okinawa was 1,800 miles from Vietnam, and the first fully equipped hospital was 2,700 miles away in Japan. Soldiers who were expected to return to duty in Southeast Asia were treated at one of these facilities or in the Philippines.

The fifth echelon comprised military and Veterans Administration (VA) hospitals in the United States. The nearest of these was at Travis Air Force Base, California (7,800 miles from Vietnam), although a significant number of casualties went on to Andrews Air Force Base near Washington, D.C. (9,000 miles from Vietnam). Soldiers who were not expected to return to duty in Vietnam were transferred to these facilities. Besides active duty facilities, the VA hospitals were a major resource for reconstructive and rehabilitative services. Between 1965 and 1969, 11,584 patients were transferred into the VA system.

Vietnam's climate favored development of a variety of tropical diseases, and the 12-month rotation schedule ensured a constant supply of nonimmune military targets for such diseases. Realizing this threat, military physicians instituted preventive measures (vaccination and prophylaxis) from the beginning of the war. Consequently, whereas disease had accounted for 90 percent of hospitalizations in the China-Burma-India theater during World War II, it accounted for only approximately 70 percent of hospitalizations of active duty personnel in Vietnam. Although the disease-to-injury admission rate for Vietnam was 4 to 1, it was 25 percent lower than that in Korea and half that of the European theater of operations after D day.

Major diseases were malaria, viral hepatitis, infectious diarrhea, fungal and other diseases of the skin, and venereal disease (usually gonorrhea or other urethritis-related diseases). Less common diseases included melioidosis, dengue, scrub typhus, murine typhus, and leptospirosis. Although plague and rabies were endemic to Vietnam, they never appeared in American military personnel. Because of its severity and its high incidence of resistance to standard drug therapy, falciparum malaria—the most common type in Vietnam—was a major medical challenge compounded by the soldiers' reluctance to take necessary prophylactic medications.

A second concern (which received publicity out of proportion to its clinical import) was drug-resistant gonococcus. Parasitic disease as a cause of discharge from military service was five times more common in the Pacific theater during World War II than during the Vietnam War. In fact, cancer was almost twice as common a cause of medical discharge as infectious disease in the latter conflict.

The World War I term "shell shock" became war neurosis, which after Vietnam became post-traumatic stress disorder (PTSD). PTSD was characterized by nightmares, flashbacks, excessive startle response, hyperalertness, sleep disorders, and detachment from one's surroundings and stayed with the patient long after the return to civilian life.

World War II's 10 percent psychiatric casualty rate dropped to 4 percent in Korea and was only 1 percent in Vietnam. During World War II, 33.1 percent of medical discharges were for psychiatric reasons. During the Korean War this dropped to 23.9 percent, and during the Vietnam War it was 13.7 percent. This surprisingly low rate was initially attributed to modern methods of combat psychiatry but in retrospect may have been factitious, as a number of veterans developed incapacitating psychiatric illnesses after discharge from the service. Between 1965 and 1970, the number of workdays lost to psychiatric illness more than doubled. PTSD became the second-worst disease in terms of lost work.

Drug abuse was widespread in Vietnam. In one study, 23 percent of soldiers interviewed said that they had used marijuana, 10 percent admitted amphetamine use, 7 percent used LSD (lysergic acid diethylamide), and 1.6 percent used heroin. In addition, there were disturbingly widespread reports of violence against both Vietnamese civilians and American officers as well as acts of disobedience, ranging from refusal to take antimalarial pills to frank insubordination during combat.

In spite of the higher hospitalization rates for medical diseases, the majority of deaths in the Vietnam War were battle related. In the European theater of operations between June 1944 and May 1945, the battle death rate was 51.9 per 1,000 average troop strength. In Korea it was 43.2 per 1,000, and in Vietnam between July 1965 and June 1969 it was 21.9 per 1,000. The ratio of wounded to killed in action was 3.1 to 1 during World War II to, 4 to 1 during the Korean War, and 5.6 to 1 during the Vietnam War. Although some of this might be due to a change in types of weapons, much of the improvement can be credited to better battlefield medicine and surgery. Partial support for this statement can be found in the fact that mortality after arrival at a hospital was 4.5 percent during World War II and 2.5 percent during the Vietnam War in spite of improvements in transport that brought many more severely wounded but still living soldiers to the hospitals.

Indeed, improved evacuation of the wounded was a hallmark of military medicine in Vietnam. Lack of roads, difficult jungle terrain (some helicopters were equipped with spring-loaded penetrators to make holes in the forest canopy), and the strategic situation made helicopter evacuation uniquely suited to Southeast Asian warfare. At its height of activity, the Army Medical Corps operated 116 air ambulances, each capable of carrying six to nine litters. During World War II the average time to treatment had been 10.5 hours, during the Korean War it was 6.3 hours, and during the Vietnam War it was 2.8 hours, with many patients being hospitalized within 20 minutes of injury. During the 1968 Tet Offensive, helicopter ambulances evacuated an average of 8,000 casualties a month.

A second hallmark of Vietnam War military medicine was an abundance of well-trained surgical specialists. American residency programs were producing large numbers of surgeons capable of complex procedures that had not been available in previous wars. Vascular surgery typifies this improvement. During World War II, only 81 attempts were made to repair major blood vessels. That number rose to 300 in Korea, but the procedure had become standardized in Vietnam, where several thousand such repairs were done. Survival in patients burned over less than 60 percent of their bodies improved dramatically. The number of amputations during the Vietnam War was less than half that of World War II or the Korean War.

Part of the improved surgical results during the Vietnam War can be attributed to a difference in ordnance in that war compared with ordnance in previous conflicts. Unsophisticated weapons and the more common use of mines resulted in more extremity wounds than in previous wars, and the environment made the wounds more likely to be contaminated. The type of wound changed as the war evolved. Whereas 42.7 percent of wounds were from small arms in 1966, that number had decreased to 17 percent by 1970. In 1966, 42.6 percent of the wounds were from mines and booby traps, a number that had increased to 80 percent by 1970. Artillery and mortar injuries accounted for 75 percent of casualties during World War II and the Korean War but were never that common in Vietnam. Injuries from purposely contaminated *punji* sticks were unique to the Southeast Asian war.

Medical and surgical improvements also decreased morbidity during the Vietnam War. Average duration of treatment was 129 days during World War II,

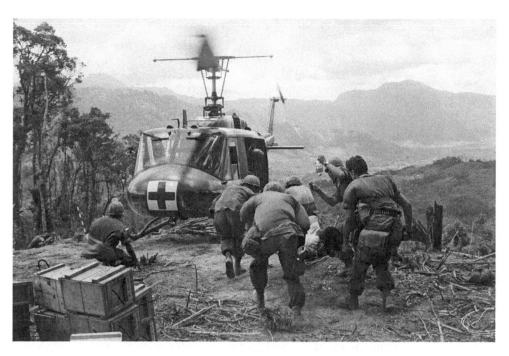

Courageous helicopter pilots took enormous risks to evacuate wounded soldiers during the Vietnam War. (Bettmann/Corbis)

93 days during the Korean War, and 65 days during the Vietnam War. Of the 194,716 wounded during the Vietnam War, 31 percent (61,269) were treated and released. Of those hospitalized for injury, 75.3 percent returned to duty in some capacity, although only 42 percent returned to duty in Vietnam. Only 3.3 percent of those injured in battle died. Of non-battle-related hospitalizations, 77.8 percent returned to duty, and only .3 percent died.

In all, improvements in evacuation and medical, perioperative, and intraoperative care led to fewer and shorter hospitalizations and improved survival in Vietnam War soldiers as compared with survival of soldiers of earlier conflicts.

U.S. forces had 47,382 killed in action, 10,811 noncombat deaths, 153,303 wounded in action (some 74,000 survived as quadriplegics or multiple amputees), and 10,173 captured or missing in action. The majority of the U.S. casualties were from the U.S. Army. Between 1961 and 1975, 30,868 soldiers died in Vietnam as the result of hostile action, and 7,193 died from other causes. Of those killed, the U.S. Army accounted for 65.8 percent, the U.S. Marine Corps accounted for 25.5 percent, the U.S. Navy accounted for 4.3 percent, the U.S. Air Force accounted for 4.3 percent, and the U.S. Coast Guard accounted for .1 percent. Of ranks (including navy equivalents), 88.8 percent were enlisted men and warrant officers, 8.6 percent were lieutenants and captains, and 2.6 percent were majors and colonels. Twelve U.S. generals died in Vietnam. In April 1995 the U.S.

Department of Defense listed 1,621 Americans missing in Vietnam and 2,207 for all of Southeast Asia.

James R. Arnold

ENTRIES

Anesthesiology

Anesthesiology is the physiologic and pharmacologic management of patients during surgery.

Use of drugs to relieve the pain and anxiety of surgery dates to prehistory. The first wartime use of anesthesia for surgery was by American surgeon Edward H. Barton in 1847 during the Mexican-American War. Military practice played a major role in the evolution of anesthesia from an adjunct managed primarily by nurses and medical students into a medical specialty. Ether anesthesia, although complicated by tracheal irritation or aspiration of vomited stomach contents, was considered by Americans too simple a process to warrant expending the resources of a trained physician. The British, however, took a different view, and London physician John Snow became the first professional anesthesiologist in 1847. Intravenous anesthesia became a standard with the invention of barbiturates in the 1920s.

World War II brought dramatic changes to anesthetic practice for a number of reasons. First, more complicated surgical procedures on more severely wounded people required better intraoperative care. Second, women, who had been primarily responsible for anesthesia, were not in the draft pool, so the military was forced to train men to do the job. Third, American military physicians were exposed to the British system in which doctors rather than nurses did the bulk of anesthesia. Finally, in an effort to attract workers during a period of frozen wages, American companies began offering health insurance, which made it possible for civilians to pay for expensive operations and the ancillary personnel necessary to perform them.

The U.S. Army instituted a series of 12-week training courses for general practitioners to turn them into anesthesiologists. These men were routinely available at the field hospital and specialty hospital level. Early in the war, spinal anesthesia and open-drop ether were common, but, as the war progressed and as American surgeons became more adept at handling critically injured soldiers, endotracheal intubation and complex monitoring became standard.

During the Korean and Vietnam conflicts, more rapid transportation of the wounded and improvement in surgical technique and in resuscitation brought progressively less stable patients to the operating room. By the Vietnam War, the combination of barbiturate induction and halothane, nitrous oxide, and oxygen anesthesia, frequently combined with prolonged artificial ventilation, had become standard. Techniques of managing shock and severe trauma moved from military to civilian practice in the latter decades of the 20th century.

Surgical and anesthetic practice changed somewhat in the Afghanistan and Iraq conflicts of the late 20th and early 21st centuries in that emphasis was placed on rapid stabilization near the front and early transport of the wounded to specialized rear-area facilities. Forward-area mobile hospitals composed of two tents and supplies carried on six Humvees could be set up in less than an hour wherever the troops happened to be. Procedures in those facilities were generally kept under two hours. Bleeding was stopped and patients were stabilized before being moved—often without closing their incisions—to larger hospitals, some of which were hundreds or even thousands of miles away. Whereas it took an average of 45 days for a wounded soldier in Vietnam to be transferred to the United States, it took only an average of four days in the Iraq War and could be as little as 36 hours. During transport, the patient remained sedated and ventilated, resulting essentially in a very prolonged anesthetic. These techniques have resulted in a dramatically lower death-due-to-injury rate than in previous conflicts and in saving lives that would have inevitably been lost in earlier conflicts.

Jack McCallum

Further Reading

Aldrete, J. A., G. M. Marron, and A. J. Wright. 1984. "The First Administration of Anesthesia in Military Surgery: On Occasion of the Mexican-American War." *Anesthesiology* 61 (November): 585–588.

Gawande, Atul. 2004. "Casualties of War—Military Care for the Wounded in Iraq and Afghanistan." *New England Journal of Medicine* 351 (December 9): 2471–2480.

Metzler, Samuel, and John Auer. 1909. "Continuous Respiration without Respiratory Movements." *Journal of Experimental Medicine* 11: 622–625.

Morton, William T. G. *Remarks on the Proper Mode of Administering Sulphuric Ether by Inhalation*. Boston: Dutton and Wentworth, 1847.

Waisel, David. 2001. "The Role of World War II and the European Theater of Operations in the Development of Anesthesiology as a Physician Specialty in the U.S.A." *Anesthesiology* 94: 907–914.

Wangensteen, Owen H., and Sarah D. Wangensteen. *The Rise of Surgery from Empiric Craft to Scientific Discipline*. Minneapolis: University of Minnesota Press, 1978.

Body Armor

Body armor in Vietnam was primarily known by the terms "flak jacket" and "flak vest." The term "flak" is derived from the German word for antiaircraft gun, *fliegerabwehrkanone*.

Flak suits were in widespread use by the U.S. Army Air Forces in 1945. These protected an airman's torso, groin, and thighs and were complemented by an armored centerpiece on which the airman sat. These suits evolved into infantry body armor during the Korean War. The M1951 flak vest represented a significant technical innovation that protected the ordinary soldier's chest, abdomen, and back from small shell and grenade fragments.

The U.S. Marine Corps' M1955 armored vest and the U.S. Army's M69 fragmentation protective vest, fielded in 1962, both offered neck protection. These two vests, along with the earlier M1951 and M1952 models, were standard for U.S. Marine Corps and U.S. Army forces in Vietnam. The M1955 armor weighed about 10 pounds, while the M69 armor weighed about 8.5 pounds. These sleeveless vests were composed of nylon filler and inserts enclosed in cloth.

Until late 1968, helicopter crewmen generally wore infantry body armor, at which time aviator body armor was introduced. Gunners wore full armor, while pilots and copilots generally wore only frontal armor. Torso armor was composed of aluminum oxide ceramics and was able to defeat high-velocity small-arms projectiles. Leg armor was made from composite steel. Full armor weighed about 25 pounds; however, new variants incorporated even lighter and stronger ceramics based on boron carbide. Body armor, fragmentation-small arms protective, aircrewmen was introduced in 1968; it became the standard-issue body armor.

Later infantry body armor developments were directly inspired by advances in aircrew armor. Special body armor was also used by naval and riverine forces. Naval and coast guard forces were issued floating body armor, while many riverine troops wore a light flak jacket composed of a special titanium-nylon composite.

Robert J. Bunker

Further Reading

Dean, Bashford. *American and German Helmets and Body Armor of World War I and Body Armor in Modern Warfare.* Baltimore: Gateway Printing, 1980.

Dunstan, Simon. *Flak Jackets: 20th Century Military Body Armor.* London: Osprey, 1984.

Katcher, Philip. *The American Soldier: U.S. Armies in Uniform, 1755 to the Present.* New York: Military Press, 1990.

Kennedy, Stephen J. *Battlefield Protection of the Soldier through His Clothing/Equipment System.* Natick, MA: U.S. Army Natick Lab, 1969.

U.S. Army. *Body Armor for the Individual Soldier: DA PAM 21-54.* Washington, D.C.: U.S. Government Printing Office, 1965.

Drugs and Drug Use

Drug use was a serious problem for U.S. forces in Vietnam, especially from 1968 onward. A Department of Defense study revealed that in 1968, slightly more than half of American servicemen in Vietnam used drugs. By 1970 that number had risen to more than 60 percent. The study estimated that by the time of American withdrawal in 1973, almost 70 percent of American servicemen in Vietnam had used some type of illicit drug. Cheap and readily available, drugs provided an escape from the anxiety and boredom prevalent among combat soldiers.

After the 1968 Tet Offensive, drug use rose dramatically. Marijuana was the drug of choice for most GIs. In 1969, 30 percent of enlisted men sent to Vietnam had used marijuana previously. That rate jumped to nearly 60 percent after arrival in Vietnam. A marijuana cigarette cost a mere ten cents in Saigon. A soldier could buy an entire carton of prerolled marijuana cigarettes in resealed cigarette packs for either $5 or a carton of American cigarettes. Smoking marijuana eventually became part of the standard initiation rite for those arriving in Vietnam. A U.S. Marine Corps colonel said, "When a man is in Vietnam he can be sure that there are probably drugs within twenty-five feet of him."

Amphetamines were also popular, although less common than marijuana. Narcotics, such as opium and heroin, ran a distant third behind marijuana and amphetamines for obvious reasons; no one wished to be caught nodding during an ambush. Binges remained fairly common in the rear, however, because of the astoundingly low prices and remarkable purity. In Vietnam soldiers could buy a gram of 95 percent pure heroin for $2. The same amount in the United States cost more than $100, and it was rarely more than 10 percent pure. Opium, available either in liquid form or rolled into cigarettes, gave the user a similar high. Although less common, opiates produced more lasting addictions than marijuana or amphetamines and led some veterans to crime to support their habits back in the United States.

The relatively high incidence of drug use among GIs in Vietnam may be seen as either a predisposition to use of drugs or as a reaction to one's environment. Easy access to the drugs may have been a determining factor. Statistics show, however, that personnel in Vietnam were much more likely to use drugs than were their comrades-in-arms in Europe, where drugs were also easily accessible. Combat stress certainly accounts for a portion of the disparity. Still, men who had used marijuana, narcotics, or amphetamines before entering the military composed the vast bulk of the user population. Many users in Vietnam did so for the first time, but for the vast majority this consequence of combat experience was not a lasting one: 93 percent of first-time narcotics users and 86 percent of first-time marijuana users stopped completely upon returning to the United States.

Benjamin C. Dubberly

Further Reading

Appy, Christian G. *Working Class War: American Combat Soldiers & Vietnam.* Chapel Hill: University of North Carolina Press, 1993.

Boetcher, Thomas D. *Vietnam: The Valor and the Sorrow.* Boston: Little Brown, 1985.

Ebert, James R. *A Life in a Year.* Novato, CA: Presidio, 1993.

Lewy, Guenter. *America in Vietnam.* Oxford: Oxford University Press, 1978.

Medevac

The term "medevac," an acronym combining the words "medical" and "evacuation," refers to the movement of casualties from the battlefield to more secure locations for immediate medical attention. Although evacuation from the battlefield for medical attention had been practiced for some time, the frontless nature of the guerrilla war in Vietnam called for exploitation of a Korean War innovation: casualty evacuation via helicopter.

The U.S. Army experimented with aeromedical evacuation from the introduction of crewed flight, but this did not come into its own until the 1950–1953 Korean War. Korea's rugged mountainous terrain and poor road network made overland movement extremely difficult. By war's end, medical evacuation helicopters had evacuated 17,700 casualties, and nonmedical helicopters supplemented that number with many more. Although the Korean War made the potential of helicopter medical evacuation obvious, the Vietnam War proved its worth.

Vietnam added dense jungle, tropical heat, and a frontless battlefield to the problems that medical evacuation faced in Korea. Although general-use helicopters provided aeromedical evacuation prior to and after their arrival, U.S. Army Medical Department air ambulance units were introduced into Vietnam in April 1962. Expanding with the surge of American ground troops, they remained in Vietnam until total U.S. troop withdrawal in 1973. Nicknamed dustoff missions, air ambulance evacuations lifted between 850,000 and 900,000 allied military and Vietnamese civilian casualties during their period of service. With their crews landing virtually almost anywhere without consideration of the dangers, medevacs provided rapid response and reduced time from injury to treatment; this helped reduce the rate of deaths as a percentage of hits from 29.3 percent in World War II and 26.3 percent in Korea to 19 percent in Vietnam.

Arthur T. Frame

Further Reading

Dorland, Peter, and James Nanney. *Dustoff: Army Aeromedical Evacuation in Vietnam.* Washington, D.C.: U.S. Army Center of Military History, 1982.

Neel, Spurgeon. *Medical Support of the U.S. Army in Vietnam, 1965–1972.* Washington, D.C.: U.S. Army Center of Military History, 1973.

Medics and Corpsmen

Medics and corpsmen have been designated as noncombatants by the military and by the rules of war in international law. In the Vietnam War, however, medics frequently carried weapons to protect their wounded and themselves, and this invalidated their noncombatant status and Geneva Convention protection. By 1969, 90 percent of U.S. Army medics serving in Vietnam were draftees. The U.S. Navy, which provided corpsmen for the U.S. Marine Corps, did not have draftees, but at least 33 percent of its recruits were motivated by the draft to join the military.

In both the U.S. Army and the U.S. Navy, medics and corpsmen had to meet required test standards. These tests were normally administered during basic training. In some cases recruits requested and received a medical military occupational specialty (MOS), but in most cases recruits were handed their medical MOS according to army or navy needs. Medics and corpsmen differed from the average draftees. They usually had some college background and were considered to be highly motivated.

Army medics were trained at Fort Sam Houston, Texas, in a 10-week, 480-hour course. Recruits were instructed in communicable diseases, sterilization, anatomy, physiology, and emergency treatment. Medics receiving orders for Vietnam were given 14 hours of battle preparedness training outside the classroom. The navy's basic medical course lasted four months and comprised human biology, pharmacology, and basic patient care, with practical experience in hospital wards. At the end of the basic course, some students took specialized training work. Those in the U.S. Marine Corps received four to five weeks of battlefield training at either Camp Lejeune, North Carolina, or Camp Pendleton, California, where they went on forced marches with full packs, fired weapons, and navigated cross-country without a compass. They also received additional training in managing battlefield casualties, triage (deciding who should receive treatment and in what order and which of the wounded were less likely to survive even if treated), and direct patient care.

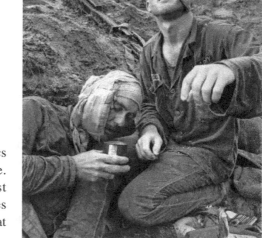

During the Vietnam War, combat medics achieved an elevated standard of care. Here a wounded medic of the First Cavalry Division (Airmobile) continues to treat a wounded soldier during combat in 1966. (AP Photo)

Combat medics and corpsmen, once in Vietnam, were normally assigned to infantry units. Under ideal conditions, each line platoon had two medics or corpsmen assigned to it. Because of the heavy casualty rate among medics and corpsmen, however, most units were understaffed. U.S. search-and-destroy tactics in Vietnam normally were centered on platoons, and line medics and corpsmen accompanied these missions. While on patrol, medics and corpsmen carried out many of the same responsibilities as the infantry. Their basic responsibility was to care for the wounded; however, medics also stood perimeter guard and participated in firefights.

Mines and booby traps accounted for 65 percent of wounds and 36 percent of fatalities sustained by Americans in Vietnam. Small arms accounted for 16 percent of wounds and 51 percent of the fatalities sustained. Because of the threat of shock, treatment during the first few minutes after injury was most critical to the survival of the wounded. Medics and corpsmen contributed to the fact that the mortality rate for wounded (1–2.5 percent) was less than in any prior American war.

Medical kits used in the field contained various battlefield dressings as well as splints, tape, tweezers, safety pins, plastic airways, aspirin, intravenous fluids, and morphine. When a man was injured, medics evaluated the wound and began treatment. If there were multiple casualties, corpsmen had to triage their patients. The corpsmen also arranged for evacuation and determined who should be evacuated first. Medics provided psychological and emotional as well as medical support and were widely respected by the troops.

The U.S. Army assigned combat medics to seven-month rotations, with the remainder of their tour in rear areas and noncombat assignments. This policy was based on studies of the psychological effect of combat on the medics. Time between patrols was normally spent at a base camp. Corpsmen performed sick call or were involved with the Medical Civic Action Program (MEDCAP), providing medical care to the rural populations at nearby villages or hamlets. MEDCAP was a part of the pacification program. Medics and corpsmen also managed base sanitation and water purification.

During the Vietnam War, medics were among the most respected soldiers on the battlefield. Of 238 Medals of Honor awarded in the war, 12 went to U.S. Army medics, and 4 went to U.S. Navy corpsmen. An estimated 1,300 medics and 690 corpsmen died in the war. Army medics were recognized with the Combat Medical Badge (CMB), an award equal in prestige to the Combat Infantry Badge.

Pia C. Heyn

Further Reading

Heyn, Pia Christine. "The Role of Army Combat Medics in the Vietnam War, 1965–1971." Master's thesis, Georgia State University, 1994.

McCallum, Jack E. *Military Medicine: From Ancient Times to the 21st Century.* Santa Barbara, CA: ABC-CLIO, 2003.

Mullins, William S., ed. *A Decade of Progress: The United States Army Medical Department, 1959–1969.* Washington, D.C.: Office of the Surgeon General, 1971.

Nurses, U.S.

U.S. military nurses arrived in Vietnam early in the conflict. In March 1962, 13 U.S. Army nurses arrived at the Eighth Field Hospital, Nha Trang. The first members of the U.S. Navy Nurse Corps were stationed in Saigon at the same time. U.S. Air Force nurses soon followed, and the number of military nurses serving in Vietnam rose steadily after 1966 to a peak of 900 in January 1969. This coincided with the number of troops deployed, which was at its highest number of 543,400 in April 1969. Nurses served as flight nurses, in hospitals throughout Vietnam, and on board the hospital ships *Repose* and *Sanctuary.*

The work of nurses closely paralleled that of physicians and medical corpsmen. Most patients were either wounded in battle or sick with infectious diseases. Care of those infected with tropical diseases was primarily supportive, providing liquids, medications for relief of symptoms, nourishment, and rest. Nurses were often infected themselves, and most days lost from work were related to tropical diseases.

Nurses received wounded personnel in the field in hospitals of varied sizes and equipped with varied resources. The wounded men had been stabilized by a medic or corpsman and then transported, most often by helicopter, to 1 of 19 medical facilities. Although physicians were responsible for the triage of wounded men, nurses often shared this task and were sometimes delegated triage decisions because physicians were needed to begin treatment or surgery.

For those whose wounds were so severe that treatment was futile, nurses focused on pain relief and psychological support. Some nurses reported that comforting the dying soldier was an essential task so that the soldier and his family would know that he had not died alone.

Most wounded had suffered either small-arms injuries or explosive injuries from mines or booby traps. Small-arms fire typically caused severe tissue damage, interfered with blood supply to the wound, and often resulted in multiple wounds. Explosive devices caused large and contaminated wounds. After surgery had been performed on the wounded, nurses were primarily concerned with prevention of infection, relief of pain, tissue regeneration, and psychological support.

The role of nurses was significantly challenged by the soldiers in Vietnam and conflicts in American culture during the 1960s and 1970s. Not only was the war unpopular, but the country was also struggling with civil rights issues and the women's movement. Alcohol and drug abuse complicated an already complex social milieu, and the traditional role of nurses in providing neutral, unconditional support was made much more difficult. Additionally, many nurses encountered the same psychological trauma as the soldiers for whom they cared.

Nurses served aboard fixed-wing evacuation flights, transporting patients, most often to Okinawa or Japan, for further treatment or rehabilitation. These nurses were trained in trauma and critical care and worked with significantly more independence than did nurses prior to the war.

The Vietnam War brought at least three changes in the nursing profession. First, nurses developed practice specialties, much as physicians had already begun to do. Nurses were particularly successful in the specialties of trauma and critical care and anesthesia. Second, the war afforded many opportunities for nurses to practice more independently and with greater professional autonomy. Nurses, physicians, and patients were able to observe the benefit of increased flexibility and effectiveness in nurses' activities. Third, in 1966 men were authorized by Congress to join the three nurses' corps. Men ultimately made up about one-fourth of the nurse corps and were most commonly found in anesthesia and surgical specialties. Men were a valuable addition to the nurse corps; however, many soldiers found that female nurses were an important factor in morale. This same phenomenon has been reported in other American wars and is probably related to the socialization of women as comforters.

Several studies and biographies of nurses who served in Vietnam reveal experiences of a more personal nature. First, women there were socially isolated, restricted to the hospital, the barracks, and occasionally the officers' club. Second, many nurses were frustrated by their inability to see a patient through his recovery. The excellent transport and treatment systems were key factors in the low mortality rate, but these denied the nurses and physicians the ability to see progress and recovery. Third, nurses, like soldiers, experienced difficulty in readjusting to life at home after their Vietnam experience.

One nurse was killed in the Vietnam War: First Lieutenant Sharon Lane was killed by hostile action while on duty at the 312th Evacuation Hospital, Chu Lai, on June 8, 1969. The contribution of nurses to the American military effort during the war was recognized in 1993 with the dedication of a statue, sculpted by Glenna Goodacre, which was placed near the Vietnam Veterans Memorial. The statue depicts three women assisting a fallen soldier.

Rhonda Keen-Payne

Further Reading

Donahue, M. Patricia. *Nursing: The Finest Art.* St. Louis: C. V. Mosby, 1985.

Kalisch, Phillip A., and Beatrice Kalisch. *The Advance of American Nursing.* 3rd ed. Boston: Little, Brown, 1994.

Kalisch, Phillip A., and Beatrice Kalisch. "Nurses under Fire: The World War II Experience of Nurses on Bataan and Corregidor." *Nursing Research* 25(2) (November–December 1976): 401–429.

Kirkpatrick, Sandra. "Battle Casualty." *American Journal of Nursing* 68(5) (July 1968): 998–1005.

Norman, Elizabeth M. "A Study of Female Military Nurses in Vietnam during the War Years 1965–1973." *Journal of Nursing History* 2 (November 1986): 43–60.

Smith, Winnie. *American Daughter Gone to War.* New York: William Morrow, 1992.

DOCUMENTS

Patrick H. Brady Medal of Honor Citation Dust Off: Army Aeromedical Evacuation in Vietnam

Casualty evacuation during the Vietnam War was difficult because of the country's poor road network and the fact that many engagements took place in roadless jungles and forests. Consequenty, the military relied upon helicopter transport to carry the wounded from the battlefield to the hospital. The slang of the time called such aeromedical evucation missions "Dust Off," and improved management of shock and multiple trauma resulted in a death rate for soldiers who arrived at a field hospital of only 2.6 percent. That extraordinary achievement depended upon the skill and courage of helicopter pilots who flew in aeromedical evacuation units. Air ambulance pilots and crewmen stood a high chance of being injured, wounded, or killed during their one-year tour of duty. Theirs was one of the most dangerous types of aviation. Of some 1,400 Army commissioned and warrant officers who served as air ambulance pilots, 40 were killed by hostile fire, 180 wounded, while another 48 were killed and about 200 injured in nonhostile crashes, many while flying at night and in bad weather during evacuation missions. The following excerpt first describes a series of missions flown by Dust Off pilot Patrick H. Brady and then provides Brady's Medal of Honor Citation.

Dust Off Wins Its First Medal of Honor

As Dust Off flew more and more missions the bravery of its pilots and crews became evident to all who fought in South Vietnam. While each of these pilots returned from a Dust Off mission something of a hero, some pilots distinguished themselves more than others. On the night of 5 January 1968 a South Vietnamese reconnaissance patrol left its camp in a heavily forested valley surrounded by mountains west of Chu Lai. An enemy force soon hit the patrol and inflicted several casualties. When the patrol limped back into camp with its wounded, Sgt. Robert E. Cashon, the senior Special Forces medical specialist at the base, tended to two critical patients and radioed his headquarters for a

Dust Off ship. Soon the aircraft arrived overhead and tried several times to land in the camp. The pilot finally had to leave because fog and darkness obscured the ground. The monsoon season had enshrouded the mountains in soft, marshmallow clouds and fog several hundred feet thick. The clouds and fog extended east all the way to the flatlands between the mountain chain and the South China Sea.

Dawn brought little improvement in the weather. Visibility and ceiling were still zero. The next crew who tried to reach the camp, at 0700, also failed, even though they had been flying in that area for five months. True to the Kelly legacy of unhesitating service, Patrick H. Brady, now a major, and his crew of Dust Off 55 now volunteered for the mission into the fog-wrapped mountains.

They flew from Chu Lai to the mountains at low level just under the cloud base, then turned northward to Phu Tho where a trail wound westward through the mountains to the reconnaissance camp.

The fog grew so thick that none of the crew would even see the rotor tips of the helicopter. To improve the visibility, Brady lowered his side window and tilted his ship sideways at a sharp angle from the ground. The rotor blades blew enough fog away for him to barely make out the trail below the ship. Hovering slowly along the trail and occasionally drawing startled enemy fire, Dust Off 55 finally reached the valley and the camp. The visibility there was so poor that the ship completely missed the camp's landing zone and set down in a smaller clearing less than twenty meters square between the inner and outer defensive wires of the camp. The outpost had earlier taken mortar rounds and was still under sniper fire. Sergeant Cashon later said that the landing area would have been hazardous even in good weather. But Dust Off 55 loaded up, climbed out through the soup, and flew the two critical patients and four others to surgical care.

Brady's sweat from the first mission was hardly dry when another request chattered in over the 54th's radio. In the late afternoon of the day before, a company of the 198th Light Infantry Brigade, 23d Infantry Division, operating on the floor of the Hiep Due Valley, came under a concerted attack by six companies of the *2nd North Vietnamese Division*. For nine hours from their well-fortified positions in the surrounding hills, the North Vietnamese rained mortars and rockets on the Americans. The enemy had covered the likely flight paths into the area with 123-mm. antiaircraft guns. Early in the assault they had shot down two American gunships. Difficult communications and the nearness of the enemy on the night of the fifth had made a Dust Off mission impossible, even though the enemy had inflicted heavy casualties on the Americans. By dawn the company had sixty wounded on its hands.

On the morning of the sixth, a Dust Off pilot WO1 Charles D. Schenck, starting from fire support base West overlooking the valley, tried to fly a medical team out to the company and bring some of the wounded back. But the vertigo he suffered from the zero visibility forced him to abort. Shortly after he returned and told Dust Off Operations Control of his failure, Major Brady and Dust Off 55 began to prepare for flight. Brady, who knew the Hiep Due Valley, listened to Schenck and the other pilots who had tried to reach the stranded company. Then he loaded a medical team in his ship, cranked the engine, and took off. Several miles from the battle area he found a hole in the soupy clouds through which he descended to treetop level. After twenty long minutes of low-level flight, Dust Off 55 neared the stricken company. Brady's surprise approach and the poor visibility threw off the enemy's aim; the helicopter landed safely. Once on the ground the medical team quickly found and loaded the most seriously wounded. Brady made an instrument takeoff through the clouds, flew to fire base West, and delivered his casualties to the aid station. He then briefed three other crews on how he would execute his next trip into the area. The three ships tried to follow Brady in, but thick fog and enemy fire made them all climb out and return to West. Brady kept going, landed, picked up a load of wounded, and flew them out to West. Twice more he hovered down the trail and brought out wounded. Although the three other ships again tried to emulate his technique, none could make it all the way. Brady and his crew evacuated eighteen litter and twenty-one ambulatory patients on those four trips. Nine of the soldiers certainly would not have survived the hours which passed before the fog lifted.

As soon as Dust Off 55 refueled, Brady was sent on an urgent mission to evacuate the U.S. soldiers from a unit surrounded by the enemy twenty-six kilometers southeast of Chu Lai. Machine guns swept the landing zone as the North Vietnamese tried to wipe out the remaining American troops. Brady tried another surprise tactic. He low-leveled to the area, dropped in, turned his tail boom toward the heaviest fire to protect his cockpit, and hovered backward toward the pinned soldiers. The ship took rounds going in and once it was on the ground the fire intensified. For fear of being wounded or killed themselves, the friendly forces would not rise up and help load the casualties. Seeing this, Brady took off and circled the area until the ground troops radioed him in a second time. As he repeated his backward hover, the enemy tried once more to destroy the aircraft. But this time the ground troops loaded their comrades, who were soon in the rooms of the 27th Surgical Hospital at Chu Lai.

After four hours of flying that Saturday morning, Brady had to change his aircraft and find a relief copilot. A few hours earlier a platoon of the 198th Light Infantry Brigade on a patrol southeast of Chu Lai had walked into a carefully planned ambush. Automatic weapons and pressure-detonated mines devastated the platoon, killing six soldiers outright and wounding all the others. The platoon leader called for Dust Off. A helicopter soon landed, but took off quickly when a mine detonated close by, killing two more soldiers of the 198th who were crossing the minefield to aid the wounded.

Hearing this, Brady radioed that he would try the mission. The commander of the first aircraft suggested that Brady wait until the enemy broke contact. But Brady immediately flew out and landed on the minefield. Most of the casualties lay scattered around the area where they had fallen. Brady's crew chief and medical corpsman hustled the wounded onto the ship, disregarding the enemy fire and mines. As they neared the ship with one soldier, a mine detonated only five meters away, hurling the men into the air and perforating the aircraft with shrapnel holes. Both crewmen stood up, shaken by the concussion but otherwise unhurt, and placed the casualty on board. With a full load Brady flew out to the nearest hospital.

When he returned to the Dust Off pad at Chu Lai and delivered his patients, he again traded his ship for another. He flew two more urgent missions before he ended his day of glory well after dark. He had flown three aircraft and evacuated fifty-one wounded soldiers. For this day's work he was awarded the Medal of Honor.

Source: Peter Dorland and James Nanney. *Dust Off: Army Aeromedical Evacuation in Vietnam.* Center of Military History, United States Army, Washington, D.C., 1984, pp. 63–66.

For conspicuous gallantry and intrepidity in action at the risk of his life above and beyond the call of duty, Maj. Brady distinguished himself while serving in the Republic of Vietnam commanding a UH-1H ambulance helicopter, volunteered to rescue wounded men from a site in enemy held territory which was reported to be heavily defended and to be blanketed by fog. To reach the site he descended through heavy fog and smoke and hovered slowly along a valley trail, turning his ship sideward to blow away the fog with the backwash from his rotor blades. Despite the unchallenged, close-range enemy fire, he found the dangerously small site, where he successfully landed and evacuated 2 badly wounded South Vietnamese soldiers. He was then called to another area completely covered by dense fog where American casualties lay only 50 meters from the enemy. Two aircraft had previously been shot down and others had made unsuccessful attempts to reach this site earlier in the day. With unmatched skill and extraordinary courage, Maj. Brady made 4 flights to this embattled landing zone and successfully rescued all the wounded. On his third mission of the day Maj. Brady once again landed at a site surrounded by the enemy. The friendly ground force, pinned down by enemy fire, had been unable to reach and secure the landing zone. Although his aircraft had been badly damaged and his controls partially shot away during his initial entry into this area, he returned minutes later and rescued the remaining injured. Shortly thereafter, obtaining a replacement aircraft, Maj. Brady was requested to land in an enemy minefield where a platoon of American soldiers was trapped. A mine detonated near his helicopter, wounding 2 crewmembers and damaging his ship. In spite of this, he managed to fly 6 severely injured patients to medical aid. Throughout that day Maj. Brady utilized 3 helicopters to evacuate a total of 51 seriously wounded men, many of whom would have perished without prompt medical treatment. Maj. Brady's bravery was in the highest traditions of the military service and reflects great credit upon himself and the U.S. Army.

Source: Congressional Medal of Honor Society. Available online at http://www.cmohs.org/recipient-detail/3236/brady-patrick-henry.php

Medical Support of the U.S. Army in Vietnam

The Office of the Surgeon General collected statistics about death and wounds during the Vietnam War. The study found that compared to World War II and Korea, more soldiers received multiple wounds from rapid fire small arms. In addition, small arms caused two-thirds of the head and neck wounds and three-quarters of trunk wounds. Head and neck wounds were particularly lethal. However, early evacuation—invariably using helicopters—the extensive use

TABLE 9.1: Prevalence of Amputation during the Vietnam War as Compared to Other U.S. Conflicts

Conflict	Total Number of Amputations	Ratio of Amputations to Total Wounded
World War I	2,610	1 to 78.2
World War II	7,489	1 to 89.7
Korean War	1,477	1 to 69.9
Vietnam War	5,283	1 to 29.0

TABLE 9.2: Percent of Deaths and Wounds according to Agent, U.S. Army, in Three Wars, World War II, Korea, and Vietnam

Agent	Deaths			Wounds		
	World War II	Korea	Vietnam[1]	World War II	Korea	Vietnam[1]
Small arms	32	33	51	20	27	16
Fragments	53	59	36	62	61	65
Booby traps, mines	3	4	11	4	4	15
Punji stakes	–	–	–	–	–	2
Other	12	4	2	14	8	2

[1]January 1965-June 1970.
Source: Statistical Data on Army Troops Wounded in Vietnam, January 1965-June 1970, Medical Statistics Agency, Office of the Surgeon General, US Army.

238 | Health under Fire

TABLE 9.3: Location of Wounds in Hospitalized Casualties, by Percent, U.S. Army, in Three Wars: World War II, Korea, and Vietnam

Anatomical location	World War II	Korea	Vietnam[1]
Head and neck	17	17	14
Thorax	7	7	7
Abdomen	8	7	5
Upper Extremities	25	30	18
Lower Extremities	40	37	36
Other Sites	3	2	20[2]

[1]For a 24-month period.
[2]Including multiple wounds.
Source: Statistical Data on Army Troops Wounded in Vietnam, January 1965–June 1970, Medical Statistics Agency, Office of the Surgeon General, US Army.
Source: Spurgeon Neel, Medical Support of the U.S. Army in Vietnam, 1965–1970. Department of the Army, Washington, D.C., 1973, p 54.

of blood, and the presence of full trained neurosurgeons in the combat zone significantly reduced the mortality rate for head wounds. The collection of death and wound statistics allowed the military medical service to develop better process and ancillary caring techniques for the wounded particularly in the areas of anesthesia, blood and plasma expanders, burn treatment, wound healing, shock, and surgical routine.

■ CHAPTER 10
Wars in the Middle East and Afghanistan

INTRODUCTION

American military intervention in the Middle East began in 1990 and remains ongoing at this time. On August 2, 1990, Iraq invaded Kuwait. In response, the United States organized an international coalition to fight Iraq. Operation Desert Storm officially began on January 17, 1991, with an air campaign that lasted over a month, and ended on February 28, after a 100-hour ground offensive by coalition troops.

Casualties for Operation Desert Storm include those individuals killed, wounded, or captured in the operation that liberated Kuwait from Iraqi occupation and defeated Iraq during the 1991 Persian Gulf War. Given the number of troops engaged, casualties for the war were extremely low, at least for the coalition arrayed against Iraq. Controversy has dogged the question of casualties on two counts. First, the percentage of friendly-fire deaths has been debated; and second, there is no agreement on the number of Iraqi soldiers and civilians killed. The U.S. Department of Defense (DOD) reported 148 American battle deaths and 145 non-combat deaths. A total of 467 Americans were wounded in action, but more than 3,000 others were injured in non-combat related accidents. Some statistics actually estimated that had American troops not been deployed, more would have died of natural causes and from accidents than those killed in the Gulf combat theater. The tactical use of air power, technological superiority, and efficient evacuation of the wounded to medical centers in Europe helped minimize U.S. combat deaths.

In addition to the official numbers of soldiers wounded in combat or accidents, the Department of Veterans Affairs (DVA) has declared that more than 180,000 veterans of the Persian Gulf War were permanently disabled from mysterious ailments, sometimes referred to as Gulf War Syndrome.

U.S. forces returned to the Middle East when the War on Terror was launched on October 7, 2001. The American intervention in Afghanistan was a response to the terror attacks against the United States of September 11, 2001. As of 2014, U.S. forces remain in Afghanistan.

A third American intervention in the Middle East, Operation Iraqi Freedom, began on March 19, 2003. The quick and decisive victory won by the United States in the 1991 Persian Gulf War, which saw few American casualties, and the low initial American casualty count for the Afghanistan War, Operation Enduring Freedom, had conditioned U.S. citizens and politicians to expect a speedy and relatively easy victory in Iraq. Although the initial combat phase (March 19–April 30 2003) produced few U.S. and Coalition combat deaths, the subsequent insurgency led to several thousand more, with the toll continuing to climb. On January 1, 2010, Operation Iraqi Freedom formally ended. However, U.S. forces remained in Iraq to provide security through December 15, 2011. Nearly nine years of conflict claimed the lives of about 4,500 American troops.

During the U.S. wars in the Middle East, the widespread use of body armor has altered the historic pattern of combat injuries. In addition, modern battlefield surgical techniques dramatically lowered the percentage of men and women who died from their initial injury. A consequence of both these trends is a large increase in the number of survivors with persistent disabilities. Unprecedented numbers of disabled veterans have required long term or permanent care, a need that has posed immense challenges on the military health care service.

Although small-arms fire accounted for most of the injuries early in the Middle Eastern conflict, improvised explosive devices subsequently caused most fatalities and wounds. These most often result in blast and burn injuries. Body armor, although relatively effective in protecting the torso, leaves the victims susceptible to extremity injuries, and there have been a large number of amputations. The American military has been active in prosthetic research, particularly at Walter Reed Army Medical Center, and has been in the forefront of research into devices such as computerized limbs and specialized artificial joints. One of the major trends resulting from the wars in the Middle East has been the diffusion of medical knowledge and procedures, particularly those related to traumatic injury, from the military service into civilian medical practice.

James R. Arnold

ENTRIES

Biological Weapons and Warfare

Biological weapons are forms of natural organisms, or modified versions of germs or toxins, that are used as weapons to kill or harm people or animals. Natural biological weapons include diseases such as anthrax or smallpox. Modified versions include toxins or poisons such as ricin or aflatoxin. Along with nuclear and chemical arms, biological weapons are considered to be weapons of mass destruction

(WMDs). The proliferation of WMDs, including biological weapons, is one of the most serious security issues in the Middle East.

By the early 1970s, several Arab states had established biological weapons programs as a means to balance Israel's nuclear arsenal as they concurrently sought to develop their own nuclear and chemical weapons programs. Biological weapons were attractive to many states because they were perceived as being less expensive and easier to manufacture. Biological agents could also be developed far more quickly than nuclear or chemical programs.

In 1974 the Iraqi government officially launched a biological weapons program, and within a year the country established facilities for research and development of biological agents. Through the 1970s and 1980s, Iraq obtained cultures and biological agents from Western governments and firms through both legitimate and illicit means. Among the biological weapons Iraq obtained were anthrax, salmonella, and botulinum. By 1983, Iraq began stockpiling biological warheads and accelerated its program, including efforts to develop new types of weapons. During 1987–1988, Saddam Hussein's regime employed biological weapons against Iraq's Kurdish minority. Large-scale Iraqi production of anthrax and aflatoxin began in 1989, and that same year Iraqi scientists initiated field tests of biological weapons. In 1990, Iraq stockpiled some 200 bombs and 100 missiles capable of delivering biological agents.

Under the terms of the cease-fire that ended the 1991 Persian Gulf War, Iraq began destroying its biological weapons capability. Also in 1991, Iraq ratified the Biological Weapons Convention. United Nations (UN) weapons inspectors were granted limited access to biological weapons facilities and were able to verify the extent of the program and confirm that some materials had been destroyed. The belief by President George W. Bush's administration that Hussein's regime had not complied with UN resolutions to destroy its WMD programs was a major justification for the U.S.-led invasion in 2003.

Tom Lansford

Further Reading

Cordesman, Anthony. *Iran's Developing Military Capabilities.* Washington, D.C.: CSIS, 2005.

Guillemin, Jeanne. *Biological Weapons: From the Invention of State-Sponsored Programs to Contemporary Bioterrorism.* New York: Columbia University Press, 2005.

Walker, William. *Weapons of Mass Destruction and International Order.* New York: Oxford University Press, 2004.

Blast Injuries

Blast injuries are those caused by explosive devices. The study of blast injuries has become particularly important in light of recent attacks by terrorists and

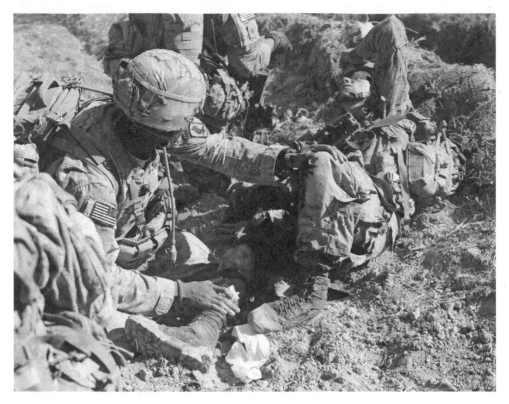

An American soldier serving in Afghanistan receives medical assistance following the detonation of an Improvised Explosive Device in October 2012. (Munir Uzzaman/AFP/ Getty Images)

insurgents. Weapons that cause blast injuries are of two general types: conventional bombs and enhanced blast explosive devices. The first generate a shock wave emanating from a point source that results in rapid increase and decrease of pressure followed by a blast of moving air and possibly by fragments from either the device itself or from surrounding structures. This effect can be multiplied if the primary blast is used as a trigger for a secondary explosion. The damage from either device is increased by reflected waves if the explosion occurs in a closed space.

Blast injuries are of four types. Injuries from direct pressure are principally the result of barotrauma and are most damaging to areas with an interface between air and fluid, especially air-containing organs, such as the ear, lung, or bowel, or fluid-filled organs exposed to the outside, such as the eye. Ear drum rupture occurs at the lowest pressure differential and is a sensitive indicator of potential damage to other organs. Eyes can bleed or rupture, as can the bowel. The most lethal injuries are those to the lung and include contusion, hemorrhage, and edema. Victims in close proximity to an explosion can also suffer traumatic amputation. Although body armor protects against flying fragments, it offers no protection from pressure injury.

The second effect is that from flying projectiles and has been the main cause of death from improvised explosive devices (IEDs) during the conflicts waged in Afghanistan and Iraq in the early 21st century. Secondary air movement from a blast can cause collapse of surrounding structures, resulting in crushing injury to those trapped within. Finally, burns, asphyxiation, or toxicity from inhaled gases or dust can also cause significant injury.

Prior to World War II, blast injury in war was relatively uncommon. Blast injuries from terrorist attacks have become increasingly common beginning in Israel after World War II and in Northern Ireland for the last four decades. In the October 1983 bombing of the Marine barracks in Beirut, Lebanon, 234 immediate blast-related deaths occurred and 122 more victims were injured, 59 percent suffering significant head trauma. The largest terrorist explosive attack in the United States was the 1995 detonation at the Alfred P. Murrah Federal Building in Oklahoma City that resulted in 518 injuries and 168 deaths. With that exception, blast injuries have been very uncommon in the United States, resulting in an average of fewer than 50 deaths a year. Blast injuries have, on the other hand, accounted for more than half the combat casualties in the Iraq War. Responsible weapons have included grenades, missiles, artillery shells, land mines, and especially IEDs. As in the Beirut experience, 59 percent of those wounded by blasts in Iraq have suffered traumatic brain injury.

Jack McCallum

Further Reading

DePalma, R. G., D. G. Burris, H. R. Champion, and M. J. Hodgson. 2005. "Blast Injuries." *New England Journal of Medicine* 352 (March 31): 1335–1342.

Mellor, S. G., and G. J. Cooper. 1989. "Analysis of 828 Servicemen Killed or Injured by Explosion in Northern Ireland 1970–1984: The Hostile Action Casualty System." *British Journal of Surgery* 76 (October): 1006–1010.

Stein, M., and A. Hirshberg. 1979. "Medical Consequences of Terrorism: The Conventional Weapons Threat." *Surgical Clinics of North America* 79 (December): 1537–1552.

Chemical Weapons and Warfare

Chemical weapons use the toxic effects from man-made substances to kill or incapacitate enemy forces. Chemical weapons range from riot control agents such as tear gas and pepper spray, which cause short-term incapacitation, to lethal nerve agents such as tabun and sarin, which can kill humans with only a minuscule exposure. The use of living organisms, such as bacteria, viruses, or spores, is not classified as chemical warfare but rather is considered biological warfare.

However, certain chemical weapons such as ricin and botulinum toxins use products created by living organisms.

Chemical weapons are typically described by the effects they have on victims. The major classes of chemical weapons are nerve agents, blood agents, vesicants, pulmonary agents, cytotoxic proteins, lachrymatory agents, and incapacitating agents. Nerve agents quickly break down neuron-transmitting synapses, resulting in the paralysis of major organs and quick death. Blood agents cause massive internal bleeding or prevent cells from using oxygen, leading to anaerobic respiration, seizures, and death. Vesicants, also known as blistering agents, burn skin and respiratory systems, either of which can be fatal. Pulmonary agents suffocate victims by flooding the respiratory system. Cytotoxic agents prevent protein synthesis, leading to the failure of one or more organs. Lachrymatory agents cause immediate eye irritation or blindness, although the effects are deliberately temporary. Incapacitating agents, also temporary, cause effects similar to drug intoxication.

The most important characteristics of an effective chemical weapon are its ability to be delivered accurately and its ability to persist as a danger to enemy troops. Throughout history, delivery methods for chemical weapons have evolved from simple dispersion, often by releasing a gas into the wind, to artillery shells or missile warheads containing chemical agents and to aerodynamic dispersal from aircraft. Since World War II, binary chemical weapons have been developed that contain two substances that are harmless by themselves but when combined form a weapons grade chemical agent.

During World War I (1914–1918), more chemical weapons were used than during any other war in history. At the Second Battle of Ypres (April 22, 1915), German troops opened canisters of chlorine gas and waited for the wind to push the gas into Allied trenches. Soon both sides were using artillery shells to deliver chemical attacks, incorporating a wide variety of chemical agents.

Although they caused a great deal of panic and disruption on the battlefield and caused more than 1 million mostly nonlethal casualties in World War I, chemical weapons were never decisive by themselves. The chemical weapons of the period were relatively weak by modern standards, and no army of the time had developed nerve agents. Although early gas masks and other countermeasures were relatively primitive, they did neutralize the chemical effects to some degree.

During World War II (1939–1945), chemical weapons were used in a few isolated instances, although both the Axis and the Allies had developed large arsenals of extremely toxic agents. Both sides feared retaliation by the enemy, and neither chose to use its massive stockpiles of chemical weapons.

In the Middle East, the first modern large-scale use of lethal chemical agents occurred during the Iran-Iraq War (1980–1988). During the 1991 Persian Gulf War, Iraq was accused of launching Scud missiles with chemical warheads against Israel, although no traces of chemical weapons were found. Iraq did not strike the attacking coalition forces with chemical weapons. Chemical weapons in the hands of terrorist groups pose a significant potential threat. On March 20, 1995, Aum Shinrikyo, a Japanese apocalyptic cult, released sarin gas on a Tokyo subway, killing 12 commuters and injuring more than 5,000. In 2002 the terrorist organization Al Qaeda released a videotape purportedly showing the deaths of dogs from a nerve agent. Al Qaeda has repeatedly announced its intention to obtain chemical, biological, and nuclear weapons.

There have been many attempts to prohibit the development and use of chemical weapons. In 1874 the Brussels Declaration outlawed the use of poison in warfare. The 1900 Hague Conference banned projectiles carrying poisonous gasses, as did the Washington Arms Conference Treaty of 1922 and the Geneva Protocol of 1929. None of the prohibitions proved sufficient to eradicate chemical warfare, however. The most recent effort to eliminate chemical weapons was the multilateral Chemical Weapons Convention (CWC) of 1993. The CWC came into effect in 1997 and prohibited the production and use of chemical weapons. Numerous nations known to maintain or suspected of maintaining chemical weapons stockpiles refused to sign or abide by the treaty.

In future Middle Eastern conflicts, chemical weapons are far less likely to be used in terrorist attacks than in large-scale military operations. Chemical weapons are not easy to use. They are difficult and awkward to store, transport, and handle; their use requires detailed and expensive planning and lead times; once released their effects are difficult to predict and control; and one's own troops require specialized equipment and extensive training to operate in a chemical environment.

Paul J. Springer

Further Reading

Butler, Richard. *The Greatest Threat: Iraq, Weapons of Mass Destruction, and the Crisis of Global Security.* New York: Public Affairs, 2000.

Morel, Benoit, and Kyle Olson. *Shadows and Substance: The Chemical Weapons Convention.* Boulder, CO: Westview, 1993.

Solomon, Brian. *Chemical and Biological Warfare.* New York: H. W. Wilson, 1999.

Torr, James D. *Weapons of Mass Destruction: Opposing Viewpoints.* San Diego: Greenhaven, 2005.

Tucker, Jonathan B. *War of Nerves: Chemical Warfare from World War I to Al-Qaeda.* New York: Pantheon, 2006.

Geneva Conventions

The Geneva Conventions are a series of four international agreements that, together with ancillary conventions, form a body of law governing war.

On June 24, 1859, the Austrian Army fought a combined French and Sardinian force near the northern Italian city of Solferino. Swiss businessman Henry Dunant found more than 9,000 wounded without adequate care in various buildings in a nearby village. His impassioned description of the carnage, *A Memory of Solferino*, became a best seller and led to formation of the International Red Cross and to a conference held from August 8 to August 28, 1864, to consider regulating treatment of war casualties. Representatives from 16 nations attending that conference signed the Geneva Convention for the Amelioration of the Condition of the Wounded in Armies in the Field, the first international humanitarian law. The United States, although a conference participant, did not ratify the agreement until 1882 after a lengthy campaign led by Clara Barton.

Several subsequent conferences have aimed at amending the original convention. In 1899, restrictions on use of asphyxiating gases and expanding bullets were added. The Hague Conventions of 1907 extended protection to maritime combatants. In 1925, poisonous gases and bacteriologic warfare were banned. In 1929, additional clauses dealing with treatment of the wounded and prisoners of war were added. In 1949, protections were added for the shipwrecked, and, in 1977, protections were extended to medical personnel and civilians and attacks on the environment were banned. The conventions' protections were also extended to participants in civil wars. Finally, in 2005, a third emblem (a red square on edge on a white background) was added to the Red Cross and the Red Crescent for use by nations not following either Christianity or Islam.

The four existing conventions are:

1. Convention for the Amelioration of the Condition of the Wounded and Sick in Armed Forces in the Field
2. Convention for the Amelioration of the Condition of the Wounded, Sick and Shipwrecked Members of Armed Forces at Sea
3. Convention Relative to the Treatment of Prisoners of War
4. Convention Relative to the Protection of Civilian Persons in Time of War

Jack McCallum

Further Reading

Bennett, Angela. *The Geneva Convention: The Hidden Origins of the Red Cross*. Phoenix Mill, Gloucestershire, UK: Sutton Publishing, 2005.

International Committee of the Red Cross. 2006. "The Geneva Conventions: The Core of International Humanitarian law." January 9. www.icrc.org/WEB/Eng/siteeng0.nsf/html/genevaconventions (accessed May 22, 2006).

Moorehead, Caroline. *Dunant's Dream: Switzerland and the History of the Red Cross*. New York: HarperCollins, 1998.

Gulf War Syndrome

Gulf War Syndrome (GWS) is the name given to a host of physical symptoms and maladies among U.S. and British veterans who fought in the 1991 Persian Gulf War. G WS is a progressive, neuron-degenerative, and immunological multisymptom condition that, apparently, is not explainable by post-traumatic stress disorder (PTSD) or other variables. GWS may afflict as many as tens of thousands of people, and some estimates run as high as 150,000. The syndrome's cause is unclear; indeed, its very existence is still questioned in some governmental and scientific circles.

Within months of returning home from participation in the Gulf War, some veterans began reporting unusual physical symptoms. Those few became, over time, thousands, and then tens of thousands. Gulf War veterans reported symptoms such as chronic fatigue, loss of muscle control, persistent headaches, sleep disorders, memory loss, chronic pain, and other chronic and disabling, conditions.

Later, medical research began to show that Gulf War veterans were developing amyotrophic lateral sclerosis (ALS or "Lou Gehrig's disease") at two times the rate of soldiers who had not deployed to the Gulf. Studies have also shown greater than normal risks for multiple sclerosis, fibromyalgia, brain cancer, and, perhaps most frightening, birth defects in children born to parents who were Gulf War vets.

Despite the American DOD and the British Ministry of Defense (MOD) years of official denial of the existence of the Gulf War Syndrome, the two organizations have now funded an enormous number of medical, military, and scientific investigations into the causes of GWS. In a comprehensive 452-page report of November 2008, the Research Advisory Committee for Gulf War Veteran's Illnesses, conducted by the U.S. Department of Veterans Affairs, declared the syndrome real. Causative agents included exposure to the drug pyridostigmine bromide, meant to protect against nerve gas and pesticides. In addition, exposure to nerve agents, smoke, and other agents may have contributed to the victims' conditions.

Some other theories have blamed vaccines. Before heading off to service in the Gulf, troops received multiple vaccinations to provide protection against a number of communicable diseases. The vaccines that may have been most problematic were those for Anthrax. However, the November 2008 report issued by the U.S. Department of Veteran's Affairs holds that there is little reason to believe that the anthrax vaccine, or depleted uranium, played a role in the syndrome.

Some troops in the field may have been exposed to repeated low-level doses of chemical weaponry such as sarin or other nerve agents or mustard gases. Repeated low-dose exposures could be a causative factor; yet, it seems unlikely that such wide-spread exposures would have been overlooked by the military.

Pesticides, both government-issue and locally purchased, were used widely by American and British troops. They sprayed them on their bodies, tents, buildings, and on prisoners of war. As a result, Gulf War vets received varying degrees of long-term exposure to organophosphate and carbamate pesticides. Studies reviewed by the Rand Corporation for the Research Advisory Committee on Gulf War Veterans' Illnesses, suggest that the pesticides could be a potentially contributing factor in GWS.

A few studies have suggested parasites like leishmaniasis as a possible culprit in Gulf War Syndrome. Many researchers are now pursuing the difficult to detect mycoplasma bacteria, while others theorized that the syndrome may be the result of some, as yet unknown, virus or bacterial agent. This theory has been given some support by gastrointestinal diseases caused during the war. Battlefield stress and PTSD may play a role in intensifying the symptoms of GWS.

Pyridostigmine Bromide (PB) was administered to coalition troops as a pre-treatment against exposure to the nerve agent soman. PB was only the first part of the treatment; if a soldier were exposed to militarily effective doses of soman, then a second treatment would be administered that was designed to combine with the PB already in the body. Because of the lack of knowledge of PB's short- or long-term effects on the nervous system, it cannot be ruled out as a possible factor.

Depleted Uranium (DU) is a by-product of the enrichment of natural uranium to produce reactor fuel and weapons-grade isotopes. In the Gulf War it was both used as a projectile and to augment armor. Some researchers claim that, between its natural low-level radioactivity and the dust and uranyl oxide gas it creates on impact, DU is a health hazard and could be a cause of GWS. However, medical and scientific research seems to show that DU is safe and causes no negative long-term health effects. All the while, other studies claim that DU is a neurotoxin.

As Iraqi forces retreated from Kuwait, they set the oil fields, containing hundreds of wells, ablaze. The fires burned for nine months. Many theorists point to those sky-darkening infernos as a possible cause for the syndrome. While many short-term respiratory problems were reported at the time, studies since have shown that even though there was a great deal of airborne particulate matter, the amount of pollutants in the air, according to Rand, was lower than recommended U.S. occupational standards.

There exist dozens of other theories concerning the cause of GWS. The interesting fact to note about GWS is that it has been clustered among American and British troops. Some researchers point to the simple facts that American and British troops used more pesticides, were involved in more combat, used the anthrax vaccine, and reported, by far, the most chemical attack warnings. They were also arrayed on the battlefield in such a way that the prevailing winds pushed the airborne clouds of dust and debris from allied bombings, much of which was dispersed as high as the upper atmosphere, right overtop of them. From there it fell like a slow dusty rain from the front lines all the way to Saudi Arabia and Kuwait.

Both the United States and the British governments met the initial GWS claims from ill veterans with skepticism. By 2004, the U.S. government, through the Research Advisory Committee, seemed to make the recognition of GWS official policy. The Committee's 2004 report admitted that between 26 and 32 percent of all Gulf War veterans do manifest a multisymptom progressive neurodegenerative condition that is neither psychiatric nor stress related. The report also supports the idea that soldiers' exposure to chemical agents and pesticides seem to be the most plausible causative factors.

B. Keith Murphy

Further Reading

Harley, Naomi H., Ernest C. Foulkes, Lee H. Hilborne, Arlene Hudson, and C. Ross Anthony. *Depleted Uranium: Gulf War Illnesses Series.* Volume 7. *A Review of the Scientific Literature as it Pertains to Gulf War Illnesses.* Santa Monica, CA: National Defense Research Institute/Rand Corporation, 1999.

Johnson, Alison. *Gulf War Syndrome: Legacy of a Perfect War.* Brunswick, ME: MCS Information Exchange, 2001.

Research Advisory Committee on Gulf War Veteran's Illnesses. U.S. Department of Veterans Affairs. *Gulf War Illness and the Health of Gulf War Veterans. Scientific Findings and Recommendations.* Washington, D.C.: U.S. Department of Veterans Affairs, November, 2008.

Wheelwright, Jeff. *The Irritable Heart: The Medical Mystery of the Gulf War.* New York: W. W. Norton & Company, 2001.

Interceptor Body Armor

Interceptor Body Armor is a form of body armor employed by U.S. military forces, first introduced in 1998. It has been used extensively in Operations Enduring Freedom and Iraqi Freedom. Interceptor Body Armor is considered a personnel protection "system," the individual parts of which work together to provide superior protection from bullets, shrapnel, etc.

The system is comprised of an outer tactical vest (OTV) and two small-arms protective inserts (SAPI). The outer vest and the inserts are made of finely-woven Kevlar KM2 fibers, which are both heat and bullet resistant. The armor was tested to be able to withstand and stop a 9-mm 124-grain full metal jacket bullet (FMJ) traveling at a velocity of 1,400 feet per second. The system will stop a variety of slower-moving bullets and shrapnel fragments and features removable inserts for shoulder, neck, throat, and groin protection. The two SAPIs that may be added to the front or back of the outer vest significantly increase the system's protective capacity. Made of boron carbide ceramic, the inserts can stop 7.62-mm NATO rifle round with a muzzle velocity of 2,750 feet per second.

Interceptor Body Armor also features numerous configurations that mimic existing backpacks and carrying systems, so soldiers can tailor their body armor for specific tasks or missions. When worn with the two inserts, the total weight of the armor system is 16.4 pounds (the outer vest weighs 8.4 pounds, while the two inserts weigh 4 pounds each). This is markedly less than the Interceptor's predecessor, the PSAGT, which weighed in at a hefty 25.1 pounds. Nearly ten pounds lighter, Interceptor Body Armor also allows soldiers considerably more freedom to maneuver. More recently, SAPIs designed for side protection have also been introduced. Heavier than the standard inserts, they weigh in at 7.1 pounds each. A complete armor system costs $1,585.

During the Iraq War, many infantry soldiers complained that Interceptor Body Armor was too cumbersome and too stout for the generally lightly-armed Iraqi insurgents they were battling. Some argued that they were unable to pursue the enemy with the full armor system and the many supplies and arms they had to carry. On the other hand, U.S. troops who principally rode in vehicles praised the system for its ability to protect against IEDs and ambushes.

Interceptor Body Armor has not been without its problems and detractors, however. In May 2005, the U.S. Marine Corps ordered the recall of more than 5,000 OTVs because they allegedly were unable to stop a 9 mm bullet, which was the requirement upon manufacture. Furthermore, many soldiers and Marines refused to wear the additional side inserts because of their added weight, making them more vulnerable to injury or death. One Marines Corps study has suggested that 43 percent of those Marines killed by torso wounds may have been saved had Interceptor Body Armor been more effective.

Paul G. Pierpaoli, Jr.

Further Reading

Savage, Robert C. Woosnam. *Brassey's Book of Body Armor.* Dulles, VA: Potomac Books, 2002.

Solis, William M. *Defense Logistics: Army and Marine Corps Individual Body Armor System Issues.* Washington, D.C.: U.S. Government Printing Office, 2007.

Persian Gulf War Veterans Health Registry

A major provision of Title VII of the Veterans Health Care Act of 1992 (Pub. L. 102–585; 106 Stat. 4943), passed by the United States Congress on October 6, 1992, and signed into law by President George H. W. Bush on November 4, 1992. Title VII established a comprehensive clinical health evaluation and registry program within the Department of Veterans Affairs (DVA) to address the health care concerns and illnesses of veterans of the 1991 Persian Gulf War.

Both the Veterans Health Care Act of 1992 and the Persian Gulf War Veterans Health Registry reflected growing governmental concerns with health issues and health benefit needs of American veterans who served in Operations Desert Shield and Desert Storm. Initial specific concerns revolved around the environmental and chemical exposure of veterans to the smoke of more than 750 oil well fires set by Iraqi forces in the theater of operations in February 1991 and other petroleum-based emissions from everyday troop operations. Health concerns over the impact of troop chemical and biological warfare vaccinations also arose. In response, the DVA quickly established a registry soon after the war's April 1991 cease-fire to begin clinical examinations of Persian Gulf War veterans concerned with war-related illnesses.

The DOD followed in December 1991 with its own registry of troops exposed to oil well fire smoke who desired examinations. During this time and into 1992, however, media outlets began reporting stories of Persian Gulf War veterans experiencing inexplicable symptoms of fatigue, joint pain, skin rashes, headaches, chronic sleeplessness, and cognitive problems. Initial investigations by researchers from the Walter Reed Institute of Research found no specific cause. The media reports, however, raised public concerns and the specter of a mystery illness, commonly labeled as "Gulf War Syndrome."

Congress responded to these specific health issues and public concerns with inclusion of the Registry under Title VII of the Veterans Health Care Act of 1992. A reinforcement and expansion of the DVA's initial 1991 program, Title VII and the Registry also increased the outreach of the DOD's limited registry beyond veterans affected by oil well fire smoke and established cross-reference procedures between both departmental registries to enhance information-sharing. Designed more as a descriptive informational database than a research program, the Registry provided for the listing of the name of each Persian Gulf War veteran who either applied for DVA services, filed a disability claim associated with military service, requested a DVA health examination, or received such an examination from the DOD and asked to be included in the Registry.

Deceased veterans whose dependents filed certain dependency and indemnity claims could also have their names listed. Title VII also provided for the inclusion of health information for a listed veteran who granted permission for such data to be included in the Registry, or the health information of a veteran who was deceased at the time his or her name was listed. Aware of veterans' ongoing health concerns, Congress required the DVA to periodically contact Registry veterans as to the status of health research reviews conducted under other Title VII provisions.

Linked to the Registry, other critical provisions under the title included health examinations, consultations, and counseling services requested by veterans, and a mandated agreement with the National Academy of Sciences to review medical and scientific information on the health consequences of Persian Gulf War service. Medical information reviewed pursuant to this provision further included the medical records of Registry veterans who granted permission for such a review, as well as the records of DOD registry participants. Finally, as a capstone to the legislation, Title VII authorized the president to transfer government-directed Persian Gulf War health research and provide annual reports to Congress.

The Registry's list has now grown to include the names of over 50,000 veterans. Implementation of the Registry and the research review provisions of Title VII also spawned numerous governmental-funded health studies and additional congressional legislation to enhance research efforts. The Institute of Medicine within the National Academy of Sciences has since explored potential health effects stemming from the use of insecticides, vaccines, nerve agents, depleted uranium, and fuels used or emitted during the war. Although research continues and much has been learned, specific or unusual causes of many veteran symptoms and illnesses have yet to be determined because of the lack of objective and timely pre-deployment and post-deployment health screening information and exposure monitoring measures.

Mark F. Leep

Further Reading

Barrett, Drue H., Gregory C. Gray, Bradley H. Doebbeling et al. "Prevalence of Symptoms and Symptom-based Conditions among Gulf War Veterans: Current Status of Research Findings." *Epidemiologic Reviews* 24 (2002): 218–227.

Guzzardo, Joseph M. and Jennifer L. Monachino. "Gulf War Syndrome–Is Litigation the Answer?: Learning Lessons from *In Re Agent Orange*." *St. John's Journal of Legal Commentary* 10 (1995): 673–696.

Institute of Medicine. *Gulf War and Health.* Volume 4. *Health Effects of Serving in the Gulf War.* Washington, D.C.: The National Academies Press, 2006.

Institute of Medicine. *Health Consequences of Service During the Persian Gulf War: Recommendations for Research and Information Services.* Washington, D.C.: The National Academy Press, 1996.

Post-Traumatic Stress Disorder (PTSD)

PTSD is a medical and psychological condition that may be caused by exposure to hostile combat situations and other traumatic events. It may be temporary or long lasting.

Various characterizations have been used to describe combat trauma over the years, including "shell shock," "war neurosis," and "battle fatigue." "Shell shock" was the most common term during World War I, while "battle fatigue" replaced it in World War II (although the term "combat exhaustion" was often preferred in the U.S. Army). Symptoms associated with combat-induced trauma can include involuntary trembling, outbursts of uncontrollable anger, nightmares, flashbacks, restlessness, depression, alcoholism, and an inability to focus. Such conditions may last for days, months, and even a lifetime.

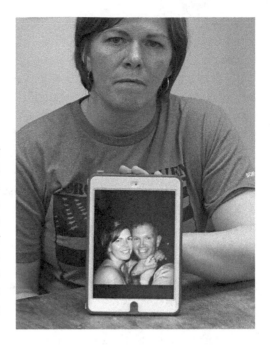

In this May 12, 2014 photo, Amy Miner poses with a photo of herself and husband Kryn Miner, an Army veteran who suffered from Post Traumatic Stress Disorder (PTSD) and who was shot to death by one of their children after threatening to kill the family. The Veterans Affairs health system confronts a difficult challenge helping veterans who struggle with PTSD after returning home. (AP Photo)

It was not until the 1980s that the United States government recognized psychic injury due to combat as a legitimate service-related disability. At the same time, such medical diagnoses became popularly known as Post-Traumatic Stress Disorder. The outcome of successful lobbying of Congress and the Department of Veterans Administration (DVA) by veterans' interest groups led to a two-year study (1986–1988), known as the National Vietnam Veterans Readjustment Study. The study examined the psychological effects of veterans who had performed hazardous duty in Southeast Asia. The study revealed that 15.2 percent of all male veterans (497,000 out of 3,140,000 who served "in country") and 8.1 percent of women (610 out of 7,200), many nurses, were diagnosed with PTSD. In 2004, DVA statistics noted that almost 161,000 Vietnam veterans were still receiving disability compensation for PTSD. By then, combat trauma was no longer cast in a negative light or lightly dismissed as in previous conflicts.

Although the short duration of the 1991 Persian Gulf War and lower levels of combat exposure in that conflict meant less psychological trauma, a 1999 study revealed that rates of PTSD among the approximately 697,000 deployed service members had increased significantly over time. A rate of 3 percent for men and 8 percent for women was detected immediately upon returning from the war. This rate rose to 7 percent for men and 16 percent for women within 18 to 24 months.

A study for Afghanistan veterans shows that 183 veterans out of 45,880 have been diagnosed with PTSD. In Iraq, a 2008 DVA study noted that almost 12,500 of nearly 245,000 veterans have visited DVA counseling centers for readjustment problems related to PTSD symptoms. Almost all have been soldiers and Marines because they have withstood the worst of the fighting, as opposed to Air Force and Navy personnel. In addition, 8 to 10 percent of active-duty women and retired military women who served in Iraq beginning in 2003 suffer from PTSD. The high percentage of women PTSD sufferers clearly reflects the increasing number of females who have participated in combat as part of the All Volunteer Forces (AVF).

A 2005 study examining PTSD in three Army and one Marine infantry units that fought in Iraq and Afghanistan, moreover, pointed out the type and percentage of soldiers and Marines who were exposed to some type of traumatic combat-related situation: (1) those being attacked or ambushed—92 percent; (2) those located near dead bodies—94.5 percent; (3) those being shot at—95 percent; and (4) knowing someone seriously wounded or killed—86.5 percent. Currently, almost 1 in 8 Iraq and Afghanistan combat veterans have sought help for PTSD.

Within the psychiatric profession, treatment for combat trauma or PTSD has moved from psychodynamic psychotherapy to biopsychiatric pharmacological application (i.e., use of drugs). Yet such treatment has not been matched by increased effectiveness capable of reducing the degree and length of time of this disorder. More troubling to the medical profession is the fact that almost 6 in 10 combat veterans remain unlikely to seek treatment out of fear that their commanders and fellow soldiers and Marines will lose confidence in them.

Charles F. Howlett

Further Reading

Ensign, Tod. *America's Military Today: Challenges for the Armed Forces in a Time of* War. New York: The Free Press, 2004.

Grossman, David. *On Killing: The High Cost of Learning to Kill in War and Society.* Boston: Little, Brown & Co., 1995.

Keane, T. M. and D. H. Barlow. "Posttraumatic Stress Disorder." pp. 418–453 in *Anxiety and Its Disorders,* 2nd Edition. Edited by D. H. Barlow. New York: The Guildford Press, 2002.

Pierce, P. F. "Physical and Emotional Health of Gulf War Veteran Women." *Aviation, Space, and Environmental Medicine* 68 (1997), 317–321.

Stretch, R. H., D. H. Marlowe, K. M. Wright, P. D. Bliese, K. H. Knudson, and C. H. Hoover. "Post-Traumatic Stress Disorder Symptoms among Gulf War Veterans." *Military Medicine* 161 (1996), 407–410.

Red Cross and Red Crescent

A humanitarian movement comprising three components—the National Societies, the International Federation of Red Cross and Red Crescent Societies, and the International Committee of the Red Cross (ICRC)—is collectively known as the

Red Cross and the Red Crescent. The Red Cross movement began in June 1859. After the Battle of Solferino, Swiss businessman Henry Dunant had found more than 9,000 wounded without adequate care. His novel about their plight became a best seller.

In 1863, Gustave Moynier helped Dunant organize the International Committee for the Relief of Wounded Soldiers, composed of other prominent citizens of Geneva, including Commander of the Swiss Army General Guillaume-Henri Dufour, with the goal of establishing a series of national relief committees. The group called an international conference in Geneva in October 1863, which included 36 attendees and 18 official delegates from 14 countries. Among the proposals from that group was the suggestion that volunteer medical personnel from all countries should wear a white arm band with a red cross (a reverse of the Swiss national flag), which had been designed by Dufour. Within a year, nine national societies had been formed.

Dunant also thought that all medical personnel on the battlefield should be treated as neutrals, and, to that end, a second conference was convened in the Swiss capital, which drafted the Geneva Convention in August, 1864, for the Amelioration of the Condition of the Wounded in Armies in the Field. The Conventions' 10 articles called for, among other changes, universal use of the red cross emblem and protection of medical personnel, hospitals, and wounded or sick combatants.

Although the red cross was never intended as a religious symbol, Islamic countries found it objectionable. During the 1876 Russo-Turkish War, the Ottoman Society for Relief to the Wounded chose a red crescent on a white background, and that emblem was subsequently adopted by the majority of Muslim nations.

The Geneva Convention elevated rules regarding care and protection of the sick and wounded from ad hoc agreements to the status of international law. The conventions were expanded in 1899, 1906, 1907, 1925, 1929, 1949, and 1977 and currently comprise four conventions and a collection of additional protocols. Dunant's committee, renamed the International Committee of the Red Cross, is the protector of the conventions and is also responsible for admitting new national societies to the movement.

In 1919, Henry Davison, the head of the American Red Cross, called an international conference to associate the various national societies. That conference resulted in the League of Red Cross Societies, subsequently renamed the International Federation of Red Cross and Red Crescent Societies in 1991. In 1928, the League, the International Committee of the Red Cross, and the various national societies joined as the International Red Cross which was renamed the International Red Cross and Red Crescent Movement in 1986.

The ICRC maintains a permanent administrative and medical staff and acts to both protect the rights of wounded combatants, prisoners, and civilians during wars and to provide medical care, sanitary services, and general assistance in time of war.

Jack McCallum

Further Reading

Vassallo, D. J. 1994. "The International Red Cross and Red Crescent Movement and Lessons from the Experience of War Surgery." *Journal of the Royal Army Medical Corps* 140: 146–154.

Rehabilitation and Reconstructive Surgery

Although a certain number of soldiers and sailors have survived their wounds for as long as wars have been fought, the percentage of those who live and the severity of survivable wounds have dramatically increased since anesthesia, antisepsis, and antibiotics entered the surgical armamentarium. The number of survivors with serious disabilities has increased as well. Rehabilitation and reconstruction are most often necessary in four general categories of trauma: amputations, burns, neurological injury, and wounds to the face and skin.

Amputations became particularly common after gunpowder weapons emerged as the primary means of warfare. These weapons were the first capable of producing enough power to regularly shatter bones and leave the fractures exposed to the outside world. Because of the high incidence of contamination in these "compound" fractures and the lack of effective treatment for the resulting infections, amputation became the standard method of treatment for gunshot wounds to the bone. Although some amputees survived 19th-century battlefield surgery, enough died to limit the demand for long-term care. By World War I, that trend had changed, and more than 8 million men came home from battles in Europe needing help to return to productive lives. That demand fueled rapid advances in prosthetic technology led by military hospitals, especially the Walter Reed Army Medical Center in Washington, D.C.

Coincidentally, rehabilitation and physiotherapy as professions had begun in the 1890s with the development of treatments based on massage, heat, and electrotherapy. These measures were outside the medical mainstream until the therapists convinced the military to use them, and electrotherapists became physiotherapists and acquired legitimacy and a professional status. Rehabilitation was co-opted as a medical specialty during the 1930s and was virtually entirely done either by physicians or therapists under their direct control by the beginning of World War II.

American government aid for veterans declined after the 1920 Vocational Rehabilitation Law, which allowed for occupational support but did not fund ongoing medical care for veterans. The situation again changed after the 1943 Vocational Rehabilitation Law, which funded medical care—both physical and

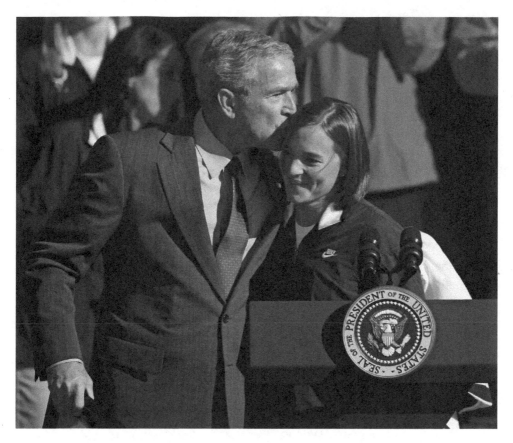

President Bush kisses Paralympian and Iraq war veteran, Melissa Stockwell, after delivering remarks to members of the 2008 United States Summer Olympic and Paralympic Teams. A staggering 45 percent of the 1.6 million veterans from the wars in Iraq and Afghanistan are now seeking compensation for disabilities they say are service-related—more than double the 21 percent who filed such claims after some previous wars. The new veterans have different types of injuries than previous veterans, in part because improvised bombs have been the main weapon and because body armor and improved battlefield care allowed many of them to survive wounds that in past wars proved fatal. (AP Photo/Pablo Martinez Monsivais)

psychological—and led to dramatic expansion in rehabilitation programs, notably in Veterans Administration hospitals.

Spinal cord injuries present a special rehabilitation challenge. Even though 45 percent of the 642 Union soldiers with spinal cord injuries documented in the *Medical and Surgical History of the War of the Rebellion* survived their initial trauma, those who were paralyzed were given supportive care only with the expectation that they would eventually die from complications such as pneumonia, urinary tract infection, or decubiti. Better wound and bladder care resulted in a few survivors during World War I and a few more during World War II. The provision of continuing medical care for disabled veterans after World War II led for the first time to several thousand long-term cord injury survivors, and the average length of survival increased from several weeks to a decade or more.

Faster, more adept surgery and better neurosurgical intensive care has also resulted in an increasing number of survivors of traumatic brain injury. The long-term sequelae of these injuries range from mood swings, anxiety, and depression to severe cognitive and motor deficits and are too often complicated by other disabilities such as loss of hearing or vision. Many of these wounds leave irreversible deficits and require multiple operations and permanent financial and social support.

Attempts at plastic surgical repair of battle injuries have been documented for centuries. During World War I, the British military enlisted artists to design and paint porcelain and metal substitutes for destroyed faces. Harold Gillies established a dedicated plastic reconstructive surgical unit at Aldershot, where he treated facial injuries. That work was carried on during World War II by his cousin Archibald Hector McIndoe at the Queen Victoria Hospital. McIndoe specialized in facial burns and treated about 4,000 airmen, most injured by ignited airplane fuel, during which time he coined the term "reconstructive surgery."

Explosives are also particularly likely to cause burns, and the most severe of those from recent American wars have been referred to Brooke Army Medical Center in San Antonio, where both the prosthetic and the plastic surgical requirements of severely burned patients are addressed before a transition to local Veterans Administration care. These patients and their families are also afforded occupational and psychiatric support.

Modern battlefield surgical techniques have dramatically lowered the percentage of men and women who die from their initial injury and have consequently increased the numbers with persistent disabilities. By January 2005, the U.S. military had issued more than 5,000 Purple Hearts to those serving in Iraq and had evacuated 14,700 people to the United States for long-term care. Although small-arms fire accounted for most of the injuries early in that conflict, improvised explosive devices subsequently assumed dominance; these most often result in blast and burn injuries. Body armor, although relatively effective in protecting the torso, leaves the victims susceptible to extremity injuries, and there have been a large number of amputations. The American military has been active in prosthetic research, particularly at Walter Reed Army Medical Center, and has been in the forefront of research into devices such as computerized limbs and specialized artificial joints.

Jack McCallum

Further Reading

Arluke, Arnold, and Glenn Gritzer. *The Making of Rehabilitation*. Berkeley: University of California Press, 1985.

Dillingham, J. R. 2002. "Physiatry, Physical Medicine, and Rehabilitation: Historical Development and Military Roles." *Physical Medicine and Rehabilitation Clinics of North America* 13 (February): 1–16.

Fauntleroy, A. M. *Report on the Medico-Military Aspects of the European War from Observations Taken Behind the Allied Armies in France*. Washington, D.C.: Government Printing Office, 1915.

Min, S. K. 2000. "A History of Maxillofacial Prostheses." *Journal of the Korean Association of Plastic and Reconstructive Surgery* 22 (July): 383–396.

Okie, Susan. 2005. "Traumatic Brain Injury in the War Zone." *New England Journal of Medicine* 352 (May 19): 2043–2048.

Peake, James. 2005. "Beyond the Purple Heart—Continuity of Care for the Wounded in Iraq." *New England Journal of Medicine* 352 (January 20): 219–222.

Veterans Benefits Improvements Act of 1994

The Veterans Benefits Improvement Act authorized the Secretary of Veterans Affairs to grant disability compensation to qualified veterans of the 1991 Persian Gulf War suffering from chronic disabilities associated with undiagnosed illnesses, including GFS. The act was signed into law on November 2, 1994, by President Bill Clinton and marked the first time in U.S. history that the DVA was given permission to provide disability compensation to veterans for undiagnosed illnesses. Since the passing of the Act, more than 3,700 Persian Gulf War veterans have received disability compensation under its provisions.

In addition to expanding the number of veterans able to receive disability compensation, the Veterans Benefits Improvement Act of 1994 included other requirements, such as the establishment of a standard procedure for completing medical evaluations of Persian Gulf War veterans, a requirement that the DVA evaluate the medical status of all immediate family members of veterans, and the launching of a program that provides veterans with easy access to current information on available benefits.

The Veterans Benefits Improvements Act of 1994 was passed in response the medical establishment's inability to diagnose symptoms and illnesses of thousands of veterans returning home from the Persian Gulf area during 1990–1991. Soldiers deployed to the Persian Gulf were reporting symptoms at a much higher rate than those who had not deployed there. Persian Gulf War illnesses still lack complete understanding. The existence of GWS has not been positively confirmed but recent studies have confirmed that almost 30 percent of Persian Gulf War veterans suffer from Chronic Multi-symptom Illness. After examining thousands of Persian Gulf War veterans with undiagnosed illnesses, a list of common symptoms was compiled to explain medically unexplained symptoms.

Research continues on the mysterious illnesses suffered by Persian Gulf veterans. In particular, researchers are studying the health effects of the many dangerous substances to which Persian Gulf veterans were exposed. Anthrax, sarin nerve gas, and DU are only a few examples from the list of substances. Some of the most common symptoms of GWS are fatigue, headaches, joint pains, muscle pains, respiratory disorders, and difficulty sleeping. Research also shows that Persian Gulf War veterans are at a greater risk for depression, anxiety, and substance abuse.

The Afghanistan War and the Iraq War have significantly increased the number of veterans needing assistance from the DVA. Wounded soldiers are surviving at higher rates than ever before due to improvements in military medicine. So far, almost 300,000 Gulf War veterans have applied for compensation and medical care. As with those of the Gulf War, veterans of the Afghanistan and Iraq conflicts suffer from unexplained illnesses. These veterans will be covered under the Veterans' Benefits Improvements Act of 1994.

Arthur M. Holst

Further Reading

Dyhouse, Tim. "$763 Billion Price Tag to Care of War Wounded," *Veterans of Foreign Wars Magazine* 94 (2007): 12.

Dyhouse, Tim. "Iraq War Vets Will Receive Benefits," *Veterans of Foreign War Magazine* 90 (2003): 12.

Law, Randi. "Gulf War Illness: An Update," *Veterans of Foreign Wars Magazine* 94 (2007): 26–27.

Veterans Health Care Act of 1992

President George H. W. Bush signed the Veterans Health Care Act of 1992 into law on November 4, 1992. It consisted of eight titles implementing a variety of new programs within the DVA to improve health care services for eligible American veterans of the 1991 Persian Gulf War as well as previous wars.

The Gulf War sparked a flurry of legislative proposals in Congress in 1991 and 1992 to address veterans' benefits. This was in large part the result of the patriotic fervor and resurgence of respect for American military personnel engendered by the conflict. The United States military personnel involved in both phases of the war, Operation Desert Shield and Operation Desert Storm, included a comparably higher percentage of reservists and National Guard troops (17 percent), and women (7 percent) than in previous American conflicts. More than 90 percent of Persian Gulf War veterans experienced service in a combat zone for the first time. The health concerns of U.S. troops included family and employment strains precipitated by abrupt calls to active duty for reservists and National Guardsmen; environmental exposure to smoke from oil-well fires; harsh desert conditions; hazards related to various military occupational specialties; vaccinations and fears of chemical and biological warfare emissions; and the emotional impact of instantaneous television war coverage on troops and their families. All played a part in heightening the potential psychological and physical health concerns within the U.S. military.

In light of these issues and in addition to the Gulf Act, Congress began passing pieces of legislation upon the conclusion of Operation Desert Storm in the spring of 1991 to address specifically veterans' health issues related to PTSD and various environmental exposures. But not until the following year did a more comprehensive health care package appear. The Veterans Health Care Act of 1992 was designed to improve and expand health care services to both Persian Gulf War veterans and other American veterans.

In recognition of the service of female Persian Gulf War veterans and a growing percentage of women serving in the military overall, Title I of the act provided for a counseling program to assist women veterans suffering from trauma associated with sexual assault and harassment while serving in the military, as well as additional women's health care and medical services. Another major provision of the act, Title VII, authorized the implementation of a Persian Gulf War Veterans Health Registry within the DVA to capture data for future research and assessments on health issues and illnesses related to service during the war. Linked to this registry within Title VII were provisions providing health examinations and consultations to veterans requesting help.

Additional titles tightened health-care sharing arrangements between the DVA and the DOD in order to expand services to veterans and their beneficiaries; revised nursing pay rates within the DVA to retain nurses and encourage recruitment; enacted drug-pricing reforms to reduce prescription drug costs for federal and nonprofit hospitals and clinics serving veterans; permitted federal grants to states to construct nursing home facilities for disabled and elderly veterans; expanded access of disabled veterans to medical treatment and care in non-DVA facilities; and applied federal judicial misconduct procedures to the Court of Veterans Appeals. The act served as an important foundation for subsequent legislation to improve health care benefits and resolve health-related issues for all American veterans.

Mark F. Leep

Further Reading

Guzzardo, Joseph M. and Jennifer L. Monachino. "Gulf War Syndrome: Is Litigation the Answer?: Learning Lessons from *In Re Agent Orange*." St. *John's Journal of Legal Commentary* 10 (1995): 673–696.

Institute of Medicine. *Health Consequences of Service During the Persian Gulf War: Recommendations for Research and Information Services*. Washington, D.C.: The National Academy Press, 1996.

Knight, Amy W. and Robert L. Worden. *The Veterans Benefits Administration: An Organizational History, 1776–1994*. Collingdale, PA: Diane Publishing, 1995.

DOCUMENT

What Was Asked of Us: An Oral History of the Iraq War by the Soldiers Who Fought It

During the U.S. wars in the Middle East, the widespread use of body armor coupled with modern battlefield surgical techniques significantly reduced the percentage of men and women who died from their initial injury. Consequently, there was a large increase in the number of veterans with persistent disabilities. Small-arms fire accounted for most of the injuries early in the Middle Eastern conflict. Improvised explosive devices subsequently caused most fatalities and wounds. Earl T. Hecker served as a surgeon at an American medical center located in German between May and October 2004. Here he operated on seriously wounded soldiers who had been evacuated by air from Iraq. The following excerpt provides some of his observations during his service.

When the improvised explosive device came on board, a whole new era of warfare and injuries came with it. Years from now Americans are going to be walking around and seeing these badly wounded people. They will ask, "Was this guy in a car accident?" No, the guy wasn't in a car accident; the guy was in Baghdad.

I remember this soldier who had an injury to the neck, and he was responsive but couldn't move his extremities. They had done X-rays at the battle site and they were preparing to ship him as a "priority one" on board the airplane, so the severity of his injury was a big deal. He needed special personnel and a nurse with him, and he was on a breathing machine or something. We got reports that he couldn't move his extremities and obviously there may be some paralysis there, quad paralysis. Shrapnel penetrated his neck and his spinal cord. I think he knew all along he was going to be a quadriplegic because he couldn't feel his arms or legs. Every morning he wanted us to show him his arms and legs. Part of my job was to notify the family, and we have a private line for those calls. I asked him once if he had a girlfriend and if he wanted me to call his girlfriend, but the answer was "No, do not call. . .just call my mother and let my mother know that I'm here."

I am a trauma surgeon, so I understand the degree of penetrating and blunt trauma in auto accidents, but this is much more. This is ten times what I've ever seen. Soldiers in Iraq are surviving horrific injuries. We see a lot of burns. It can be body burns: 10 percent, 50 percents, 80 percent body burns. We've had gasoline trucks blown up and the driver or the support staff brought in. This one individual had a greater than 50 percent burn over his total body. You add the age to that and that gives you an idea of what his mortality is going to be or what his survivability is going to be. If he has a 50 percent third-degree burn and his age is twenty, he has a 70 percent chance of dying. If you have a 50 percent burn and you're fifty years of age, you're going to die. This person had facial burns and body burns. He had his flak jacket on, so he didn't burn his chest, but he burned his arms and legs and face.

We had one fellow who had his legs blown off and we had to do further amputation. It's horrific. The tissue damage was so severe that it became gangrenous. There was no blood supply and we had to do a higher amputation. We had called his father, and his father came to visit him. He died, though. There were a lot of things that went bad.

These kids are really putting themselves on the line and you feel bad that you can't do more for them. You do as much as you can and later understand fully the severity of their illnesses and what's going to happen to them down the road. I'm not talking about this week. I'm talking about a month, two months, six months. . .a year. What's going to happen to them?

They deserve a better life afterward and to be able to take care of their families, take care of themselves, be productive, be a part of society. I'm not convinced that all these guys are going to be a part of society anymore. I think they're going to be withdrawn. Psychologically they'll be withdrawn because of the trauma of what they've gone through. I think physically they won't be able to get in and out of the car. They won't be able to go shopping. They won't be able to play with their kids the way normal individuals play with their kids. I don't know if they're going to live up to their expectation on what they're going to do in life anymore. Were they going to be a mechanic? Were they going to be an engineer? Were they going to be a doctor? What were they going to be when then finished the military? Maybe you have to think about a different profession, a different job. Will he ever get married? I don't know. This is the secret side of the war. Nobody knows about it. Nobody talks about it. Nobody addresses it. Nobody looks at it.

I've been to Normandy. I've been to Flanders Field. I've been to all these places. The soldiers are dead. They're dead. But this in an injury war. This is not so much a death war. Maybe that's the way we should look at it. Not dead but injured, an injury war. I saw injuries that I'll never forget. People don't get that. They really don't. I don't know what it's going to do to our society. If people understood that this is a war about catastrophically wounded young people, then maybe they'll appreciate what these kids really did for them and for their country. Right now it's absolutely hidden. I don't think most people think about these kids at all. Out of sight, out of mind.

Some of these people are the lost generation. They're gone. It is a sad way of putting it. I don't know. Some of these soldiers are never going to be the same again. Ever. I feel bad for them and I get upset. They're just lost.

Source: Trish Wood. *What Was Asked of Us: An Oral History of the Iraq War by the Soldiers Who Fought It*. Introduction by Bobby Muller. New York: Little, Brown and Co., 2006, pp. 194–197. Copyright © 2006 by Trish Wood; Introduction copyright © 2006 by Bobby Muller. By permission of Little, Brown and Company.

Index

About the Editor

JAMES R. ARNOLD is the author of more than 20 military history books and has contributed to numerous others. His published works include *Jeff Davis's Own: Cavalry, Comanches, and the Battle for the Texas Frontier* and *Napoleon Conquers Austria: The 1809 Campaign for Vienna,* which won the International Napoleonic Society's Literary Award in 1995. His two newest titles are *The Moro War: How America Battled a Muslim Insurgency in the Philippine Jungle, 1902–1913* winner of the 2011 Army Historical Foundation's Trefry Award, and *Napoleon's Triumph: The Friedland Campaign, 1807.*